Foundations of
Stuttering

Foundations of Stuttering

MARCEL E. WINGATE

Academic Press
San Diego New York Boston London Sydney Tokyo Toronto

Academic Press
a division of Harcourt, Inc.
525 B Street, Suite 1900, San Diego, California 92101-4495
http://www.academicpress.com

Academic Press
Harcourt Place, 32 Jamestown Road, London NW1 7BY, UK
http://www.academicpress.com

Library of Congress Control Number: 2001094340

International Standard Book Number: 0-12-759451-5

PRINTED IN UNITED STATES OF AMERICA
01 02 03 04 05 06 SB 9 8 7 6 5 4 3 2 1

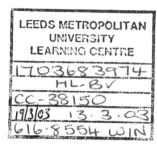

To my most memorable professors

George Lovell — Grinnell College

Roger Loucks — University of Washington

CONTENTS

PART **I**

Orientation

1 Introduction

Describes the objectives of the book. Discusses two general conditions that obstruct progress in the field. Draws the important distinction between facts *of* stuttering and facts *about* stuttering, to be elaborated in Chapters 3 and 4.

2 Stuttering as Object

Highlights obstructions posed by the various "definitions" of stuttering and the orientations they represent. Reports a pertinent study that illustrates the provinciality and untenability of such definitions.

3 Stuttering as Subject: Study of "The Thing Caused"

Addresses the facts *of* stuttering—namely, the criteria essential in identifying it. Contrasts these features to the many subsidiary phenomena that are typically the focus of description and explanation.

4 Facts About Stuttering

Describes the facts *about* stuttering—conditions well-documented to be importantly associated with stuttering, and which are therefore significant to understanding its nature.

PART **II**

Impedimenta

5 Excess Of Testimony

Illuminates the principal subjective contributions that constitute a distorting background in efforts to explain stuttering.

6 Deceptive Concepts

Presents a critical analysis of the principal explanatory concepts that have dominated the literature of stuttering for the past sixty years.

7 A Matter of Words

Discusses the careless, and in certain sources the contrived, use of terms; a major basis for the continuing confusion in the field.

8 Two Faces of Normal

In the literature of stuttering, "normal" has been construed essentially in the statistical sense, ignoring the basic reference of the term. This bias, although perhaps to some extent inadvertent, is often exploited to claim stuttering to be within normal limits.

9 Speech Minimized

The casual lay attitude toward speech, conditioned by one's long-term experience with it, subverts an adequate appreciation of its dimensions, even in sources studying it professionally.

PART **III**

Substance

10   Fluency

Sources in the literature of stuttering, preoccupied with "disfluency," remain unaware of the actual nature of fluency. This chapter presents a comprehensive analysis of fluency, and a system for recording its observable features. The system of analysis is illustrated in graphic "Fluency Profiles," half of which represent speech samples of notable American personages.

11 Normal Speech Processes

Discusses the various dimensions of ordinary spontaneous speech production, with special note made of features especially pertinent to the foci of Chapters 10 and 12.

12 Speech and Stutter

Review and discussion of linguistically relevant findings about stuttering, relating this material to pertinent content of the preceding two chapters.

13 Neural Background

A brief exposition of central nervous system structures and the tentative evidence for their involvement in speech production, with certain implications relevant to stuttering.

PART **IV**

Denouement

14 Derivations

This chapter presents a substantial revision of the traditional orientation to the "management" of stuttering. The core of revision is derived, in considerable measure, from the substance contained in the preceding chapters of the book.

PREFACE

This book presents a new departure in the literature of stuttering. Its objective is to establish a rational and scientifically defensible foundation for the study and management of the disorder, based in the fact that stuttering is manifestly a disorder of speech.

The literature of stuttering consists heavily of lore, competing "theories," conjectures, and rationalizations, within most of which there are recurring inconsistencies and contradictions. Moreover, the substance of this literature is oriented almost entirely to explanation of stuttering as a psychological problem.

The major theme of this book emphasizes and interrelates, largely from the literatures of stuttering, psychology, psycholinguistics, and neurolinguistics, matters that support the analysis of stuttering as anomaly of speech production. Subordinate to this major theme is a critical analysis of much of the literature in the field, which, although widely accepted, lacks scientific orientation—and in certain instances, ordinary credibility.

The first four chapters, constituting Part I, develop some very fundamental considerations regarding extant circumstances in the field. The first two chapters address the persisting preoccupation with cause, which, expressed in provincial and largely subjective explanations, is a pervasive condition that obstructs progress in the field. Within this context one finds a substantial effort to evade, distort, and even deny objective specification of the disorder; efforts that are couched in provincial beliefs. The next two chapters center around objective identification and description of stuttering, and certain well-supported facts about the disorder that are significant to understanding its nature.

The five chapters of Part II bring into focus the several major forces that obstruct a fully objective, scientifically oriented study of the disorder.

The four chapters of Part III, approximately half the book, present pertinent content from literatures in psychology, linguistics, psycholinguistics, stuttering, and neurolinguistics that support a credible analysis of stuttering as a disorder of speech production. Particular attention is directed to appraisal and discussion of fluency, and to central dimensions of speech as produced. The topic of fluency, which should be the principal reference in any discussion of stuttering, has been badly neglected in the literature of the field. Also, typically, the topic of speech production receives minimal, and quite peripheral, attention.

The content of the final chapter develops a rationale and strategy for "management" of the disorder that is based largely on the material presented in the previous chapters.

Completion of the manuscript for this book was assisted by encouragement and support of the administration at Washington State University, through our department chair Gail Chermak; I very much appreciate that affirmation of interest. I am especially indebted to two professional colleagues, Colleen Wilcox and Robert Potter, for their many valuable suggestions, made in the course of their diligent reviews of each chapter as each was created.

Marcel E. Wingate

FIGURES

TABLES

PART I

Orientation

Science is itself an honest, open, intelligent habit of mind that concerns itself variously with learning about empirical reality. All of us must concern ourselves with the acceptance of relevant empirical facts and at the same time must not be seduced by theories from a sister science which subserves the purposes only of that specific scientific discipline.

D. C. O'Connell and S. Kowal, *Temporal Variables in Speech*

CHAPTER 1

Introduction

Myself when young did eagerly frequent
Doctor and Saint, and heard great argument
About it and about; but evermore
Came out by the same door where in I went.

The Rubáiyát, Quatrain Twenty-Seven

The literature on stuttering is enormous, far-reaching and, in certain respects, complex. It is complex largely because it extends unequally in so many different directions. This condition is one that leads aspiring authors of texts either to attempt an omnibus coverage of the field or, in the other direction, to favor some particular formulation. Both kinds of endeavor fall short of what this field of interest sorely needs—a focus on the core findings about the disorder, and a critical assessment of extant concepts and rationale.

The intent in preparing this book was not simply to summarize or encapsulate all that one can read about stuttering. It is, rather, an effort to extract from this literature major dimensions central to progress in understanding the disorder; a distillation that will bring into focus the range of information about stuttering that can be shown—reasonably, credibly, and reliably—to be substantial, well-established, and stable, and that can be defended as contributing positively to understanding the basic substance of the disorder.

In the course of presenting this material, matters that have not been considered elsewhere in the literature will be developed in considerable detail. Topics that, in previous sources, have received less attention than they would seem to merit will be addressed with more care, and relatively less time will be devoted to substance that has been discussed at length in a number of other sources. The significant material from the latter category will be presented by synopsis or distillation, and the reader then referred to sources that contain more detail or elaboration. Also, much that has been written about stuttering will be intentionally ignored—in particular, no effort will be made to present the various purported "theories" of stuttering and their presumably related therapies. Enough sources have already paid too much attention to the distracting topic of theories, and to the supposedly associated therapies that typically are simply pragmatic techniques retrofitted to a contended position. One can find such material in many readily available sources; therefore, the topic will be considered in only a very general sense in Chapter 3.

PROBLEMS: OVERVIEW

In the course of pursuing the objectives of this book, it will be necessary to identify and discuss certain major problems of the field of stuttering, problems that have seriously impeded progress toward understanding the disorder and dealing with it realistically. Students of stuttering must be able to fully appreciate the serious obstacles to an objective understanding of the disorder that are posed by certain pervasive problems, affecting what is said, written, and accepted in the field. Most of these problems are extensive in influence, yet are rarely recognized or, at best, acknowledged only superficially.

Interestingly, most of the problems have surfaced, or at least substantially expanded, in the twentieth century. Notably, their effect has been most pronounced within the latter half of the twentieth century, an era in which most other fields of inquiry have been characterized by a sophistication in the methods of science. Ironically, this is also the era in which speech pathology emerged and developed as a professional specialty, with a focus on stuttering playing an oversized role for many years (see later in this chapter).

On the whole, the problems that confound the study of stuttering are interrelated or overlapping. The most broadly invasive ones, such as an unscientific attitude, unwarranted generalization, and unsubstantial or indefensible concepts, are so insinuative that they go unchallenged. In fact, it seems that, more than being simply tolerated, these problems have not actually been recognized as such. One or more of them will be found to surface in many contexts; in this book they will, for the most part, be addressed as they arise. Certain of the problems have sufficient presence that they are best discussed as focal topics, problems such as the excessive role of testimony, the distortions of "normal," and the cavalier indifference to speech as a subject. Such issues will receive separate, lengthier treatment in the chapters of Part II.

THE BASIC PROBLEMS

It is important that the reader be aware that all of the various problems to be considered arise from an underlying flaw; namely, a preoccupation with explaining the cause of the disorder. Although this grand determinant has existed for centuries, it has enlarged dramatically in the twentieth century. The preoccupation with cause[1] emerges in almost everything written or said about stuttering in professional as well as lay sources; it is clearly and pointedly reflected in the many "definitions" of stuttering that have been offered from within the profession, a condition that is addressed in Chapter 2.

An intimately related problem, denotable separately from the one above although subsidiary to it, is the one posed by the excessive amount of literature dealing with stuttering. There is a long history of writings on stuttering, extending far back into the pre-Christian era.[2] In any long-term review of the recorded interest in disorders of speech, one will find that, except perhaps for the long-expressed interest in the speech of the deaf, stuttering has always attracted far more attention than other speech defects. Prior to approximately the middle of the eighteenth century, stuttering was often considered along with other disorders of speech. Subsequently, it came to receive proportionately greater attention or to be more often treated independently, a phenomenon that expanded as the early decades of the twentieth century passed.

The modern-day preeminent interest in stuttering can be documented quite impressively from the time that speech pathology began to emerge as a profession. At professional meetings in the early years of what was to become the American Speech and Hearing Association (ASHA), stuttering was the predominant topic of the papers presented and program discussions (Paden, 1970; Moeller, 1975). Moreover, continually over the years that have followed, attention to stuttering has always been disproportionate relative to other topics dealing with speech anomalies. Considering the relatively low incidence of this anomaly vis-à-vis other speech disorders, attention to stuttering has been especially disproportionate in professional sources. Moreover, in lay sources, the number of articles and books on stuttering far outdistance publications about other disorders of communication.

Table 1.1 shows the number of convention papers and journal articles devoted to each of 11 categories of professional interest in the first 31 years of the ASHA's existence. Clearly, the interest in stuttering far exceeds all others, comprising almost a third of all contributions. This trend continued through the next 18 years, as revealed in Table 1.2, which reports only articles that appeared in the two journals of the American Speech and Hearing Association. Although the percentage of all contributions on stuttering in Table 1.2 is halved in comparison to the data in Table 1.1, articles on stuttering still continued to

TABLE 1.1   Level of Professional Interest in the Various Areas of
Speech and Hearing Disorders, 1926–57*

	Convention papers	Journal articles
Aphasia	67	47
Articulation disorders	60	54
Audiometry	110	72
Cerebral palsy	64	41
Cleft palate	49	34
General speech pathology & therapy	129	81
Service programs	118	0
Speech and language development	0	35
Stuttering	201	205
Voice disorders	55	42
Average for all areas other than stuttering	70	44

Data from Paden (1970, table 3, p. 51).

TABLE 1.2   Level of Professional Interest in the Various Areas of Speech
and Hearing Disorders, 1958–76

	JSHD	JSHR	Total
Aphasia	53	60	113
Articulation disorders	121	89	210
Audiology/audiometry	166	331	497
Education & therapy (hearing disorders)	111	13	124
General speech pathology & therapy	53	5	58
Psychoacoustics	0	196	196
Speech and language development	89	147	236
Speech & voice science	0	235	235
Stuttering	103	186	289
Voice	104	37	141
Average for all areas other than stuttering	77	123	201

appear more often than any other category. The comparison is extended to a more recent date in the content of Table 1.3. Note, first, the much expanded list of categories, reflecting the diversification in the field occasioned by increasingly varied sites of employment for speech and hearing personnel (hospitals, medical clinics, preschools, etc.). However, even within this substantial expansion of categories, the attention to stuttering in these two sources is considerable.[3] These data do not include (comparable) figures to be distilled from the pages of the *Journal of Communication Disorders*, in print since 1969; nor books on the subject; nor the considerable amount of publication activity to be found in other sources within the broad periphery of an immediate

TABLE 1.3 Level of Professional Interest in the Various Areas of Speech and Hearing Disorders, 1977–90

	JSHD	JSHR	Total
Acoustic immittance & psychoacoustics	142	115	257
Aphasia, apraxia & agnosia	97	57	154
Articulation, resonance and phonological disorders	113	97	210
Assessment of hearing	54	37	91
Assessment, Screening, treatment & diagnosis of speech & language	285	218	503
Audiology	116	241	357
Aural rehabilitation, habilitation education, and conservation	83	85	168
Hearing loss, deafness, and otic pathologies	172	180	352
Hearing aids, prosthetics, and cochlear implants	102	51	153
Language disorders, learning disabilities, & mental retardation	172	254	426
Other disorders	83	112	195
Speech & language development, including anatomy and physiology	193	171	364
Speech production & perception and auditory processing	187	138	325
Stuttering and fluency disorders	237	73	310
Voice and laryngeal disorders	75	91	166
Average for all areas other than stuttering	134	132	266

interest in disorders of speech. Moreover, 1977 saw the appearance of a new journal, the *Journal of Fluency Disorders*, which is devoted almost entirely to stuttering, in which an average of 32 articles a year have been published.

The problem presented by this profusion of material is not simply one of excess. The excess contains a great deal of redundancy, with many different (although very often the same) writers saying the same things repeatedly, sometimes with only minor variations on the theme. In addition, the voluminous writings on stuttering have an appalling range of quality, even within "the literature of the field"—which includes the professional journals. Writings range from the level of anecdote and vicarious testimony to the level of laboratory research. Much of the literature is superficial, misleading, internally inconsistent or contradictory, sometimes sensational, occasionally maudlin, and too frequently touting one or another personal or thematic bias. At the extreme, no little amount of the literature on stuttering, at all levels, can be dismissed as inconsequential; some of it as ridiculous.

It is pertinent to note here that one of three major considerations that motivated the founders of the American Speech and Hearing Association to establish a professional organization was their concern about the unscientific level of some of the articles and books then being published in the field (Paden, 1970). However, this problem has continued to plague publications addressed to stuttering.[4]

The literature of stuttering must be read carefully, circumspectly, and critically. The unsophisticated reader will not, of course, be likely to detect departures in logic that involve specialized or esoteric material, but it is very possible for even the uninitiated to detect inconsistencies and contradictions in much of what has been written by maintaining a skeptical and analytic attitude. I have found that upper-division undergraduate students, unsophisticated in regard to stuttering, generally have been able to identify contradictions and inconsistencies in sources assigned to them for that purpose. Actually, one might well prepare oneself to assume the proper orientation by frequently rereading selections from Bergen Evan's illuminating book, *The Natural History of Nonsense*. Similarly, Andreski's *Social Science as Sorcery* could also be used as an appropriate primer.

FACTS: OVERVIEW

In addition to being fully aware of the substantial problems extant in the field of stuttering, anyone who wishes to undertake study of the disorder objectively should also be knowledgeable about what can be supported as facts of the disorder. Here one faces another problem, namely, what are the trustworthy facts regarding stuttering?

As I have noted elsewhere (Wingate, 1983), what is to be accepted as fact is a very critical matter, especially in a field like stuttering. Well-supported, credible facts are vital in moving toward understanding a subject. In this field, where there is so much variation among reports and findings, anything that is to be considered a fact should have a very substantial base. To date there is a notable amount of unevenness and inconsistency in what has been offered, and accepted, as fact.

The literature of stuttering contains frequent reference to facts regarding the disorder. Occasionally one even finds a specific effort to list the "known" facts. Table 1.4 presents nine such lists, which span dates between 1913 and 1982. Many of the items presented there have appeared as isolated references in other literature sources.

Two Kinds of Facts

A first step in considering stuttering facts is to differentiate facts *about* stuttering, and facts *of* stuttering. Most of the items contained in the lists of Table 1.4 are appropriately considered to be facts *about* stuttering, that is, they are observations made about a recognized phenomenon, whose identity is conveyed in the term by which it is known. The identity of the phenomenon rests in observations of a special kind. They too are facts, but of a different order, appropriately considered as facts *of* stuttering. The facts *of* stuttering consist of observations by which the phenomenon is recognized; they are intrinsic to its identity.

There are very few facts *of* stuttering, and they are considerably more defensible than many reported facts *about* stuttering. Actually, the facts *of* stuttering can be dealt with as one basic fact having several necessary descriptive dimensions, as follows. Stuttering is a *speech disorder*; it is a unique anomaly in the flow of speech characterized by iterative and/or perseverative speech elements involving word/syllable-initial position. This description will be elaborated and discussed as the substance of Chapter 3, and will receive much attention in later chapters as well.

The facts about stuttering listed in Table 1.4 exemplify the discordance in accepted knowledge regarding stuttering. In general, one could reasonably expect to find considerable agreement among several separate compilations of the facts regarding something—anything—that are presented by presumably

TABLE 1.4 Concurrences in Nine Separate Lists of Stuttering Facts

	Bluemel (1913)	Travis (1933)	West (1943)	Bender (1943)	Reid (1946)	West (1958)	Karlin (1959)	Sheehan (1970)	Andrews (1983)
Childhood onset		X	X		X	X	X	X	X
Onset is gradual						X			
Onset rate >15 years	X								X
More males than females	X		X		X	X	X	X	X
Heredity			X		X	X	X	X	X
Sinistrality			X			X			
Twinning in family			X		X	X			X
Neuromuscular incoordination			X						
Slow diadokinesis			X						
Metabolic differences			X			X			
Frequent URI			X						
Not in diabetics			X						
A convulsive phenomenon						X			
Range of intelligence							X		X
More in special classes		X							X
Held back in school		X							
Speech delay			X		X	X			X
Linguistic factors					X				
Not final consonant (C)	X								
Vowels (V) difficult also	X								
More with C with short V	X								
Repeat word just stuttered	X								
Voice lacks inflections			X						
Not when alone	X			X				X	X
Stuttering in thought	X								
Not when singing	X			X	X				X
Not in choral speaking	X			X	X				X
Other ameliorating conditions									X
Recovery		X					X	X	X
Various treatments successful				X					
In most cultures								X	
Incidence/prevalence		X		X	X		X	X	X
All social levels							X		
Diverse forms	X								
Variability			X	X	X				
Increased by fear						X			X
Distraction								X	
No Native Americans					X				
Position in family					X				

knowledgeable sources. It is quite sobering, then, to find that the agreement among these several lists is spotty and, overall, not very substantial. Moreover, the disagreement only hints at the extent to which these observations vary in their substance. The extent of discordance itself could raise serious reservation about whether many of the items appearing in these lists identify acceptable facts regarding stuttering. Actually, many of the items in the first eight lists do not meet minimal criteria for status as fact; the three items at the bottom of the list are prime examples of this fault, but half a dozen others are similarly limited. Overall, the discordance reflects inadequate scope; this is due in some measure to the vintage of some lists, but more potently to the limitations of personalized interest. The ninth list is derived from a source that, generally speaking, is more adequate in scope. Most of the items in that source are at least reasonably well documented and, moreover, based on research findings. At the same time, several items presented as facts by the latter source are not included in this table because the breadth of their support is too narrow.[5]

It is especially pertinent to emphasize here that none of the sources include the three most thoroughly supportable and significant facts about stuttering, of which anyone involved in the field should be clearly aware, namely: (1) its cause is unknown, (2) its essential nature[6] is not understood, and (3) there is no known cure.

Observations made *about* stuttering do not tell us anything, directly, of the disorder itself. They must be recognized as *ex post facto* observations, whose meaning and potential value emerge only in reference to the acknowledged entity—stutter occurrences. They can contribute significantly to the effort to understand the disorder, but their substance must first be carefully assessed. Through use of adequate and justifiable criteria, observations about stuttering can be assayed and arranged in at least a rough order of relative merit, after which their significance for stuttering can be appreciated. A systematized arrangement of this kind can itself serve as a reference to which other less compelling discoveries may be meaningfully linked, through rational and defensible analysis, into a network of interrelationships that should contribute powerfully to understanding the nature of stuttering. We will deal with these issues in appropriate later chapters, including a defensible distillation of facts *about* stuttering as the subject matter of Chapter 4.

It is relevant to mention here an issue that will be addressed in a more appropriate context in Chapter 7. The issue is grounded in the principle that reporting and discussing facts *about* stuttering presupposes the facts *of* stuttering, realistically and accurately referenced. It is a principle to keep in mind throughout all discussions regarding stuttering.

A GENERAL PROFILE

Beyond the three basic facts about stuttering noted earlier, readers should be apprised of several notable circumstances that have characterized stuttering over its lengthy history. First, and of fundamental significance, it has always been identified in terms of the same, repeatedly observed, anomalies of speech.[7] Second, in spite of the extensive attention it has received, the essential nature of the disorder (what underlies those anomalies) remains an enigma. Third, attention to stuttering has been characterized by a preoccupation with notions regarding its cause, and proposals for its cure. Fourth, accounts of its cause have been predominantly conjectural, even when linked to objective observations—and in most instances the linkage is very tenuous. Fifth, the conjectures regarding the nature of stuttering have reflected influential beliefs and concepts unique to the historical era in which the conjectures have been espoused. Sixth, so many explanations of stuttering, especially in the twentieth century, have attributed it to, or have emphasized, psychological factors. Seventh, accounts of cause have been unduly influenced, in many instances determined, by stutterers themselves—especially certain stutterers who have attained some prominence or authority, and who have then proffered their personal views as essential truth in explaining the cause and nature of the disorder. Eighth, treatment efforts have been almost entirely empirical, that is, based on commonsense, practical, *ad hoc* procedures. In other words, the various "theories" of stuttering (if one must call them so) have rarely led to a specific therapy method (see Wingate, 1977b).

The "notable circumstances" listed above are addressed from several directions in the pages of this book. Because stuttering is so obviously a disturbance in speech, the underlying theme throughout the book is that the study of stuttering must be approached fundamentally in reference to what is known about speech and its production. This orientation is a departure from typical approaches to the subject, in which attention to stuttering in the context of speech has been, for various reasons, largely incidental.

The subject matter sequence considers, first, presumptions about stuttering and the premature explanations they generate (Chapter 2); followed by exposition of matters that should be the focus in a scientifically oriented study of the disorder (Chapter 3); then a review of the more reliable facts about stuttering (Chapter 4) that contribute in various ways to understanding the nature of the disorder. The five chapters of Part II discuss circumstances that, in differing but significant ways, have hindered progress toward understanding the nature of stuttering. Importantly, a lack of adequate attention to speech per se is a common dimension of all these circumstances. This problem is given special attention in Chapter 9, which becomes a prelude to the chapters of Part III. The chapters of Part III deal pointedly with fluency dimensions of normal speech, with normal speech production and vagaries thereof, and with matters pertinent to stuttering as disorder of speech. The single chapter of Part IV addresses matters distilled from the previous chapters for their significance in appreciating the nature of stuttering and pertinent implications for its management.

SYNOPSIS

The subject of stuttering is widely acknowledged to be confusing and difficult. A substantial part of this condition is due to the extensive literature about the disorder, so much of which is not scientifically oriented or supported, but is instead replete with conjecture, fabrication, and an extensive body of substance best described as lore.

The objective of this book is to undertake a new departure in approach to the study of stuttering. It is an approach that will ignore much of the material standardly incorporated in books on the subject, critically review significant substance in the relevant literature, and discuss pertinent content not previously considered.

NOTES

1. Following a presentation I gave at Northwestern University in 1989, in which I made a point of criticizing this preoccupation, a colleague in the audience rose to assert, "You can't talk about stuttering without talking about cause!"

2. The interested reader is referred to Wingate (1997) *Stuttering: A Short History of a Curious Disorder*.

3. It is notable, consistent with the issue being drawn here, that less than one-fourth of the articles appeared in the *research* journal.

4. For recent examples, see Perkins *et al.* (1991) and the statement by Bloodstein (1990).

5. A criticism raised in an article (Wingate, 1983) published with the paper by Andrews *et al.* (1983).

6. By "essential nature" I mean what underlies the overt phenomena, what subtends those characteristic anomalies of the speech sequence that identify stutter in observation.

7. The facts *of* stuttering. Regarding its lengthy history, see, in particular, Wingate (1997).

CHAPTER 2

Stuttering as Object

The study of the causes of things must be
preceded by a study of the things caused.

Hughlings Jackson[1]

The title of this chapter was chosen to emphasize the fact that, in the
lengthy record of attention to stuttering, the principal abiding objective
has been to advance some explanation of its nature. In essence, stuttering has been addressed primarily as a puzzling object, a sort of riddle that
entices a ventured explanation—the ventured explanation being the objective.

PREMATURE EXPLANATIONS

Explanations of stuttering have proliferated in the twentieth century, especially
following the eminence achieved by psychology during the early decades of
the century. The widely disseminated, captivating ideas from a wide range of
psychological writings provided a font that infused so many attempts to explain
stuttering, centered around some psychological notion. Some of these notions
came from a lay source, reflecting a "psychology of the masses" that came to
be called "Pop-Psych."[2] However, many accounts—the more influential—have
been mounted by persons having formal study in psychology, some of it fairly
extensive.[3]

As noted in Chapter 1, this preoccupation with explaining the cause of
stuttering is the fundamental problem in the field that, although extant for
centuries, has proliferated in the twentieth century. This condition is singularly

revealed in the many definitions of stuttering, each of them reflecting the bias of some purported "theory." We will presently consider a representative sampling of such definitions, but for the time being the following statement from a layperson who had a special interest in the disorder captures the essence of the situation.

The author of the following quotation is a recovered[4] stutterer who, curious about the disorder for a long time, decided to learn something about it from presumably knowledgeable sources. His efforts were reported in a valuable little book titled *Stuttering: The Disorder of Many Theories*[5] in which he relates:

> Not long ago, I decided to satisfy my curiosity by looking into the voluminous scientific [sic] literature that has grown up around stuttering. I had no trouble finding explanations of why people start to stutter. Indeed, I found a grab bag of competing and often contradictory explanations—some of which bore a suspicious resemblance to the old wives' tales I remembered from childhood. But the first, and possibly the most significant, thing I learned was that nothing about stuttering is as simple as it seems—for the reason that nothing about speech is as simple as it seems (Jonas, 1977, p. 8).

Note especially his mention of "voluminous" literature and his comment about the extent of contradiction he found within that literature. To have called it scientific was generous. In addition to noting his remarks regarding the many explanations of stuttering, I should also draw attention to the latter part of the final sentence, for that passage brings into clear relief an important matter to which we will devote considerable attention in later chapters, especially those of Part III.

Jonas' description of what his search revealed is easily corroborated by what one will find in a number of publications that have appeared both before and after Jonas' inquiry. The position statements of 25 authorities compiled by Hahn (1956) and the 14 contributions contained in two symposia edited by Eisenson (1958, 1975) exemplify sources that would yield an assessment comparable to that made by Jonas.

Contrary to Jonas' use of the term "theory" in his book's title, none of these attempted explanations of stuttering deserve to be called a "theory." They are, at best, hypotheses—more properly, guesses—for they are, in substance, of the order of conjecture comparable to the guesses laypersons make about many minor and quite ordinary uncertainties, which they unwittingly aggrandize with the word "theory."

Not only are the many accounts of stuttering essentially simply guesses; they are conceptually insular and ideationally autonomous. They are guesses that survive by ignoring what is inconsistent with or contradictory to their focal themes. As noted in Chapter 1, I do not intend to develop here an individual criticism of these many positions. It is sufficient to emphasize that all of them are simply points of view, and that they are both provincial and dogmatized—which is a good reason that so many of them exist, and why they attract and retain personalized commitment. These are features well known to characterize systems of belief. Small wonder that one hears so frequently the complaint that the topic of stuttering is confusing.

Among the many sources that offer an explanation of stuttering, it is rare to find an explicit statement of the viewpoint made early in the narrative. Most often one finds a sort of "preamble": frequently in the form of various generalized statements and allegories, sometimes featuring selected "facts" about stuttering, sometimes vague and tangential discourse.

The facts *of* stuttering typically receive minimal consideration: if they are mentioned at all, reference to them is very often cursory, superficial, or clouded by use of inaccurate and misleading terminology, such as "repetitions and hesitations," and often with considerable generalized reference to normal speech and such "normal nonfluency"[6] as it may contain. In sum, the typical accounts of stuttering give little attention to the critical features of the disorder but instead devote extensive effort to spinning some typically loose web of interpretation and conjecture.[7]

GIVING THE ANSWER BY QUESTION

One particular approach to introducing an explanation of the disorder is the technique of asking, "What is stuttering?" In such context,[8] this is the classic rhetorical question—one that is posed only as a device for proceeding to give the answer—which the person posing the question has well in mind and now is about to reveal. Standardly one finds that, soon after posing the question, the author then confidently proceeds to tell the reader his version of what stuttering *is*. And here, as will be clarified below, the latitude contained in the verb "is" obscures a significant issue: namely, that "is" has several connotations, two of which have crucial roles in this context. At one level, "is" indicates denotation of something observable and describable, based in direct observation. In considerable contrast, "is" also refers to the essential substance or inherent nature of something. The rhetorical question in regard to stuttering embodies the latter meaning of "is."

Most often this intended explication of what stuttering *is*, in the sense of "essential substance," soon moves to a definition of the disorder, one to which the person posing the question subscribes or of which, in certain instances, he may actually be the author. And here, as will shortly be documented, one encounters the fundamental problem in the field of stuttering—the preoccupation with cause. This problem encapsulates a number of other, more focal, problems in the field, to be considered in the chapters of Part II.

A straightforward, sincere ordinary question (one posed in the expectation of a reply) in the form of "What is __[something, anything]__ ?" is not regularly a singular question. It may pose one or more, and typically more than one, of three implied questions—questions that, individually, are substantially different in the level and character of the answer sought. The three implied questions ask for information addressed to: (a) identification, (b) classification, and (c) the nature of the "something." A reply to the original query may answer any one, or all three, of the implied questions, depending on pertinent circumstances. For instance, if a person is asked a question regarding something about which he has reason to believe the questioner knows very little or nothing, the reply should, and most often does, address all three implied questions. Clear examples occur commonly in areas in which the questioner's knowledge is limited or the subject matter is esoteric, but the person to whom the question is addressed is knowledgeable. For instance, to a marine biologist, "What is plankton?" "What is a coelocanth?"; to an astronomer, "What is redshift?" "What is a supernova?"; to a poultry specialist, "What is candling?" In such instances, the questioner may know hardly more than the name of the referent in question; it is expected that the answer will address all three dimensions of the original question: identification, classification, and nature.

On the other hand, if it can be assumed that the person asking the question is not completely naive, then the reply can assume that the questioner has knowledge of at least the descriptive, observable aspects of the referent, and very likely its classification as well. Therefore, these dimensions do not need to be addressed in the reply. Examples of the latter type of query are: "What is wind?" and "What is fog?"

The rhetorical question, in contrast, is not a straightforward, sincere question that seeks an answer in reply. Instead, as noted above, the rhetorical question is employed as a device for *supplying* an answer, already formulated. At the same time, the rhetorical question typically illustrates a query of the assumed-knowledge type; that is, the question contains the assumption that the audience recognizes what is under consideration, that they can identify the subject in question at least by its characteristic features and, most likely, in regard to its classification as well. In such instances the objective of the rhetorical question is simply to provide an entree for supplying the answer to the remaining dimension of the question—namely, regarding the *nature* of the subject. In the specific instance of "What is stuttering?" the rhetorical question contains the assumption that the audience already knows the identification, and classification, of stuttering—namely, that it is a unique defect of speech.

The author of the question, well able to assume this audience familiarity, intends to give an explanation of the source—the nature, the *cause* of the disorder.

KNOWING THE REFERENT

It is germane to note—indeed, to emphasize—that this routine assumption of audience sophistication is entirely justified. There is, in fact, extensive evidence that laypersons know the classification of stuttering (a speech disorder) and, furthermore, are well able to identify its characteristic features (elemental repetitions and prolongations). Moreover, they know all this at least as well as professional persons.[9]

In view of the overwhelming evidence that stuttering is readily identified, and has been for centuries (Wingate, 1997), it is a major irony of the field of stuttering that many professional persons, especially certain notable figures, cling tenaciously to a contention that stuttering is not reliably identifiable. The scope of this irony prompted West *et al.*(1957)[10] to remark that "everyone but the experts knows what stuttering is." West's quip was appropriately sarcastic, and as pertinent today as it was when he made it, in view of the sort of claims that persist. He was poking fun at the waste in time, energy, and paper that has resulted from the rhetoric and quibbling generated by certain professional sources who, at that time and since that time, have argued about the identification of stuttering (see, for example, Perkins, 1983; Bloodstein, 1990).

Fundamentally, it is a paradox to find that persons vested in the mantle of "expert" in a field should aver that the subject of their presumed expertise is not reliably identifiable. Experts in a field should be well able to identify its subject matter, distinguish it from possible resemblances, recognize instances in which clear identification may be uncertain, and be able to explain why occasional uncertainty may arise. In his tongue-in-cheek remark, West implied that, in spite of all the claims, contentions, purported "evidence," and argument circulating in this little constricted tempest regarding identification, the "experts" should know, at least as well as the laity, what stuttering *is* in the descriptive sense.

A full appreciation of West's intended humor is dampened upon realization that there is a dark side to this policy of disclaiming reliable identification of stuttering. Much of this effort, pressed by certain sources in particular, has been undertaken, indefensibly, from a serious intent to actually deny the reality of stuttering.[11] Such contention has been mounted largely from the claim that stuttering cannot be objectively distinguished from "normal nonfluencies." Actually, this claim is simply an aggrandizement of certain instances in which some individual irregularity in fluency may not be clearly discerned as either stutter or non-stutter. This matter is discussed in Chapter 3. However, such isolated occurrences do not indicate, as their supporters intend to claim, that stuttering is not reliably identified, and that therefore stuttering is not an actuality but is instead a misperception and an inaccurate judgment.

On the whole, solid support from many sources reveals that reliability of stuttering identification is very high, both within and among judges, and whether they be professional or laypersons. Significantly, a similar level of evidence is contained in the extensive reports of research, having varied orientations, in which demonstrating reliability in identification of stuttering is a basic requirement of the experimental procedure.[12] Even more compelling is the finding of high levels of reliability for subject selection that are reported in most of the research addressed specifically to the claim that stutter identification is unreliable! This particular circumstance embodies what is undoubtedly the most remarkable internal contradiction one is likely to encounter anywhere, as follows. Many of the publications making the complaint that stuttering is not reliably identified, also: (a) select subjects on grounds of whether or not they stutter, (b) make comparisons between stuttering and non-stuttering individuals, (c) raise some theoretical issue in which instances of stuttering are focal, and (d) make recommendations for the management of stuttering. None of these actions are justifiable if one cannot reliably identify stuttering.

Probably the most penetrating counter to the claim regarding unreliability of stutter identification was supplied by Wendell Johnson himself, who wrote, in reference to research previously undertaken:

> the chief implication of this analysis was that what we think of as stuttering reduces, on the level of fact and experience, to stutterings—and that stutterings can be counted. (Johnson, 1955, p. 198)

This statement is a forthright, open acknowledgment regarding identification of stuttering: to be able to count things, one must first identify them.

THE DEFINITION DIVERSION

Other clear evidence that the "experts" do know what stuttering is, in terms of its identification, is clearly revealed, although by default, in the kinds of definitions discussed below. These "definitions" of stuttering, which are not admissible as actual definitions, exclude entirely the matter of description of stuttering and instead present simply *a statement of presumed etiology*. By omitting a descriptive statement—saying only "Stuttering is ... —, " the authors of these definitions implicitly reveal that they consider a description of the referent to be unnecessary; undoubtedly because it can readily be assumed, as emphasized in West's remark and as confirmed by extensive evidence, that everyone knows what stuttering is—in terms of identifying it.[13] Therefore, a descriptive portion of the "definition" statement is unnecessary, and becomes superfluous.

Before proceeding to consider these etiologic types of "definition," it is pertinent to point up the function of definitions. As I noted some years ago in regard to this topic (Wingate, 1964), the objective of a definition is "to determine and state the nature and limits of" the referent, with the clear implication that the definition reflects confirmable reality. One can expect that, in a reputable dictionary, this objective will be fulfilled. Among the statements reproduced below, all but the last one are inadmissable as definitions; the first seven items are nothing more than expressions of conjecture.

The eight statements were taken from sources that are identified at the end of the chapter; the first seven also have appeared in other writings by the same authors. In the following reproduction of these definitions, the critical initial noun phrase—"Stuttering is–"—has been left out, substituted by the blank space. That phrase was omitted to emphasize what should readily become obvious, namely, that except for statement #8, a reader ordinarily (unprepared by context) would have no idea, from the statement itself, what is being "defined."

1 _____ a morbidity of social consciousness, a hypersensitivity of social attitude, a pathological social response

2 _____ the result of a conflict between opposed urges to speak and to hold back from speaking

3 _____ the disorganization of normally fluent speech that is a consequence of conditioned emotion

4 _____ a symptom of an emotionally disturbed personality that profoundly affects the physical, mental and emotional life

5 _____ a habit of making elaborate preparations for speech on the assumption that it is a difficult and treacherous process

6 _____ an anticipatory, apprehensive, hypertonic avoidance reaction

7 _____ a psychoneurosis caused by a persistence into later life of early pregenital oral nursing, with oral-sadistic and anal-sadistic components

8 _____ to speak or say with involuntary pauses, spasms, and repetition of sounds and syllables

It is particularly germane to criticism of the literature of stuttering to point out that, of all these definitions, statement 8 is the only one obtained from a source that has no connection to the field of stuttering. This eighth item, a real definition, was copied from *Webster's New World Dictionary of the American Language*.[14] The other statements are quotations from speech pathologists in the field of stuttering, taken directly from the works cited.

TESTING THE DEFINITIONS

As noted above, it seems obvious that, with the initial noun phrase omitted, even somewhat sophisticated readers would not be able to name the referent of those statements, created by professionals in the field. In contrast, a real definition from a reputable source of definitions should elicit correct identification of the referent. There is good reason to believe that laypersons can be expected to name many things, events, etc., when given a standard, reputable definition of the item. To examine this inference, the following inquiry was undertaken.

Definitions of 38 words[15] that refer to some human action or condition, were copied from the same source as definition 8 above: *Webster's New World Dictionary of the American Language*. These definitions and the eight items above were then prepared as a list, with the eight "stuttering" definitions inserted at intervals among the others, placing definition 8 as the last insertion. Seventy percent of the real definitions defined referents of orofacial activity, identified in Table 2.1.

The list of statements was presented to two groups of college students: 80 individuals in two upper-division classes on stuttering and 60 primarily sophomore-level students in an introductory speech pathology course. The task was explained to the subjects, who were then given, as examples, the definitions (and then the answers) for the words "cry" and then "run." They were told that some of the task definitions had been drawn from various sources and that therefore the same term ("answer") might be appropriate to more than one definition. This qualification was included because there was more than one definition of stuttering—and, for that reason more than one definition of "kiss" and "smile" was also included. The students were instructed to not "dwell" on any item, to guess if they were uncertain or could not give a sure answer within a relatively brief time, and then go on.

The findings of this little test confirm what was expected. Students in both courses were well able to supply the correct terms for the real (dictionary) definitions. Overall, 72% of the words the subjects gave as the referents of these definitions were the actual words intended, including the two separate defini-

TABLE 2.1 Words for Which Definitions Were Given
in the Naming Referents from Definitions task*

1. sniff	21. smile
2. guess	22. growl
3. kiss	23. kiss
4. [#1]	24. lie
5. hiccough	25. [#5]
6. smile	26. paralysis
7. ringworm	27. cough
8. schizophrenia	28. sneeze
9. allergy	29. laugh
10. cold	30. [#6]
11. stumble	31. pause
12. [#2]	32. snort
13. grimace	33. [#7]
14. groan	34. sneer
15. rash	35. spit
16. [#3]	36. jump
17. snore	37. squeal
18. pinkeye	38. [#8]
19. "raspberry"	39. sigh
20. [#4]	40. yawn

*Numbers in brackets represent the definitions for "stut-
ter" as discussed in the text.

tions of "kiss" and "smile." By accepting synonyms or credible alternatives
(e.g., "scream" for "squeal," "moan" for "groan") the success rate rose to 96%.
It is of particular significance that the *Webster's* definition of "stutter" elicited
the correct answer 95% of the time.

Most often the subjects did not give terms (answers) for the professional-
source "definitions" (of stuttering) that were under scrutiny—answers were
given for only 22% of the total possible opportunities. This finding itself gives
clear confirmation of the deduction mentioned above—namely, that readers of
such "definitions" would be unable to discern the intended referent. In fact,
these readers clearly had little idea of what the referent might be. Not surprisingly, there was a notable variety to the terms given in the relatively few

attempts to supply a referent for these "definitions." Eighty-two percent of the terms given were different; the remaining 18% were terms that appeared more than once. An unexpected, but very notable, aspect of these answers is that they typically reflected the generally negative aura of the professional statements. Fifty-four percent of the answers given suggested internalized struggle ("frustration," "conscience," "anxiety"); another 30% clearly reflected altercation ("argument," "aggression," "fighting"); the remainder indicated uncertainty ("confusion," "indecision"). Speech-related words were given only for the two professional-source statements that contained some reference to speech (#3 and #5). Notably, these statements too elicited a variety of terms: "speechless," "tongue-tied," "stage-fright," "mumble," "stumble," "yell" [sic], "pause," and "hesitation."

The findings yielded by this little study add substance to the criticism and rejection of the kind of "definitions" under scrutiny here, and repudiation of the rationale and motivation for them as well. As noted earlier, the etiology of stuttering is unknown. Anyone in the field, including the individuals responsible for these statements, would have to acknowledge that fact. It is, therefore, misleading, and scientifically unjustified, to offer as a definition of the disorder a statement that is simply an etiologic conjecture.

The definition by Wendell Johnson, listed as #6, has been by far the most influential of all "definitions" of stuttering. It encapsulates a conjecture about the nature and source of stuttering that, as the definition reflects, is purely psychological in substance. Heavily interpersonal or interactive in theme, it is the font of the long-term and widespread preoccupation with explaining stuttering as "learned behavior." It also underlies other accounts that emphasize the role of personal interaction, essentially with parents, as the source of stuttering. Although the extensive influence of this conjecture may have crested, there are still many who accept its tenets and implications. For instance, a 1981 survey of almost 2000 students of communicative disorders in universities of 33 different American states revealed that the majority accepted most of the assumptions of Johnson's position (St. Louis & Lass, 1981).

The seven statements presented here in illustration are not exhaustive. There are others of the same ilk, sometimes in sources that are not as provincial in origin. In addition, there are those other definitions that, although noting one or another actual (or possible) descriptive aspect of stutter occurrence, go on to add some subjective element(s). This practice is exemplified in the several definitions offered by Van Riper over the years, his last one (Van Riper, 1971b, p. 15) being: "a stuttering behavior consists of a word improperly patterned in time *and the speaker's reaction thereto*" (italics added). The first half of the statement is inadequate; the second half is not defensible. As a whole, it is not an acceptable description, let alone a definition.

Then there are the statements that define stuttering in terms of "any one or more" of a variety of items, which then proceed to give a list of such items from which to choose. The classic example was published by the Speech Foundation of America (1962), in which "stuttering may be revealed by any *one or more* of the following" (italics added). Of the six different "characteristics" listed, only one mentioned speech; the remaining five were all possible psychological states.

Objectivity Evaded

Some years ago I attempted to bring the definition of stuttering into a realistic focus by discussion of a hierarchy of features as known from the long-term observations and reports of their relative occurrences in cases of stuttering (Wingate, 1964). The hierarchy emphasized the speech features[16] as the criterial aspects, with other potentially concurrent motor acts clearly subsidiary, and emotional factors acknowledged as possibly associated.

That attempt at a "standard definition" faced a mixed reception. Evidently well received by some, it was clearly ignored, or dismissed by others. The heavy preference for etiologic constructions has persisted, being either too solidified or too appealing. Some could not relinquish an established conviction; for instance, Bloodstein (1981) and Selmar (1991), both of whom reproduce the essence of the Johnson definition, #6 in the list presented in this chapter. In fact, Selmar recites that definition verbatim, adding that it "enables us to understand why stuttering occurs" (p. 3). Some other authors were compelled to elaborate other qualitative dimensions; for example, Perkins et al. (1991) define stuttering as "disruption of speech that is experienced by the speaker as loss of control" (p. 735). This definition, although not etiologic, is even more vaporous than any of those listed earlier.[17]

The ambience in the field of stuttering, created and supported by the extensive, freewheeling preoccupation with cause, has severely obstructed progress toward understanding the disorder itself. The current preoccupation is saturated with psychological beliefs and reflections that, clearly appealing and captivating in either their over-simplification or over-complication, have led nowhere in developing a consistent, meaningful, and credible conception of the disorder.

At base, these foci that address stuttering as some sort of a psychological problem have remained tangential to the central issue; in fact, they have distracted from it. In contradiction of the orientation well represented in the etiological "definitions," and in the current preoccupation with an "interaction" rationale derived from them, no one would presume to identify anyone as stuttering who does not evidence a certain type of anomalies in his speech—a truism perennially evident but steadily ignored. Ironically, this reality was emphasized, although evidently inadvertently, by the person who was the major force in the (still-active) movement to claim stuttering to be a psychological problem, and whose "definition" (#6 in the list) epitomizes the etiologic effort—Wendell Johnson. In his widely read "An Open Letter to the Mother of a Stuttering Child" (Johnson 1949),[18] he challenged "any expert" to pick out the 10 stutterers to be included in a (demonstration) group of 100 persons. The expert would be permitted to use

> any tests whatever, except that he may not hear anyone speak, nor may he obtain any information about each individual's personality and mental ability so long as this information in any way relates to the question of *how the person speaks or used to speak*. (p. 3, italics added)

Johnson's challenge clearly acknowledges, indeed indirectly emphasizes, that identification of stuttering requires a speech sample, which can be expected to reveal certain characteristic features. As emphasized earlier in this chapter, stuttering is a *speech* problem. Moreover, it is a unique, discriminable anomaly of speaking. To ignore, minimize, subordinate, controvert, evade, or confound this reality yields only protracted confusion. "Stutter" has meaning only in reference to speech.[19] Whatever else may be evidenced by, or claimed for, someone who stutters is tangential. This is not to say that any "whatever else" is immaterial, or to be ignored, but simply that these peripherals must be accorded their proper place—as subsidiary to the speech features.

In the past half century, but especially in more recent times, certain sources have actually expanded the inaccuracy embodied in the etiologic definitions by claiming that stuttering is a "syndrome." The notion of syndrome permits inclusion of a range of contended attributes. This position is weak for many reasons. At base it violates the meaning of syndrome, since all the features included in description(s) of the purported "syndrome" of stuttering do not regularly occur with stutters. Like the definition statements of the "any one or more of the following" variety, noted earlier, the syndrome notion accords the "whatever else" more status than the stutters.

Realistically, in so many cases of stuttering there is not enough "whatever else" to make a fuss about—unless added through descriptive license. In contrast, it is the certain unique anomalies in the speech sequence that have always constituted the designation "stuttering," as attested over many centuries and from many different sources (see Wingate, 1997).

IN BRIEF

The field of stuttering, especially in the twentieth century, has been plagued with too much absorption in various fabrications that are presumptively called "theories" of stuttering. Each of these formulations constitute little more than assumptions and conjectures regarding the nature of the disorder, while at the same time minimizing or ignoring its describable reality. Typically, these positions have been expressed in some confounding "definition" of the anomaly. In a field that remains in an essentially pre-scientific state of development, these conditions only encourage proselytism, along with further speculation.

It is past time to accept Hughlings Jackson's dictum —to abandon the preoccupation with cause, with its elaborate rambles and fanciful embellishments. It is time, instead, to direct attention to *the thing caused.*"

Literature Sources of the Definitions of Stuttering

Numbers correspond to the list presented earlier in the chapter. See the reference section for full citations.

A. From professionals in the field of stuttering:

1. Fletcher (1958)

2. Sheehan (1953, 1958a,b)

3. Brutten & Shoemaker (1967)

4. Mable Gifford (1958)

5. Bloodstein (1984)

6. Johnson (1948, 1956, 1963)

7. Coriat (1958)

B. From a lay source:

8. *Webster's New World Dictionary of the American Language*

NOTES

1. quoted in Beveridge (1961). Hughlings Jackson was an outstanding British neurologist of the late nineteenth century whose work in aphasia underlay his insightful concepts of "propositional" speech, and its contrast, "automatic" speech—concepts relevant to the content of Chapter 12.

2. An especially pithy article by this title appeared in the October 7, 1966 issue of *Time* magazine.

3. In regard to these accounts, the following comment by Anthony Standen (1950) is especially pertinent: "Psychologists pay lip service to the scientific method, and use it whenever it is convenient; but when it isn't they make wild leaps of their uncontrolled fancy, and still suppose themselves to be on objective fact."

4. The matter of recovery is addressed in Chapter 4. The term "recovered," in reference to stutterers, is often placed in quotation marks because in many cases a residual tendency remains. Additionally, some individuals are so described because, even though some stutter remains evident, their speech is nonetheless markedly improved. See illustrations in Chapter 10.

5. Originally published in *The New Yorker* magazine, November 25, 1976. The insertion "[*sic*]" in the second line of the quotation is added.

6. But see discussion in Chapter 10 regarding "normal nonfluency."

7. This description applies well to the current efforts to emphasize "interactions" as central to the disorder; efforts that are essentially reproductions of the claim conceived and fostered by Wendell Johnson.

8. The same approach is employed in oral presentations.

9. In fact, there is impressive evidence that laypersons can discriminate stuttering even from written transcriptions of speech (Wingate, 1977a).

10. West *et al.* (1957, p. 15).

11. This position, initiated by Wendell Johnson, is still actively pursued by his followers.

12. It is pertinent to note here that reliability values reported by many sources are, overall, around .90 or better, a highly respectable figure.

13. *And*, it should be added, *no one* knows what stuttering *is* in the sense of its nature.

14. Similarly adequate definitions will be found in other, non-provincial, sources; such as medical dictionaries, or the *Diagnostic and Statistical Manual of Mental Disorders*.

15. Two of the words ("smile" and "kiss") could support two separate definitions. This was done so that definitions other than the test definitions would also suit the instructions that "the same term may be appropriate to more than one definition."

16. A fault in this part of the definition was to allow possible inclusion of one-syllable words, even though qualified and uncertain. This matter has since been corrected, as repeated in the present work (see Chapter 3).

17. Which is sufficiently unrealistic that it has elicited appropriate criticism (Smith, 1992; Wingate, 1997, p. 155).

18. Published originally in the April 1941 issue of *You and Your Child*, it subsequently appeared in a number of other sources, as late as 1986 (see Wingate, 1997). The clear acknowledgment in this statement that stuttering is identified only in respect to speech stands as an example of the adage that "the truth will out." The adage is also pertinent to Johnson's acknowledgment, reproduced earlier in this chapter, that stutters can be counted (therefore, realistically identified). The adage is par-

ticularly well borne out in the description of stuttering contained in the report by Johnson and Brown (1935), which is reproduced early in Chapter 12, and certain related matters are considered briefly in Chapter 14.

19. One might note that certain reports have claimed stuttering in writing, in type-writing, or some other acts [even (male) urination; Paget, 1902]. Such references are allegorical only; they are meaningful only because of an intended simile to actual stuttering—in *speech*.

CHAPTER 3

Stuttering As Subject

Study of "the thing caused"

$\mathcal{T}$o address stuttering as the *subject* of study requires that the analysis begin by determining and specifying its cardinal features. Such procedure is the standard approach to any serious, especially scientifically oriented, inquiry about phenomena. In scientific inquiry, such careful analysis is required as the necessary foundation for working toward understanding what is being studied.

The initial step in determining the cardinal features of stuttering is achieved quite easily inasmuch as everyone already has a pretty good idea of what stuttering is, descriptively. In specialized areas of study, knowing what is evident to everyone provides a good place to start, but such knowledge must be objectively and rationally refined. A professional approach to the study of any phenomenon must go beyond what is clearly evident to ordinary awareness; it must undertake to identify more carefully, to analyze further, to delineate and specify rationally and critically.

Descriptively, stuttering refers to a unique interruption in the flow of speech in which the speaker is temporarily unable to proceed normally. This evident inability is reflected in two kinds of occurrence: (1) iteration (repetition) of speech fragments and (2) a brief interval of inaction. Typically, "speech fragments" refers to elements of less than a full syllable; the "interval of inaction" reflects a steady state condition.[1]

THE CARDINAL FEATURES

It seems clear that the ready recognition of stuttering is based on the two features that characterize the disorder descriptively. Each of these two features can be described by several terms, all of which (for each feature) are interchangeable because they have the same reference, based ultimately on pertinent direct observation. The reader should become familiar with the terms *iteration, oscillation,* and *clonic,* which describe one characteristic marker of a stutter event; and the terms *perseveration, protraction, fixation,* and *tonic,* which describe the other characteristic marker.

Of these various terms, clonic and tonic will be found more often in the literature of stuttering. Derived from medicine, they were first used in reference to stuttering by a Frenchman, Serre d'Alais, early in the nineteenth century. They were widely adopted in that role because they succinctly encapsulate the specific quality to which each of these terms refers. Clonic is the adjective form of "clonus," which describes the rapid, involuntary, repetitive movements of muscle groups. Tonic is the adjective form of "tonus," which refers to continuous muscular contraction. Thus, clonic has the significance of "iterative"; tonic carries the meaning of "steady state." The fact that these terms are borrowed from the field of neurology should not prejudice their use in reference to stuttering; that is, they need not carry neurologic implication. They are simply appropriately descriptive of the cardinal features.

At this point it becomes appropriate to call attention to several terms that will be used with special reference throughout this book, and that come into direct focus in this chapter. The term *"stutter event"* will be used to refer to the peripheral essence of stuttering—namely, the inability to proceed in the speech sequence. Stutterers refer to this event as the experience of being "blocked." The terms *"stutter"* and *"stutter occurrence"* will be used to refer to what is directly observable—namely, the cardinal features (clonic and tonic). The cardinal features are the classic *markers* of a stutter *event*—they point out the inability to proceed, described prosaically as the "block."

The iterative marker occurs, classically, as the repetition of the simplest elements of speech: something less than a full, or completed, syllable. This may take the form of a repeated phoneme ("speech sound") or the phoneme and some amount of indefinite sound—thus, repetition of t t t or tuh tuh tuh in an attempt to say "table." Clearly, this marker is a kind of repetition, but it is critical that one be careful to specify it as an *elemental* repetition. There are certain other, longer, forms of repetition that occur in speech, but these are not at all distinctive of stuttering. Too much of the literature in the field is either careless about these distinctions, or intentionally disregards them. We will consider these longer, ordinary, kinds of repetition in Chapter 10. The specification "elemental" faithfully describes the kind of repetition in speech that characterizes stuttering; it carries, in more familiar words, the sense of what is intended in the terms *iteration, oscillation,* and *clonic.*

The perseverative marker can involve only the simplest elements of speech—namely, a phone. In this case, the element is protracted, extended beyond its ordinary, or normal, duration. In these markers the phoneme is unreleased, or if released is followed by some amount of indefinite sound, which is itself extended. For example, t--- or tuuuh. Literature references to this marker standardly employ a lay term, "prolongation," which carries the sense of what is represented in the terms *perseveration, protraction, fixation,* or *tonic.*

The terms most widely used to speak of the two cardinal features, in both lay and professional writing and discourse, are the words "repetition" and "prolongation." Both of these words are vernacular terms, and, unfortunately, they have been used regularly in the field of stuttering in their full lay sense. To meet a basic respectable standard of professional usage they require refinement, particularly the word "repetition." This word is a generic, broadly inclusive term. It has a place in general discussions of speech, if properly employed in carefully limited designation, but it is thoroughly unacceptable for use in the kind of specific reference needed in the study of stuttering. In contexts addressed to stuttering, any appearance of this term must be severely qualified. Its continued bland use in reference to stuttering continues to confound and obstruct progress in this field.

"Repetitions" includes all kinds of repetition: monosyllabic words, polysyllabic words, phrases, sentences, etc.—essentially, variations in length. These repetition variants will be found in the speech of stutterers, but they also occur with surprising frequency in the speech of normally speaking individuals, a matter to be addressed in considerable detail in Chapter 10. Such repetitions are not at all distinctive of stuttering. They may sometimes occur in the vicinity of stutter events, but they are not intrinsic to, nor even integral with, the stutter. Later in this chapter we will discuss their occurrence in such circumstances.

The word "prolongation," on the other hand, is not so inherently misleading. Even though it too is a class term (like "repetitions"), it does not span as many differentiable categories, and it is more readily qualified. At the same time, other terms, noted earlier, offer more specificity and convey better the appropriate sense of "steady state." These terms are considered again in the section addressed to "the protractive marker."

THE ITERATIVE MARKER

Of the two cardinal features of stuttering, the repetitive marker is evidently more readily discerned than the other, as suggested by a number of observations, presented below. This most obvious, and seemingly the most prevalent, feature of stuttering is a certain unique type of repetition; a type that involves only very elemental aspects of the speech sequence—namely, *phones* (often referred to as "speech sounds"). The essential character of the repetitive feature is that it involves something less than a full, or completed, syllable. It may involve only one phone, or perhaps two in sequence, but only infrequently more than two, depending upon the structure of the word attempted. For example, in the unsuccessful attempt to say "spoke" (/spok/)[2] the characteristic repetitive feature may involve only the /s/, or it may include /sp/, or it may include a bit of indefinite vowel-like sound, as in /spə/. The /ə/, a phonetic symbol known as the "schwa," has the sound rendered in ordinary script as "uh." It is often described as the "neutral" or "indefinite" vowel. If a stutter includes a vowel-like component it is almost always the schwa, or something perceivable as schwa (see later in this chapter at discussion of Table 3.1 examples). In rare instances, the vowel-like element may resemble the intended vowel (in this case /o/), although, as will be discussed in more detail in Chapter 12, the intended vowel is not "full." The essential point here is that the cardinal repetitive feature of stutter involves less than a completed syllable; in the example used here, the complete syllable is a whole single-syllable word, "spoke" (/spok/). The foregoing specification marks the critical distinction between elemental repetitions and the other repetitions—of monosyllabic words, polysyllabic words, and phrases (and, of course, anything longer). The critical distinction is that the latter forms have complete syllabic structure.

As noted earlier, the specification "*elemental* repetition" faithfully describes the kind of repetition in speech that characterizes stuttering, carrying, in familiar words, the sense of what is intended in the more esoteric terms *iteration, oscillation,* and *clonic,* each of which conveys quite pointedly the special nature of the referent. Since being introduced early in the nineteenth century to designate the iterative feature of the disorder, the term "clonic" was widely used in description of stuttering for well over a century, evidently because of its succinctly appropriate meaning. However, it appeared quite often with the word "spasm," which, because of its neurological implication, was considered to carry that bias. Therefore, spasm was not favored by sources becoming absorbed with psychological explanations of the disorder, a persuasion gaining momentum in the second quarter of the twentieth century. Thus, the especially well-suited term "clonic" lost favor too.[3] Nonetheless, it remains a most appropriate designation for the cardinal iterative feature of stuttering.

It is necessary to reemphasize that, in regard to the repetitive hallmark of the disorder, it is absolutely essential that this feature be understood to denote *elemental* repetitions, the kind that are the essence of stuttering, as denoted above and exemplified below. It is important to emphasize this specification again because, as noted in the introduction to this section, this classic cardinal feature of stuttering has been blurred by the frequent indiscriminative use of the generic word "repetition(s)" in discussions of the disorder. It also bears restating that, for a level of fluency analysis intended to be careful and discriminating, this generic term is not only inadequate; it is discursive, misleading, and confounding.

The fact that identification of stuttering does not depend upon assessment by "experts" has been clear for a long time,[4] a matter for which the reader can undoubtedly supply his or her own confirmation. Repetitions of speech *elements* as a cardinal feature of stuttering, and their recognition as such by most everyone, is pointedly reflected in various circumstances, including occasional cartoons found in lay sources. Two cartoon examples are worth noting.

One cartoon, which appeared in a popular American magazine, clearly illustrates the extent to which stuttering is widely recognized. The cartoon shows two young men; one is standing, the other is seated. The man standing is wearing a T-shirt with the words "Speech Therapist" printed on it. He is holding one hand to his chin and his face shows a quizzical expression as he regards the other fellow who, seated facing him, is also wearing a T-shirt, on which is printed "W– W– W– W– W– ..." The cartoon has no caption or other words; its message is conveyed directly, without need for explication. There can be little doubt regarding what the cartoonist had in mind. There is also little doubt that he could be quite certain the cartoon would be readily understood by a large unseen lay audience.

A second example is supplied by "Ziggy," a nationally syndicated cartoon figure. In this item, which appeared in a stutterers' self-help journal, "Ziggy" is depicted in the act of changing a daily calendar; the next day is "M– M– Monday."[5]

Figure 3.1 replicates the logo adopted for the First International Conference on Stuttering Problems. The suggested sound of a woodpecker hard at work represents a classic analogy to the distinctive audible iteration that is the more obvious of the two criterial hallmarks of stuttering.

This iterative cardinal feature of stuttering is also reflected in the many instances in which the word "stuttering" is used metaphorically. In particular, the frequent, almost standard, reference to the "stutter" of a machine-gun, or similar weaponry discharge.[6] In a lighter vein, those who follow American

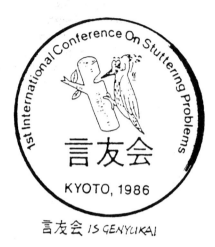

言友会 *IS GENYUKAI*

FIGURE 3.1 Logo of the First International Conference on Stuttering Problems.

football hear frequently a reference to the "stutter-step" of a ball carrier. One can comfortably assume that both the commentator and his audience recognize the nature of the movements so described. In another vein, one's visual imagery can quickly raise the appropriate scene suggested by Kipling's description of the "stuttering" of a small railroad engine, and thereby share the picture Kipling intended to represent.

The literal sound of the word "stutter" also suggests this cardinal feature of elemental repetition. That is, the word "stutter" is onomatopoeic, a term meaning that the sound of a word resembles the object of its reference. Just as "boom," "whirr," "splat," and many other words sound like what they mean, so does the word "stutter" resemble, in particular, this cardinal iterative feature of the disorder. Significantly, an analogous structure is found in the words for stuttering in many different languages; they too are typically onomatopoeic.[7]

Another linguistic support for such identification will be found in the etymology of the words for stuttering in many languages, as it is in English, where our word is derived from German *stossen*, meaning "to knock or push"—thus suggesting both cardinal features.

THE PROTRACTIVE MARKER

The second cardinal feature of stuttering is not as dramatically obvious as the first. However, it is at least as significant; in fact, as developed in the following section, it comes closer to epitomizing the actual stutter event.

Like the repetitive feature, the protractive feature also involves the simplest elements in speech: phones. Moreover, this feature is especially criterial inasmuch as a protraction involves only a single phone. In a protraction the phone is unreleased; for example, in the attempt to say "soap" (/sop/) one will most likely hear /s:::/ in which the /s/ is unreleased or, if some vowel-like sound (almost always /ə/) follows the /s/, that sound will be extended (/sə:::/).

The term "prolongation" has long been used to indicate the protractive feature. The word "prolongation" does not pose the problem of reference presented by the word "repetition"; the occurrence signified by "prolongation" is already a simple structure. Since one can only prolong a single phone, it is not necessary to add the specification "elemental." At the same time, the word prolongation can be, minimally, confounding since this word can include under its rubric a very normal kind of speech event, ordinarily referred to as a "drawl." In almost all instances, however, differentiation presents no notable problem, especially because drawls do not involve word/syllable-initial position. The distinction between prolongation and drawl centers on the aspect of its position in a syllable in relation to the syllable nucleus: a prolongation involves initiation; a drawl involves termination. Actually, some stutterers may occasionally use a drawl as a verbal adjustment to obscure or manage a stutter.

A remaining reservation about "prolongation" is that it may be construed to indicate or imply conscious intention, whereas the terms *protraction*, *perseveration*, *fixation*, and *tonic* are either more neutral in this respect or tend more to imply involuntary.

The description of these two cardinal features is not complete without adding that each of them may be either silent or audible. Their audible versions are the more obvious, but the silent instances are readily discernible, especially when they are of the protractive type. In fact, the silent form of protractions have been known by the special reference of "postures," which convey the sense of "steady state."

The Central Dimension

Clearly, the two cardinal features are descriptively different, well attested by evidence that the repetitive feature is much more compelling than the protractive. For instance, elemental repetition obviously underlies the onomatopoeic structure of the words for stuttering in many languages; it is also quite clearly the reference in metaphorical uses of the word "stutter." At the same time, the protractive feature also is clearly discernible in stutter occurrences. Although less often readily noticed, prolongations are in many instances considerably more dramatic than elemental repetitions. Importantly, both features are widely recognized, by lay and professional persons alike, as aspects of the same phenomenon.[8]

The implicit recognition that both cardinal features are aspects of stutter occurrence is based in the awareness that these two features reflect the same condition—*an inability to move ahead in the speech sequence in spite of the evident intent to do so*. Observationally this condition, if not considered obvious, is certainly readily inferred. The inference that the person is somehow stopped from moving on in the speech sequence is corroborated by the complaint of stutterers that, in a stutter occurrence, they feel "blocked." In fact, this testimony, supported by the observational inference that the speaker seems prevented from proceeding, has occasioned use of the term "block" to refer to the stutter occurrence.

It is critically important to realize that this inability to proceed in the speech sequence is inability in the sense of *the execution of a complete verbal unit*; that is, the inability to produce a normally structured syllable.

Description of stutter as a failure of transition between phones, specifically between consonant and vowel, was first presented in two publications in the nineteenth century. However, the significance of that analysis remained unrecognized until recently, even though similar observations were made by several authors during the first half of the twentieth century. This characterization of stutter, which epitomizes it as a phonetic transition defect, was refined (Wingate, 1988) by specifying that the transition failure uniquely involves *syllable-initial consonant and syllable nucleus*. This description assumes particular significance relative to certain substance in the linguistics literature—namely, the syllable-structure hypothesis—and evidence of syllable asymmetry. These matters are discussed in Chapters 11 and 12.

Stutter, the inability to continue in the anticipated speech sequence, is a syllabic disruption, and is clearly distinct from certain other phenomena that reflect, instead, an evident lapse in immediate recall of a particular word, or an attempt to select the best word for that occasion, or to create the most proper phrase, etc. The latter kinds of lapse in verbal continuity are of an entirely different kind. Occasionally they may occur in the vicinity of a stutter, but they are not, of themselves, intrinsic to the stutter. This issue is considered later in this chapter.

It is widely believed that stutterers are keenly aware of their stutters. However, evidence from research as well as from casual report reveals that stutterers do not routinely notice their stutters, "especially the little ones," as remarked to me by several stutterers with whom I have discussed the matter. In some instances in which a stutter is obvious, stutterers may remark that they can't say the word, or that they know what they want to say but can't say it. Such a report seems to well reflect what a stutterer must experience as being "blocked." Although these remarks seem to make sense and have been readily accepted in their lay expression as indicating trouble in making the appropriate sounds, the limitation may well extend beyond articulation. The "can't say it" part is obvious to an observer as well; however, the "know what I want to say" part deserves special analysis. This matter will be considered in Chapters 12 and 13.

The inability to proceed in the speech sequence is, at least in its peripheral aspect, *the essence of a stutter event*.[9] The cardinal features of that event, the iteration and protraction, are best considered as *markers* of that event; they indicate instances of the event. From this perspective the two features, and their observable difference, can be analyzed further. The protractive feature, which is in substance a direct expression of inability to proceed, should be recognized as the focal hallmark of the stutter event—it epitomizes the "block." In this light the repetitive feature, although apparently the more obvious historically, would be considered subsidiary, more as an iterative, unsuccessful and abortive attempt set off by the "block."

THE REMAINING DESCRIPTOR

Stutters do not occur randomly. A substantial body of information pertinent to this truism will be considered at length in later chapters, in which the considerable evidence regarding the loci of stutter occurrence is addressed. While the literature to be considered there, especially in Chapter 12, is of great significance to understanding stuttering, one will not often find within that literature any special mention, let alone appropriate emphasis, of the fundamental and critical non-random aspect of stuttering that will be brought into focus here.

This most significant non-random aspect of stuttering is that *stutters occur only in (word/syllable) initial position*. It is curious that the matter of initial position has been so neglected.

For the time being, we will speak in terms of *word*-initial position rather than, more correctly *syllable*-initial position, because words are invariably the referent for this phenomenon. One finds, in the extensive literature of stuttering, a great deal of attention to the topic of "difficult words," or "difficult sounds" (or, as interpretive embellishment, "feared" words or sounds). Although such discussions dwell extensively on the matter of words or sounds, the critical, yet typically unacknowledged, dimension of such references is word-*initial* position. When purportedly difficult sounds are claimed in testimony or report, those sounds are ones that occur in word-initial position, and *pari passu*, when words are claimed as difficult, they are words that begin with some particular sound. The crux of this issue is that the preoccupation with certain words or certain sounds has diverted attention from what is actually the most important aspect of these observations—the matter of their locus of occurrence, in word-initial position.

Although typical reference to this well-known fact of stuttering states it in terms of *word*-initial position, it is more accurate (and comprehensive) to point out that stutters occur only in *syllable*-initial position, since the block occasionally occurs in the initial position of an internal syllable of a polysyllabic word. In addition, it must be fully appreciated that the initial-position aspect of stutters is integral with the cardinal features; that is, "*stutter*" *refers to elemental repetitions and prolongations as features of syllable-initial position.* The corollary of this truism is that stutters do not occur in word-final position.[10] The following example should illustrate this fact vividly. If a stutter occurs with the word "pat" (/pæt/) the stutter, either clonic or tonic, will involve the phone /p/ but not the phone /t/. In contrast, if a stutter occurs with the word "tap" (/tæp/), which is phonemically the reverse of "pat" (/pæt/), the phone /t/ will be involved in the stutter, but not the phone /p/.[11]

This fact of stuttering has special significance for psycholinguistic analysis of the disorder, and will be considered further in Chapter 12, which addresses more fully the other non-random dimensions of stutter occurrence. However, we should at least note at this point that the fact of initial position bears importantly on the whole matter of "difficult sounds," especially in regard to their purported significance in explanations of stuttering. The matter of difficult sounds will be considered in several contexts of later chapters, especially Chapter 6, and again in Chapter 12.

ILLUSTRATION

As noted several times in this chapter, the literature of stuttering regularly fails to distinguish the kind of repetition in speech that characterizes stuttering from other kinds of repetition—forms that are found in the speech of all speakers (see Chapter 10). Not only is there too-frequent casual use of the all-encompassing, non-specific class term "repetition(s)," but frequently one also finds that certain sources make the effort to include full-syllable monosyllabic words in designations of stuttering. Such practice flaunts the well-recognized classical features of stutter, as reviewed above. It also ignores the fact that there is a remarkable difference between, for instance, /p p p–/ or /pə pə pə –/ and /pæt–pæt–pæt/. The critical issue here is that the repetition of complete syllables is not a criterion of stuttering. Moreover, repetition of complete syllables is not intrinsic to stuttering even when they occur in close proximity to stutters. They may have some sort of relation to stutter occurrence, but they are not the same as the stutter, nor are they a part of, or integral with, the stutter. Of course, this is also true for repetition of longer verbal units—polysyllabic words and phrases.

The sixteen examples appearing in Table 3.1 are presented to illustrate a representative variety of fluency departures that may be evident at the locus of a stutter event. In each item the target utterance, rendered there in IPA symbols, is, "He said we can take it back." Note that in each item, regardless of whether it is simple or seemingly complex, the stutter event—the "block," the inability to move on—is at the same locus, as indicated by the arrow. Where present, the stutters are manifested, in varying extent, to the left of the arrow indication.

TABLE 3.1 Illustrations of Stutters (Items 1–11) and Several Occurrences Likely to be Ambiguous Under Certain Circumstances (Items 12–16)

locus of the
stutter event

1	hi sɛd wi kæn t t t tek ɪt bæk
2	hi sɛd wi kæn tə tə tə tek ɪt bæk
3	hi sɛd wi kæn t::::::ek ɪt bæk
4	hi sɛd wi kæn tə::::::ek ɪt bæk
5	hi sɛd wi kæn kæn ətek ɪt bæk
6	hi sɛd wi kæn kæn t:ek ɪt bæk
7	hi sɛd wi kæn ə ə ətek ɪt bæk
8	hi sɛd wi kæn ə ə ə tek ɪt bæk
9	hi sɛd wi kæn wi kæn t::ek ɪt bæk
10	hi sɛd wi kæn wi kæn tə tek ɪt bæk
11	hi sɛd wi kæn rɪlɪtek ɪt bæk
12	hi sɛd wi kæn kæn tek ɪt bæk
13	hi sɛd wi kæn wi kæn tek ɪt bæk
14	hi sɛd wi kæn ə tek ɪt bæk
15	hi sɛd wi kænə tek ɪt bæk
16	hi sɛd wi kæn:: tek ɪt bæk

The first four items exemplify classic stutters, as described earlier in this chapter: silent or audible elemental repetition, respectively, in items 1 and 2; silent or audible prolongation in items 3 and 4.

The frequent appearance of /ə/ in the items of Table 3.1 reflects the extent to which this sound is reported to occur in stutter. Recent research suggests that what is perceived as /ə/ at the locus of stutter may often be a low-quality fragment of the intended vowel, and also that there may be different basic types of fragments.[12] If substantiated, this finding would have special significance for understanding the stutter event and, as well, distinguishing these sounds from those of similar impression that occur in normal speech. For the present, however, we will have to deal with these indefinite sounds as "/ə/," especially as there is no better way to transcribe them.

Items numbered 5 through 10 illustrate various other repetition forms that in some cases attend a stutter; some with monosyllabic words, or short phrases, and/or the schwa. Note that all of these intrusions, the verbal repetitions and the schwa, occur *before* the actual stutter. The last six items represent instances involving an initial experience of being blocked, or in some cases a pre-science[13]—some level of awareness—of the impending block. The insertions (repetitions or schwa, or both) may occur as an adjustment to this experience, a way of making another "run" to surmount the block. For that reason, such adjustments have come to be known as "starters." Example 5 represents such an adjustment, in which the /ə/ serves as the effective starter.

In many instances, of course, the insertions may not occur as starters, that is, running onto the next word; they may occur as a delay while attempting the word in sequence. In item 6 the word repetition did not serve a starter role, as revealed in the brief silent protraction of /t/. In item 7 the source of the initial occurrence(s) of /ə/ is uncertain, but the third occurrence served as a starter. In item 8 the adjustment attempt was abortive; note the iteration of /ə/. In examples 9 and 10, repetition of the short phrase, occasioned by the incipient block, had no value in dealing with the stutter event; a brief stutter was manifest.

Item 11 is a special example in which insertion of the word "really" illustrates the occurrence of a "pet" starter. Some stutterers make (varying) use of a favorite word or phrase as a starter, in addition to forms exemplified in the foregoing items of the table. Some of these favorites, like "really," fit rather smoothly into many verbal contexts and thereby may be quite successful as adjustment—and sometimes concealment.[14]

If the interval between insertion and potential stutter is brief, whether or not a starter is attempted, and is not followed by some evidence of stutter, the insertion will have succeeded in yielding what at least may appear to be a normal speech event. Evidences of stutters, mentioned here, are often less obvious than can be recorded graphically, as in this table. Frequently occurring minimal indications of this sort are: signs of excessive effort in initiating the word, or some minor accessory feature (see next section) that may be evident in the brief silent interval just before the word is uttered.

One must keep in mind that the kinds of insertions just discussed can sometimes masquerade as normal phenomena because insertions like these may occur as benign events in a stutterer's speech, just as the same sorts of insertions occur in a normal speech sequence, where they represent a "filler" during a momentary reflection, distraction, search for the correct word, etc. Under certain circumstances in a stutterer's speech, it may not be possible to determine whether such insertions are a normal event or an adjustment to a stutter. The remaining examples in the table (items 12 to 16) can be used to illustrate when uncertainty about identification might arise.

Uncertainty is least likely to occur if one has a clear idea of the criteria for stutter, discussed earlier in this chapter. Uncertainty about stutter identification has been created as a potential problem by sources pressing the issue that identification of stuttering is unreliable, reviewed in Chapter 2. That essentially false issue has been expanded into the implied requirement that one must be able to correctly categorize every instance as either stuttered or normal. Under most circumstances, such as deciding whether someone stutters, such requirement is of little practical consequence, since an adequate speech sample will contain enough occurrences about which one will have no doubt. In fact, this bit of reality provides the key for explaining the internal contradiction in the "unreliability" position reviewed in Chapter 2—namely, that while claiming unreliability of stuttering identification, those same sources had made practical determinations based on identifying stuttering—in the procedure of selecting individuals who stuttered, and comparison individuals who did not.

Returning to the illustrations of Table 3.1, note first that, as with the examples in the upper part of the table, items 12 to 15 also contain word, phrase, and schwa insertions. There are, however, notable differences. In the latter there are no suggestions of the cardinal features and no other clear indications of difficulty in moving forward. Again, the repetition of complete single-syllable words or short phrases occurs often in normal speech. The brief silent intervals in items 12 and 13 are nondistinctive; and they are unlikely to be made more notable because of the word or phrase repetition preceding them. The schwa, as in item 14, also appears very frequently in normal speech. The /ə/ as addition to "can" in item 15 happens to be particularly characteristic of schwa occurrences in normal speech (Wingate, 1984b). The brief extension of /n/ in item 16 is also a kind of occurrence observed occasionally in normal speech. Although extended, it is not describable as a prolongation primarily because it is in word (syllable)-final position.

If occurrences like those in items 12 to 16 were observed in the speech of someone who did not evidence instances of examples 1 to 11, the last five items (12–16), if noticed at all, would almost certainly be accepted as unremarkable, that is, as normal irregularities. However if, in contrast, the individual's speech sample contained instances of examples 1 to 11 that were noticed, one would likely be uncertain about whether the occurrence of instances like those in 12 to 16 were simply a normal irregularity or an instance of a successful adjustment to a stutter event. In such cases the uncertainty remains unresolved. In most practical circumstances, as noted above, resolution is not critical.

The matter of uncertainty about some instances of disfluency presents no significant issue; certainly not the false issue that has been made of it—namely, the claim that such uncertainty is evidence that stutters and "normal nonfluencies" cannot be reliably differentiated. To the contrary, this uncertainty helps make the point that repetitions of a monosyllabic word, and certainly of longer syllable sequences, are not instances of stutter.

Words employed as "starters" are probably best classified as a special kind of accessory feature. This category, discussed in the next section, includes a number of other actions that may accompany stutters. Certain of these other actions also seem to function as adjustments to an impending block or to the initial experience of one. At the same time, some accessory features impress one as being of a quite different nature (to be discussed below).

ACCESSORY FEATURES

In some stutter occurrences certain acts other than the cardinal features are also evident. It is important to emphasize that such acts are not regularly observed to accompany stutters, which is the principal reason for their designation as "accessory." They do not appear routinely in cases of stuttering, nor in all instances of stutter by any one person who may evidence some of such features. Their occurrence is clearly something of an individual matter, with variation from person to person and, as well, in their appearance in the speech sequences of any particular individual.

The topic of accessory features receives a great deal of attention in the literature of stuttering, most often, however, under names other than "accessory features." One will most likely encounter the term "secondary features" (often abbreviated to "secondaries"), a term based in a persuasive point of view presented in 1932 by C. S. Bluemel (see below). Certain other terms that have been widely used, notably "avoidances," are considered in following paragraphs.

In contrast to the term "accessory features," in which the word *accessory* means simply "something extra," all of the other terms used to indicate such actions have surplus meanings. For instance, from the beginning, "secondary" meant second in time, that is, secondary *to*, or following upon the primary (first) features, the clonic and tonic markers. However, in actual usage it soon came to carry the added meaning of "stemming from," or "built upon," the so-called primary stuttering (the speech features). "Secondary" has never been used solely with the much more appropriate and defensible meaning of "second in importance." In consequence, the term gained an expansive, although erroneous, significance.

Unfortunately, the extensive consideration accorded the topic of accessory features is made up predominantly of anecdote, hypothesis, hearsay, and lore. For instance, there are no actual data bearing on the frequency with which these features appear, either in general or in respect to individual cases. Moreover, one will not find in extant literature any comprehensive, or even reasonably representative, list of these features. Typically, the whole matter is presented in general terms that describe the purported origin and role of actions of this sort, with few, often no, actual examples. This matter will be elaborated later in this section. Nonetheless, attention to the occurrence of these phenomena has gained a most prominent place in the literature of stuttering, to the point of eclipsing attention to the speech features themselves.

These other acts, which have some temporal concurrence with stutters, constitute a major complicating impediment in the study of stuttering, for they have provided attractive substance for misguided attempts to explain the disorder. A fundamental error, intrinsic to views proposed regarding the nature of these acts, is that presumption and belief have been mixed in with observation, with no provision for an intervening step of careful analysis and rational reflection. The first dimension of this error is that, in spite of the extensive variety reportedly observed in this aggregate of accessory features, they have all been assumed to be of similar substance, to have a common origin and the same function.

The actions encompassed in this aggregate of special features vary considerably in respect to their observable characteristics, ranging from simple muscle twitches to the utterance of word sequences. An especially representative sample of such actions, obtained from a number of relevant sources, is presented in Table 3.2. In view of the extensive range of these features, the reader might surmise that there would also be at least some range in conception of their origins. Such is not the case. In spite of the "great variety" that is not

TABLE 3.2   Accessory Features Obtained from Literature
Review

Action	Sources noting*
Eye blink	a, c, g, i, j, k, l, q, r
Eye close	a, c, k, l
Stare	f
Pupil dilation	i
Looks sideways	a, q, r
Forehead movement	i, r
Perspiration	i
Grimace	a, c, d, g, p
Lip raise	q
Lip tremor	a, c, d, m, o
Pressing lips	h, q
Distorts mouth	i, n, r
Protrudes tongue	g, n, r
Jaw drop	q
Jaw tremor	a, m, o
Grits teeth	l
Sharp inspiratory gasp	b, j, n
Forcible inhalation	h, r
Forcible exhalation	h
Holding breath	a
Talk on residual air	p, r
Bobs head	d, n, r
Hand to mouth	o
Pull at hair	o
Sudden movements of extremities	d, g, r
Clenching fist	f
Tapping/stamping foot	f
Sounds/noises	a, c, f
Words/phrases	e, f, j, o

*The letters listed under this heading represent the sources in
which the item was noted.

only claimed but routinely emphasized in the literature, they are nonetheless assumed to be of a kind, to reflect the same underlying process. Moreover, this assumption involves a substantial, but clearly unrecognized, inconsistency, as follows. In one line of discussion, any or all of the accessory features are explained as reactions to the occurrence, or threat, of stutter, in which case they are, by this very account, implicitly separate from (i.e., different than) the stutters. However, in another line of discussion the accessory features are lumped together with the cardinal features (the stutters), and then all together are spoken of as the "symptoms" of stuttering. Remarkably, both lines of discussion regularly appear together in the same literature sources in which this topic is addressed and in which, moreover, the two lines not only are not differentiated but instead are treated as integral. This inconsistency is one of a number of such lapses in conception to be found in the literature of stuttering. The matter of "symptoms" is considered in the next section of this chapter.

The idea that accessory features occur as reactions to stutters stemmed principally from the personal reflections of a stutterer, C. S. Bluemel (Bluemel, 1932).[15] Bluemel, a psychiatrist who achieved a certain prominence in the early days of the fledgling professional association in the United States, proposed that for some indefinite period of time in early childhood a stutterer evidences only the cardinal features, the speech anomalies, which Bluemel called "primary stuttering." In his account, the child is essentially indifferent to these unique anomalies in his speech during this early period. However, according to Bluemel, the child eventually comes to view his stuttering as undesirable, after which he begins to react to and then to struggle with the problem. As a result, purportedly, the child acquires other acts that reflect the struggle. Bluemel spoke of this now elaborated disturbance in fluency as "secondary stuttering," a description that thereafter was accorded conceptual status.

As noted earlier, "secondary" quickly accrued surplus meaning. Use of the word in this connection should properly be phrased as secondary *to* stuttering, because these other acts, presumably occurring in reaction to the stutters, are thereby identified as separate from the stutters, and are therefore also subsidiary in importance. However, note that in the usage advanced by Bluemel, and accepted uncritically thereafter, "secondary" still does not mean second in importance, nor even any longer secondary *to* stutters: it now encompasses the accessory features *and* the cardinal features, an amalgamation given a status of its own—"secondary stuttering."

Bluemel's personal account, accepted enthusiastically by the unsophisticated membership of a new association, was attended by several other serious problems, which also have persisted. Such problems—for instance, the presumption that stuttering regularly develops (i.e., becomes worse)—will be addressed in the section of Chapter 4 that reports findings regarding recovery. It will be considered again later, especially in Chapter 14. Our immediate concern, addressed to beliefs regarding the accessory features, is that the notion of secondary stuttering encouraged and inflated the role claimed for reaction. This easily grasped notion, which held special appeal in an era when psychological explanations of individual differences were burgeoning rapidly, overwhelmed contrary evidence that existed even then. The notion went on to accrue not only vigorous support but eager embellishment in many subsequent explanations of stuttering.

Bluemel's exposition engendered the belief that accessory features are all of a kind, stemming from the same base, namely, personal reaction to stutters. At the same time, it underlay the later developing belief that the accessory features have a common substance with the speech features—that they are all "symptoms."

Significantly, the notion of "primary" and "secondary" stuttering actually did not fare well in efforts at practical application. Among other limitations, this testimonially based conception incorporated a critical role for "awareness." But how is one to determine if someone, especially a young child, is aware of stutters, without asking for some testimony? Someone's awareness of an immediate circumstance is impossible to assess observationally. This, and other, serious limitations notwithstanding, the general primary–secondary notion has continued to have a certain currency, under the persisting presumption that the acts that sometimes accompany stutters function as reactions to stutter.

As proposed originally by Bluemel, some of these actions give the appearance of struggle, suggesting that the stutterer is struggling to overcome, or work through the "block." That suggestion is credible for some accessory features. In certain stutter occurrences, what one observes is very reminiscent of the experience of attempting to manage a door or drawer that is unexpectedly stuck. Acts that fit this analogy are credibly described as struggle. However, many accessory features do not convey this image of struggle.

The belief that all accessory features are reactions to stutter is often expressed in the notion of "vicious circle," a catch phrase used to summarize the idea that stuttering "grows" via the sequence: stutter → reaction → struggle → stutter → reaction → struggle → stutter → reaction, etc. This notion is an outstanding instance of the lore in this field. Not only is the idea of vicious circle contradicted by extensive evidence, it flouts even common sense. That is, if stuttering did routinely develop according to such a progression, one could expect that the typical stutterer, beginning to stutter somewhere around 3 years of age, should be practically mute by age 8. Clearly, this does not happen. In fact, as documented in Chapter 4, the "progression" is in the other direction: stuttering is much more likely to dissipate as the child grows. Moreover, even when stuttering has become "chronic," it occurs in only a small proportion of what the person says, as documented in Table 4.1.

This major legacy of the primary–secondary scheme, the contention that stuttering regularly develops and goes through stages of worsening, continues in vogue despite substantial evidence to the contrary, as well as the fact that certain early influential supporters of the notion eventually repudiated it (in particular, Van Riper, 1971b). The effort to understand stuttering will benefit if the terms primary and secondary are abandoned, and if the notion they reflect be recognized as a major unproductive diversion in the study of the disorder.

The term "secondary" in particular has lived on, consolidating in one or another form of expression in the subsequent literature. One finds, as might be expected, frequent use of the word "secondaries" to indicate accessory features, but there are other terms that carry even more surplus meanings, for instance, "expectancies," "postponements," and "avoidances." The latter term, in particular, has had an especially remarkable career.

The notion of avoidance had humble beginnings, evidently originating in the testimony of some stutterers that they would like to avoid stuttering. However, avoidance was pushed into explanatory prominence by Wendell Johnson, beginning with introspective reflections published in 1936 (Johnson & Knott, 1936) and subsequently elaborated into the contention that stuttering consists simply of efforts to avoid stuttering (Johnson & Moeller, 1956).[16] From this position, accessory features came to be discussed as "avoidances," with the explanation that these acts are acquired as attempts to avoid stuttering. Although this account is often expressed, and has been widely accepted, as the true explanation for accessory features, the account has always been confounded. In the first place, to merit designation as "avoidances," each of these acts should enable a stutter to be avoided. But common observation clearly reveals that accessory features cannot be said to achieve this result. Except for the possible successful employ of a "starter," the accessory features are notable failures in the presumed objective of avoiding stuttering—because the stutter occurs anyway. The issue is expanded in those cases wherein the stutterer is said to evidence a sequence of several accessory acts, each one purportedly having been added because the preceding one(s) was not successful. In such instances, if one accepts that each act is built on the failure of the one(s) preceding it, one finds then only a series of failures; that is, all of the acts have failed to avoid a stutter, so none of them can have been an avoidance. Even if it is contested that they are to be considered only as *attempts* to avoid, they are still failures.

But more *non sequiturs* arise. The typical discourse addressed to accessory features acknowledges their concurrence with a stutter, thereby tacitly admit-

ting that these features fail as "avoidances." Another highly significant inconsistency in the notion of accessory features as avoidances is the recognition,
made in a number of sources, that in any number of cases accessory features
are present at the onset of stuttering; which has to mean that "secondary
stuttering" is co-occurring with "primary stuttering" from the beginning. The
ultimate inconsistency in this standard treatment of accessory features (that
they are due to reaction) is to also contend that they are *part of* the stutter
occurrence.

There are some things a stutterer may do that could sensibly be called
avoidances—essentially because of achieving that result. The simplest of these
is to just stop talking! Some stutterers do make that particular adjustment.
Other adjustments of this kind are: to speak in a dialect; or rephrase, if sensing
possible trouble; or pretend to reflect; or feign a cough or yawn; or talk while
moving, to generate a "beat"; and so on. Some stutterers employ any one, or
more, of such adjustments—or something similar. The simple but required rule
here is that only an adjustment by which a stutter *is* avoided may sensibly be
called an "avoidance." Any adjustment failing such result requires a different
description. Certainly the interpretation of "avoidance," more so even than
"struggle," cannot be claimed summarily as explanation for accessory features.

Somehow, in spite of its illogic, the notion of "avoidance" seems to have had
a special appeal, and, as noted earlier, it has found extended employment. It
came to be an explanatory principle in other more elaborate ways than as a
misnomer for accessory features, turning up as the central dimension of several
"theories" of stuttering. In fact, as noted earlier, the position espoused by
Wendell Johnson presents avoidance as the sole actual substance of the disorder, as epitomized in definition 6 in Chapter 2. The progression of "avoidance"
from a simple, generalized reflective testimony to the level of theoretical construct will be considered in some detail in Chapter 6.

OBJECTIVE REVIEW OF ACCESSORY FEATURES

The items listed in Table 3.2 were recorded from exploration of a sizable (48)
sample of literature sources that had seemed likely to contain information of
this sort. As noted earlier, the kinds of actions listed in Table 3.2 cover a
considerable range. However, the number of items found is unexpectedly small,
especially in view of the claims so often made regarding the "hundreds" or
"myriads" or "an almost incredible variety" of such features. In fact, one source
(Froeschels, 1921) claimed that patterns of these features run into "many
thousands." The claim, repeated by the same author several times (Froeschels,

1956, 1961) has also been cited frequently in other sources. Such claims have no notable documentation; no support for them was discovered in at least the sizable literature search undertaken for the assessment presented here.

Nonetheless, claims of "myriads" of accessory features have been widely accepted. This acceptance seems to be almost entirely a product of the frequent restatement of such claims, attended occasionally by a few dramatic examples, and the lore that has resulted. Perpetuation of the belief is also supported by less forthright statements that nonetheless encourage these claims.[17]

In contrast to such images, not only did the present substantial literature search yield just this rather small number of items, but actual examples were found in only a small number of the sources explored—just 17 of the 48 reviewed, of which 3 were studies addressed specifically to accessory features. In other words, although most of the sources explored did contain discussion of accessory features, including the familiar account of their purported role, many still gave no examples and only very occasionally were more than two examples given. Additionally, it was of particular interest to find that five of the eight sources, whose titles would lead one to expect specification, contained only general discourse but no mention of any examples. Also, among sources giving examples, there was a notable preference for naming, or emphasizing, the larger body actions. Although the smaller acts are acknowledged to occur much more frequently than the larger ones, the latter not only create a more dramatic impression for readers but also are seemingly more amenable to explanation as being voluntary, and therefore open to the presumption of being acquired (i.e., learned) reactions.

The last two items in Table 3.2 are intentionally separated from the others in reflection of certain qualitative differences from them, a matter to be taken up soon. The first 24 items are listed in a sequence that approximates the entries in Table 3.3, to which comparisons will be made shortly.[18] The lower case letters appearing in the second column of the table are codes used simply to represent each of the 17 sources that yielded the items listed. The letters indicate the distribution of each item and the frequency with which each was mentioned in each of the sources coded. Note that most of the items are mentioned in only a few sources, and that, in contrast, a few items are mentioned often.

Three of the sources yielding these items were studies purposely undertaken to identify observable phenomena of stuttering (Barr, 1940; Lohr, 1969; Conture & Kelly, 1991), which is why they are featured here. Barr's study, of 10 young adult subjects, was the more comprehensive in respect to the range of features observed; Lohr's data were obtained from 17 subjects comparable to those participating in the Barr study. The principal findings of both studies relative to accessory features agree well. Barr's report indicated that for all of

TABLE 3.3 Motor Tics*

Simple motor tics
(sudden, brief, meaningless movements)

Eye blinking
Eye movements
Nose twitch
Grimacing
Mouth movements
Lip pursing
Teeth clicking
Jaw snaps
Head jerks
Shoulder shrugs
Arm jerks
Finger movements
Abdomen tensing
Kicks
Rapid jerking of any parts of the body

Complex Motor Tics
(slower, longer, more "purposeful" movements)

Sustained "looks"
Facial gestures
Biting
Touching objects or self
Throwing
Banging
Thrusting arms
Gestures with has
Gyrating and bending
Dystonic postures
Copropraxia[†]

---

*Data from Leckman and Cohen (1988).
[†]Obscene gestures.

her subjects six of these features—eye blink, eye close, eyebrow movement, lip tremor, jaw tremor, and holding breath—occurred in more than 25% of the subjects' total stutters. Comparably, Lohr observed that four of these features— eye blink, eye close, lip tremor, and jaw tremor—were characteristic of all her subjects. The Conture and Kelly study was unique in respect to comparing stutterer and nonstutterer youngsters age 3 to 7, 30 in each group. They reported 21 nonspeech acts of the face/head and upper body that occurred in the spontaneous speech of both groups. Three items—eye blink, eyes turn left, and upper lip raise—were significantly more frequent among the stutterers; two acts, lip press and jaw drop, approached significance.

It is of particular interest that eye movements are so prominent among the features reported in each of the three studies, just reviewed, addressed specifically to recording accessory features. This consistent finding assumes notable significance in view of the frequency with which eye movements are reported in sources giving a more generalized, informal statement regarding stutter occurrences, as compiled in Table 3.2. The extent to which eye movements figure so prominently in these various reports recalls findings from certain other studies,[19] undertaken for different purposes, that also revealed notable anomalies of eye movement to be associated with stutter.

If one reflects carefully on the variety of features listed in Table 3.2, it seems inescapable that they are not likely to be all of a kind. They vary on several obvious dimensions: notably, location, complexity, and quality. The last two items involve voicing, distinguishing them from the remainder, which are more properly considered as motor acts. The penultimate item includes references that were not made clear in the sources noting them— for example, "snorts" and "grunts" are most likely to be "noises"—however, "sounds" might also have referred to the foregoing and, in addition, to phonemes, especially the schwa. Whether or not some of such acts are purposeful is a matter about which it is wasteful to speculate here, but one should acknowledge that they might be either. The last item, "words/phrases," seems to be generally of a different order than the other items. One may infer that, in general, utterance of words or phrases are likely to constitute purposeful acts. Moreover, at least certain such verbal features are credibly reported, by certain stutterers, to have been used intentionally as fillers or starters. Nonetheless, it remains plausible that not all of such actions are purposeful.

Separation of the items involving voice from those identifiable as motor acts per se does not imply that the latter are homogenous in significance. Even among these motor acts there are evident differences, such as: the locus of the act, the range and extent of movement, the muscle mass involved, possible purposefulness, and other aspects. Those that are seemingly more complex might encourage description as purposeful and, therefore, in this context, as struggle. In contrast, the very small, limited movements have very little of a credibly purposeful quality about them.

Further review suggests a likely overarching dimension for the entire list, namely, involuntary–voluntary. Certain actions, such as blushing, perspiration, and pupillary dilation are clearly involuntary, as are actions described as "tremor." At the other extreme, it would seem that the use of words or phrases is most likely to be, at least at some level, voluntary. To the extent that any accessory feature might be voluntary, it seems explainable as an intended adjustment, either immediately preceding, or concurrent with, a stutter. Verbal features provide the classic illustration, especially in view of testimony describing certain of them as adjustments. However, the picture is not so clear for many of the other items since, in unspecified circumstances, such acts could occur quite involuntarily, and not as expressions of adjustment. Also, a certain number of the items in Table 3.2 are only grossly descriptive, items like: "pressing lips," "distorts mouth," and "grimace." More careful observation and recording of such items might well have provided a more certain reflection of their character—for instance, information pertaining to the context in which the lips were pressed. In accord with a number of other observers, I have frequently noted a stutterer to make oral movements, often exaggerated, that were clearly inappropriate to the phoneme presumably being attempted—for example, pursing the lips when intending to say "coat."[20] In a similar vein, certain items in Table 3.2 describe actions that are clearly inconsistent with speech production effort, such as: "grits teeth," "protrudes tongue." While one might claim such actions to be odd, "bad habits," they seem to have more the character of some error of organization or of transmission in a neural activating system. Then there are those little essentially muscle-twitch acts, such as eye blink, the most impressive of all in terms of the regularity with which they are observed; these acts clearly have no discernible relevance to speech attempt. These small acts, more persuasively than any others, seem aptly described as involuntary, as well as irrelevant to speech intent.

Another matter pertinent to understanding accessory features is that, on the whole, stutterers are not very aware of such features as they may evidence, an observation clearly reflected in the fact that widely employed therapy procedures, such as the use of a mirror, have as one goal to help stutterers identify the accessory features they may evidence. Special note should be made of the observation, reported regularly, that stutterers are typically unaware of their accessory features, particularly the simpler ones.

Two behavioral observations, unrelated to stuttering, are relevant to the matter of accessory features. It is noted routinely in cerebral palsy patients that intended movements, especially if attempted with something more than the usual effort, are very often accompanied by extraneous movements, a phenomenon referred to as "overflow." A similar phenomenon is found among normal children when in the process of learning certain skills. An example most likely to be observed is of kindergarten age children learning to cut with scissors. A variety of extraneous movements frequently accompany the scissors manipulation. Most often these extraneous movements involve oral structures (tongue, lips, jaw), but sometimes the head and even the shoulders. Early efforts in learning to print, and then to write cursively, also are activities likely to be associated with similar extraneous movements. Again, these movements are unintentional, unrelated to the actions undertaken, and clearly are not learned. They are most like "overflow."

ACCESSORY FEATURE PARALLELS

The accessory features in stuttering bring to mind another area of anomaly that contains at least remarkable parallels to accessory features—namely, the area of movement disorders, especially tics.

The literature on tics is extensive, and no attempt will be made to even summarize the generally relevant dimensions. The immediate objective here is to afford the reader some awareness of phenomenal aspects of the disorder. These characteristics merit the attention of students of stuttering because of their many compelling parallels to the accessory features.

Tics are a type of hyperkinesia, at this time quite well differentiated diagnostically from several other forms of movement disorder. Tics are identified as abnormal involuntary movements that caricature normal motor acts. On the whole, they are considered to be unintended acts, even though some may have the appearance of being purposeful. They are described in terms of anatomical location, number, frequency, duration, intensity, and complexity.

Phenomenal classification identifies two major types—motor tics, and phonic tics—each class having the subdivisions of "simple" and "complex." Tables 3.3 and 3.4 reproduce illustrations of these types. Relative frequency of tic forms follows the sequence of the headings in the two tables, with simple motor tics being the most common, and complex phonic tics the least frequently observed. Moreover, the latter, the most dramatic form, rarely if ever occur in the absence of simple phonic tics and motor tics of one form or another. In fact, the presence of complex phonic tics occasions a diagnosis of Tourette's syndrome, which lies within the spectrum of tic disorders. In frequency of occurrence, the loci of motor tic appearances follows a rostral–caudal (see note 17) pattern of frequency; those of the face and head are by far the most frequently occurring. (See Jagger *et al.*, 1982; Leckman & Cohen, 1988; Lees, 1985.)

Comparison of Table 3.3 to the motor items of Table 3.2 reveals some striking similarities, not only in terms of characteristics but also in respect to their relative frequency of occurrence. These similarities serve to raise question as to their similarity in nature. All forms of tic, including those involving coordinative movements, are reported to be involuntary. Accessory features, in

TABLE 3.4   Examples of Phonic Tics*

Simple Phonic Tics
(sudden, meaningless sounds and noises)

Throat clearing
Coughing
Sniffling
Spitting
Screeching
Grunting
Gurgling

Complex Phonic Tics
(sudden, more "meaningful" utterances)

"Shut up"
"Stop that!"
"Oh okay"
"How about it"
"Okay honey"
[echolalia][†]
[coprolalia][#]

---

*Data from Leckman and Cohen (1988).
[†]Repeats utterances heard, or said
[#]Obscene words or phrases.

contrast, have been presented as essentially voluntary acts. As noted earlier, certain of the larger motor accessory features may seem purposeful, and they have been routinely interpreted as such, although they may not be. However, the nature of some other accessory acts, even ones that might seem complex, remains questionnable. In addition, there are those accessory features that are either very likely to be, or most certainly are, involuntary.

Comparison of phonic tics (Table 3.4) to their accessory feature counterparts in Table 3.2 (the last two items) cannot be as direct as for the motor items, due primarily to inadequate specification in the "phonic" items of Table 3.2. However, some amount of comparison between these two data sets can be undertaken, allowing that I draw upon personal, and vicarious, experience. Most of the phonic tic examples seem clearly to be of a different order than counterpart accessory feature examples of which I am aware, directly and indirectly. In respect to counterparts of simple phonic tics, for instance, I have not observed, nor heard of, such acts as spitting,[21] screeching, or gurgling to accompany stutters. In contrast to the given examples of complex phonic tics, the verbal accessory features I have observed, and otherwise know of, have generally seemed more ordinary in quality and more relevant to the situation. Terms like "well," "really," "lemme see," and "y'know," even though stereotyped, are at least not odd; they even could be intentionally appropriate. On the other hand, I recall certain verbal features that, in most instances, could not fit sensibly into the utterance; one example is /ɪzə/ ("is a"); another is /ənɛn/ ("and then").

These comparisons of accessory features with tics broach an area of inquiry that merits being pursued, to an expected benefit for understanding stuttering. This initial analysis itself holds certain values. For one, it yields further grounds to reject the belief that accessory features are all of a kind. For another, it demonstrates the need for careful assessment of accessory features, one that is balanced and based on inquiry and analysis rather than supposition. Third, indirectly but compellingly, it confirms the cardinal features as the phenomenal substance of stuttering, as follows. Persons evidencing motor tics are not mistaken as stutterers, even though any number of their tics are not distinguishable from motor accessory features. The reason tiqueurs are not misidentified as stutterers is simply, but critically, that tiqueurs do not evidence the cardinal features of stuttering.

It is appropriate to note, in this section, that there are certain characteristics found to be common to stuttering, motor tics and Tourettes syndrome. All three disorders appear in childhood, are more common in males than in females, wax and wane over the course of their expression, and increase in intensity under emotional stress. These commonalities do not suggest any similar specificity of origin, but they do indicate semblances in neurologic anomaly.

"SYMPTOMS" OF STUTTERING

An issue raised several times in earlier parts of this chapter was concerned with the widespread practice of treating the cardinal features and the accessory features, together, as *symptoms* of stuttering. The result of such practice is that the cardinal features have become reduced in significance, obscured within a mass of accessory features reputedly numbering at least in the "hundreds." In contradiction of this practice, it is especially worthwhile to call attention to pertinent, representative findings, reported separately over a long time-span by three individuals whose works have held a notable prominence in the field. Early in the century, Froeschels (1915), in addressing the matter of the purported thousands of "symptoms" evidenced by many hundreds of stutterers, reported that the clonic and tonic features were "the only symptoms common to all." Two decades later, Van Riper (1937a), reviewing the "almost incredible variety of such symptoms" to be found among stutterers, also found that "the tonic and clonic blocks alone were experienced by all." More recently Sheehan (1974) noted that, "Of all the diverse symptoms of stuttering mentioned in the literature ... only two have been found to be common to all stutterers: 1) tonus ... and 2) clonus."

In effect, the perfect agreement among these three sources indicates that the reported myriad accessory features are superfluous for the identification of stuttering, and are essentially of no consequence relative to the effort to explain stuttering as caused by reaction of some sort.

The reason for the perfect agreement revealed in these three sources is not hard to find—and the same level of agreement will be found among any other sources that might undertake similar review. The reason clonic and tonic (or their synonym descriptors) are the only features to be found in all cases of stuttering is simply because, as emphasized earlier in this chapter, these cardinal features are the sole definitive dimensions of stuttering—they are the *sine qua non* of stuttering. In contrast, the accessory features are just that—accessory. They are not unique to, and certainly not distinctive of, stuttering. In fact, in at least very many instances of stutter they are not observed.

There is another, equally significant correction to make regarding the so-called symptoms of stuttering. Fundamentally, it is incorrect to speak of stuttering "symptoms."[22] Symptoms are surface indications of some condition that cannot be observed directly. There are, thus, no symptoms of *stuttering*; stuttering is stuttering! Stuttering is very obvious, clearly open to direct observation. It has no symptoms, just as there are no "symptoms" of limping, of sneezing, of tremor, of shivering, of fever—and so on. These occurrences, as with stuttering, do not have symptoms—they are themselves symptoms. Stutters, the cardinal (or speech) features, may properly be viewed as symptoms only if they are considered to be signs of something that is not evident, some condition underlying the stutter event. One might possibly contend that, at least peripherally, they are symptoms of the stutter *event*, the inability to proceed. But the latter is readily inferred; in fact, seems rather obvious. "Symptom" has a more profound significance.

Similarly, the accessory features too are properly considered as symptoms only if construed as signs of something not evident. However, that "something" is certainly not stuttering. Again, peripherally, some of the accessory features might be called symptoms of struggle, but this also seems inappropriate because at least certain accessory features give a clear impression of struggle—so they *are* struggle, not symptoms of it. Those accessory features that are not readily explained as an adjustive effort might be spoken of as symptoms, but they too are not symptoms of stuttering. They may well have some sort of close connection to stutters but such relationship is unclear. As a category, these features are not a part of stuttering, principally because actions designatable as accessory features can, and do, occur independently of the speech features, the stutters. The reader is reminded that a tiqueur is not misidentified as a stutterer, in spite of the fact that certain tics are in many important respects parallels (even phenomenal duplicates) of certain accessory features.

A BRIEF SUMMARY

This chapter has been addressed to observations and analyses that show stuttering to be describable principally in terms of two essential, omnipresent, *cardinal* features, which have been known for a very long time by the terms "clonic" and "tonic"—terms for which there are several other good synonyms that are even more explicit, such as "iterative" and "protractive." In some cases of stuttering one may also observe, in addition to the cardinal features, certain subsidiary acts, aptly designated *accessory* features, that vary in respect to their character, frequency of occurrence, and their essential nature. Although these actions may appear in the vicinity of stutters, their relationship to stutters is, in general, unclear.

Contrary to descriptions in wide usage, it is improper to speak of *symptoms of* stuttering; stuttering is itself a symptom, of some condition that is as yet unknown.

NOTES

1. "Inaction" is what observers regularly perceive, and also is the experience reported most often by stutterers. However, rare testimony has reported awareness of subtle muscular activity during these episodes. See relevant discussion in the section of Chapter 5 headed "Only the Stutterer Knows."

2. The diagonal lines mean that the enclosed letters are transcriptions in the symbols of the International Phonetic Association.

3. Actually, the demise of "clonic" followed after Wendell Johnson, editor of the *Journal of Speech and Hearing Disorders* from 1943 to 1948, prohibited use of the word "spasm" in manuscripts submitted to the journal—the only relevant professional organ during that time.

4. As noted in Chapter 1.

5. The "Speech Therapist" cartoon appeared in the June 1980 issue of *Playboy*. The "Ziggy" cartoon was published in the summer 1985 issue of *Look Who's Talking* (Vol. 2, no. 2).

6. In fact, *Webster's New World Dictionary of the English Language* uses "machine guns" to illustrate the meaning of "stutter." As to "other weaponry discharge," see, for instance, in "An Anthem for Doomed Youth" (Wilfred Owen, 1918):
   What passing bells for these who die like cattle?
   Only the monstrous anger of the guns.
   Only the stuttering rifles' rapid rattle
   Can patter out their hasty orisons.
   The sounds of other military weaponry embellish the illustration. The slower cadence of certain heavier guns led to one type being called "pom-poms"; a heavier type "ack-ack." In contrast, the ultra-rapid fire of machine pistols occasioned the name "burp guns." The cadence of ordinary machine-guns and rifle fire already had an appropriate epithet—"stutter."

7. For a range of examples see Van Riper (1971) and Wingate (1976, 1997).

8. Well exemplified in the observation that when someone attempts to imitate stuttering the performance clearly includes both features.

9. As emphasized in Chapter 1, no one knows what stuttering "is" in the sense of its fundamental nature. However, from observational inference, consistent with stutterers' personal report, it seems evident that the stutterer is somehow stopped from proceeding.

10. This inverse way of stating the fact is the only mention of it that appears in the lists of "facts" recorded in Table 1.4 (the 19th item in the first column, from Bluemel).

11. As produced in these two words, the example phonemes occur as allophones, differing by virtue of positional influences which may well be critical. However, the differences are not evident to the speaker, nor to casual review.

12. See Howell & Williams (1988) and Viswanath & Neel (1995).

13. The matter of prescience is discussed in Chapter 6.

14. The word "really" is used here because it stands out in my recollection of one young adult stutterer who used it very skillfully—except that it's so frequent, and sometimes inappropriate, appearance was revealing.

15. At this point, we encounter the first reference, in this book, to the influence of testimony, a topic given separate attention in Chapter 5.

16. This position is repeated in many other publications and presentations by Johnson, and other followers of the Iowa School.

17. For instance, Bloodstein's (1995, p. 19) statement that "It is difficult to catalog all of the acts or tensions that may become associated with stuttering."

18. A sequence identified in biological and medical literature as "rostral-caudal," meaning literally, "beak-to-tail," but in figurative usage meaning "proceeding from head-first."

19. See, for instance, Jasper and Murray (1932), Murray (1932), Moser (1938), Kopp (1963), and Brutten et al. (1984).

20. Clear examples are evidenced by several stutterers appearing in a videotape prepared by Ehud Yairi at the University of Illinois at Urbana-Champaign several years ago. The actual objective of the tape was to illustrate the remarkable effect on stuttering of the ameliorative conditions.

21. Occasional, unintentional "spray," perhaps, but not expectoration.

22. The related inaccuracy of "syndrome" has been discussed in Chapter 2.

CHAPTER 4

Facts About Stuttering

Facts are the air of the scientist. Without them
you can never fly. Without them your 'theories'
are useless efforts. Yet while studying, experi-
menting and observing, try not to stay on the
surface of facts. Try to penetrate to the secret of
their occurrence, persistently search for the laws
that govern them.

> Ivan P. Pavlov, *Bequest to the Academic*
> *Youth of Soviet Russia, 1936*

*D*iscussion in Chapter 1 drew the distinction between facts *of* stuttering,
which identify its observational reality, and facts *about* stuttering, which
are of a different order, pertaining largely to information regarding the
disorder that indicates something about its underlying substance.

Each of the various facts to be presented in this chapter makes a unique
contribution to the study of stuttering, which will be noted in some extent as
each one is reviewed. All of these facts, conjointly, have a common, fundamental significance for the disorder: they are obvious testimony to the reality of
stuttering. That is, facts *about* stuttering follow from, and have substance only
in reference to, an existing, recognized entity—stuttering—an entity that is
well known by the three essential facts *of* stuttering, noted in Chapter 1 and
discussed at length in Chapter 3—namely, iterative and protractive markers in
syllable-initial positions.

Facts about stuttering represent a range of observations, reports, and inquiries regarding the disorder that arise from many different sources over a long period of time. Some observations that have been offered as facts about stuttering are not acceptable as such. In Table 1.4, for instance, certain items listed there are even erroneous, such as the "No Native Americans." This item was an unsupported claim, presented by Wendell Johnson as evidence for his conjectural, but highly persuasive, "evaluation hypothesis," which was accepted so widely as true. However, the claim is soundly contradicted by broadly based relevant findings.[1] Many of the other items appearing in that table lack adequate support, as reflected in the table entries. However, some of the items listed in Table 1.4 have a status sufficient to be included among those to be reviewed in the present chapter, and will have the notation [‡].

The facts about stuttering to be presented in this chapter have met the criterion of substantial confirmation, with a record sufficient in breadth to give assurance of future replication,[2] even though the facts vary in terms of the extent of their existing, and potential, confirmation. This variation will serve as reference for presenting the items sequentially in an order based upon a generalized assessment of their relative substantive support.

The narratives addressed to each of the facts will not develop the individual topics in great detail nor be encumbered with extensive reference citations. The objective of each narrative is to give a summary statement that will convey the essential substance of the fact. Certain appropriate references will be cited, which the reader can consult for pertinent sources, providing entry into literature relevant to topical explorations.[3] A number of the facts are interrelated, or overlapping, and these connections will be noted.

FOR CENTURIES

Stuttering is an ancient disorder (see Wingate, 1997). Wherever sufficient cultural records are found, reference to stuttering appears; for instance, in ancient Egyptian hieroglyphs, wherein the iterative hallmark of stutter is prominently evident. Early Greek writings make note of it, and in that era Aristotle made pithy observations about the disorder, and remarkable analysis of its surface phenomena. As the extent of cultural records increased, one finds a generally proportional reference to stuttering, with considerable expansion in the late eighteenth and nineteenth centuries. This trend continued into the early twentieth century, burgeoning near mid-century, coincident with the growth of the national professional association in the United States.[4]

A major significance in this fact of stuttering's antiquity is that, not only has stuttering existed for a very long time but also, over this time, it has been recognized in very different cultures, in good and bad times, and in individuals of widely different stations in life. It is particularly important to note, in specific regard to the issue of the identification of stuttering that, over this very long span of time, evidently everyone has known what everyone else has been talking about.[5] The significant corollary of this fact is that, over the same time-span, there has been only minuscule reference to any of the extensive "normal nonfluencies" of ordinary speech (see Chapter 10), even though there is every reason to assume that these aspects of normal speech have been as prevalent in earlier times as they are now.

THE AMELIORATIVE CONDITIONS

A certain number of alterations in mode of oral expression have long been recognized to have a clearly beneficial effect on a stutterer's speech, for which they are identified as "the ameliorative conditions." The effect of several of these modes is well documented, reliable, and dramatic. Two conditions head the list: singing, and speaking to rhythm. These two are followed closely, in their effect, by choral speaking, auditory masking, and delayed auditory feedback.

There are certain other circumstances that have been reported to exercise a notably beneficial effect on a stutterer's speech, but it seems more appropriate to consider these reports as essentially tentative since their documentation is, on the whole, not as broadly based as for the conditions in focal review here. Nonetheless, some mention should be made of such tentative items, which will be noted whenever appropriate, since they have credibility within the context of the present topic.

Readers interested in more detail regarding the ameliorative conditions than will be presented here are referred to Chapters 7 and 8 in *Stuttering: Theory and Treatment* (Wingate, 1976).

SINGING[‡]

It has long been reported, and from many sources, that stutterers do not stutter when they sing. It is a phenomenon well known to many laypersons, and related through commonplace episodes. This effect has a remarkably absolute quality: the dramatic, abrupt change in the oral expression of a stutterer from speaking to singing gives an impression of an effect that is controlled by a switch—"on" or "off." Importantly, the effect is not limited to instances of

singing a familiar song; the change also is induced when the person sings any
words (phrases, sentences) to some adaptable tune, or even to an unrecogniz-
able tune.[6]

As might be expected, various explanations have been advanced to account
for this remarkable phenomenon. Unfortunately, the explanation given most
often is that the effect is due to "distraction." The implausibility of this account,
in general, is discussed in Chapter 6. Certain other attempts at explanation
offer some strained rationale, such as that the stutterer, when singing, thinks
of himself as a different person. It seems pointless to mention other equally
fanciful reflections. The change must be due to some performance difference(s)
between the activities of singing and speaking. Certain differences of this sort
have been identified, but essentially by persons interested in singing, who
worked with normal speakers. An obvious difference is that, in singing, there
is a clear emphasis on voicing, as expressed through the vowel forms of the
lyrics. The extent of this difference is well reflected in Figure 4.1.

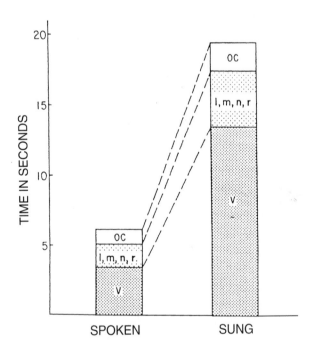

FIGURE 4.1 Composition of spoken and sung versions of the same utterance. V =
vowels; oc = consonants other than /l, m, n, r/. Data from Vennard & Irwin (1966).

SPEAKING TO RHYTHM

This condition has an ameliorative effect directly comparable to singing: the effect is immediate, dramatic, and thorough as long as it is maintained. The rhythm effect has been recognized for at least two centuries, and has been documented extensively. Rhythm was incorporated into treatment programs throughout the nineteenth and early twentieth centuries. It was denigrated during the 1930s and 1940s[7] by certain influential stutterers within the profession, and this condemnation resulted in it being disavowed for some 20 years. However, interest in rhythm gradually reappeared, and for a time it was subject to a notable amount of a certain type of experimental inquiry. During this period, rhythm was once again incorporated into a number of treatment programs, ones that were at that time cast largely in learning theory form. The research activity during that period yielded a fair amount of valuable information regarding the rhythm effect. For instance, it was found that, although a variety of rhythm patterns can yield a positive influence, a regular rhythm (the original form) is not only simplest to produce but is also, understandably, the easiest to follow and, most importantly, has the most marked and reliable effect.

Still, the principal agent of the rhythm effect, if there is a principal one, remains unknown. Possibly, the effect may have several concurring dimensions. Regularity of pattern seems an evident contributor; many bodily activities find natural expression in, or are enhanced by, rhythmic (recurring pattern) expression, epitomized in sea chanteys and other work songs. In speaking to rhythm, the individual evidently is guided to align syllables, principally stressed syllables, with the "beats" of the rhythm. The guiding rhythm probably induces other changes in the production of speech, prominent among which is an emphasis on voicing, expressed through the concentration on syllable nuclei—the vowel forms (vowels, diphthongs, and the occasional triphthong). Thus, there emerge certain similarities between the evident effects of rhythm and of singing. One can gain an appreciation of how the features noted above emerge when speaking to rhythm, by reading aloud poems having a clear meter.[8]

It is of particular interest that the use of rhythm was introduced by an eighteenth-century British elocutionist whose focal interest in the art of speaking centered around, in his words, the "rhythmus" of the language.[9] Students of stuttering should make the effort to become familiar with the accumulated knowledge regarding rhythm and stuttering. A reasonably comprehensive review is presented as Chapter 7 (and pp. 209–212) in Wingate (1976); later publications should be sought in appropriate journal sources. Students should also become knowledgeable about aspects of speech involved in what Thelwall called the "rhythmus" of the language (see Wingate, 1997, pp. 43ff).

Choral Speaking[‡]

The effect of this condition is not quite as dramatic in impression as are the first two, principally because in those two conditions the stutterer performs solo. Nonetheless, the influence of choral speaking is substantial, and the effect is well documented.

The explanations offered for the effect of this condition include most of those proposed to account for the first two, especially "distraction," which is as vacuous here as it is in its other offerings. Except for distraction, these other facile explanations have attracted little attention, and do not merit being considered here; the interested reader will find a review of these explanations in Wingate (1976, pp. 196–205). In contrast, the explanation of "distraction" has been glibly offered, and as superficially accepted, for many years. It will be discussed at some length in Chapter 6.

A particularly relevant publication, which came to my attention only recently, presents an analysis of choral speaking that offers a link to the effect of rhythm. Boomsliter et al. (1973), in a study of "unled choral reading" with normal speakers, found evidence in support of their hypothesis that speakers synchronize their speech by conforming to basic (prosodic) timing patterns of the language, of which the native (normal) speaker is inherently (but not consciously) aware. These patterns in the language are conceived as being organized in terms of linguistic stress patterns. Notably, this analysis is very consonant with Thelwall's emphasis on the "rhythmus" of the language (see above).

Auditory Influences

Masking

The "masking" of speech is effected when a continuous source of sound is sufficiently loud that the individual cannot hear his speech in the usual manner, that is, via the airborne sound waves created by his voice. Auditory masking is usually arranged in experimental circumstances, or for illustration, by delivering "white noise" into the subject's close-fitting earphones.[10] Importantly, the white noise must be louder than the level of ordinary conversational speech so that the subject cannot hear himself in the usual way. Since we naturally listen to ourselves speak, this condition (louder white noise) induces what is called "the Lombard effect," in which the subject speaks more loudly than usual, in an effort to once again hear himself speaking.

In many respects, the Lombard effect duplicates conductive (airborne) hearing loss, one symptom of which is that the affected individual speaks loudly. Interestingly, there is impressive evidence that stuttering is considerably less prevalent among the hearing impaired.

The amelioration of stuttering under auditory masking is comparable to the effect produced by the three ameliorative conditions reviewed above. Explanations for this effect include, but range beyond, the explanations already mentioned. Among the latter are accounts that invoke some psychologically based reflection, such as that the stutterer is less reactive to his speech because he cannot hear it; among other accounts there is recourse to a "feedback" rationale (see below). Once again, however, a most obvious dimension of the induced change is the increased level of voicing. There are also certain related effects, such as a more monotone type of speech. A review of this material is presented in Chapter 8 of *Stuttering: Theory and Treatment* (Wingate, 1976).

Delayed Auditory Feedback (DAF)

This condition came into the field of stuttering largely by happenstance. In the course of adjusting some audio equipment, an electronics engineer noticed that a very brief delay in hearing oneself talk distorted one's speech in certain ways, of which the most compelling was a form of repetition. This result was reported in an article bearing the unfortunate title "Artificial Stutter" (Lee, 1951) in which "aluminum-num" was reported as the kind of repetition induced. The title was unfortunate because this kind of repetition, sometimes observed under delayed feedback, is very unlike stutter. As discussed in Chapter 3, stutter involves a word-initial syllable, not a word-final one. However, a number of sources, unaware of or indifferent to this critical difference,[11] elaborated the error and proceeded to present stutter as some anomaly in the speech "feedback" system. This conception was undoubtedly influenced by historical events of the time: it was the era of early efforts at space venturing in which the concept of feedback in mechanical control systems was widely recognized and understood.[12]

Curiously, DAF came to be employed in the effort to treat stuttering. The rationale for this endeavor was not at all clear; it might have occurred as another happenstance. Since stuttering was at the time presented as some anomaly of feedback,[13] how could one expect it to be improved by further disturbance in feedback? Interestingly, DAF was shown to have an ameliorative effect on the speech of at least some stutterers. Once again, it seems most likely that the beneficial effect was due to certain changes induced in the subject's manner of speaking.

As with masking, the DAF effect requires the use of microphone and ear-phones, because many speakers can rather easily ignore the delayed speech unless forced to hear it by increasing the signal volume. Therefore, speakers are induced to speak more loudly (as with masking). In addition, DAF induces the speaker to "stretch" syllables—essentially the syllable nuclei, the vowels—in the effort to adjust to the "extended" speech as heard.

It should be mentioned that DAF is not the straightforward influence pre-sented by masking, or the other ameliorative conditions. Even normal speakers differ in their tolerance of, and adjustment to, DAF. Some few persons are able to ignore it even when the volume is above conversational level; others are so unsettled by the delay that they cannot continue speaking. The most common effect is that the person speaks more slowly, in a sort of monotone, and more loudly. An objective, pithy discussion of DAF will be found in Lenneberg (1967).

Summation

The several conditions that clearly ameliorate stuttering appear to be somewhat diverse in nature, yet they all produce the same result: speech without stutter. The source, or sources, of the effect are not very well understood. Various explanations have been offered, but the nature of the influence is still unclear. The most promising lead seems to be that, despite the apparent variety of the conditions, all of them produce alteration in manner of speaking, in which voicing is the most prominent dimension.

THREE IN ONE

Three important facts about stuttering are interrelated to the extent that it is difficult to speak of them separately. These three facts are: (1) childhood disorder, (2) remission, and (3) prevalence. Their interrelationship is captured by pointing out that prevalence of stuttering is some function of age because many stuttering youngsters no longer stutter as childhood passes.

CHILDHOOD DISORDER[‡]

Occasionally stuttering is described as a disorder of childhood, which might imply the fact of remission. However, such characterization overlooks the clear evidence that many persons who stutter are well beyond childhood. Nonetheless, to call stuttering a disorder of childhood emphasizes the fact that, by far, most persons who stutter are children.

Typically, stuttering begins in the early years of speech acquisition, between approximately ages 2 and 5. It seems to first become manifest after the child has begun to use connected speech,[14] and the onset is almost always gradual.

Readers should be aware that for many years following establishment of the American professional association (in 1925), especially following Bluemel's statement in 1932 (see below), standard doctrine about childhood stuttering held that it regularly—actually, *universally*—"develops," becoming more severe as the child grows. It was claimed that stuttering worsens as the child, reacting to his stutter, struggles with it and soon enters into a "vicious spiral" of reaction, struggle, more reaction, more struggle, etc.[15]

The claim that stuttering develops was initiated and then promoted by certain stutterers within the profession who presented it as their personal story and seemed to believe that they represented all stutterers. The contention and belief that early stuttering becomes worse originated in a 1932 convention program presentation by Sidney Bluemel, a psychiatrist who stuttered, wherein he presented the ideas of "primary" and "secondary" stuttering, the latter purportedly the outgrowth of the former.[16] The notion that stuttering develops was pressed enthusiastically and soon became widely accepted in the field, in spite of not only a notable lack of supporting evidence but, as well, the existence of sensible and impressive evidence to the contrary. The persuasion that stuttering develops was abetted by a substantial lapse in reasoning. Regarding the latter, if stuttering were to develop according to the supposed "vicious spiral," one should expect that, with stuttering onset occurring during ages 2 through 4, the child should stutter so badly by age 8 or 9 as to then be essentially mute. Even in that era it should have been abundantly clear that such progression did not happen (see the following section on remission/recovery). However, the unsupported claim that stuttering routinely "develops" was allowed to persist, even enlarge, especially through efforts made by certain sources to describe (regular) "stages" of stuttering development (see especially Bloodstein, 1960). Although Van Riper[17] was for some time among proponents of the notion of "stages," he eventually repudiated the confabulation, acknowledging that "it was all sheer folly" (Van Riper, 1971b, p. 101).

The notion that stuttering develops became established, and grew, by ignoring (in fact, suppressing) one highly important fact about stuttering—its remission. This antilogy is starkly epitomized in Wendell Johnson's influential work *The Onset of Stuttering* (Johnson & Associates, 1959). The stated objective of that endeavor was to document how and why stuttering develops, and the plethora of data collected and published therein was so interpreted by the author. However, the pertinent critical data contained within that extensive presentation contradicted the interpretation expounded. In clear contrast to the contention of the narrative, the most critical, and most impressive, of the reported findings revealed that, over the approximately 2½ years of the study, 91 of the 118 little stutterers had recovered or were "much better," and another 13 were "somewhat better." In dramatic contrast, just three were listed as "somewhat worse," and only one child was said to be "much worse." In other words, in only 3% of these youngsters did their stuttering, to *any* extent, become worse over the span of two and a half years!

The above findings of this extensive, and often-cited study contained clear evidence that stuttering had not developed but, to the contrary, had most often become at least much improved. Importantly, these data were completely ignored, actually subverted, passed over in Johnson's continuing narrative that spoke only of the presumed reasons that stuttering "develops." In spite of the compelling data indicating substantial remission of stuttering, there was no mention at all of either remission, or of recovery.

REMISSION/RECOVERY[‡]

These terms have a similar, but not identical, meaning. "Remission" implies improvement in a condition for which no responsible agent may be evident. The extent of improvement may vary, from partial to complete, and such qualification typically is stated. The word "recovery" implies that improvement is complete, that is, a return to original status. However, common usage often adds some qualification of extent, such as "partial," or "full." "Recovery," compared to "remission," also often implies the contribution of some influence(s) or responsible agent(s).

In the literature of stuttering, one finds more frequent use of "recovery," possibly because this term allows mention, or claim, of some external contribution to the improvement, such as sometime treatment experience or the patient's independent effort to improve. However, "remission" carries the correct meaning for those many instances in which youngsters gradually no longer stutter: it is very likely to be as correct for many other cases as well.

As noted above, the contention that stuttering develops was encouraged to persist because the fact of remission, which contradicts the belief in "development," was clearly ignored. Intermittently over many years, various sources have consistently reported clear and substantial evidence that stuttering does not regularly—nor even very often—get worse. Actually, in many cases it does not even persist. It is sobering to note that impressive evidence of this fact was published, in a pertinent professional source (Byrne, 1931), the year *before* Bluemel (1932) set the "development" juggernaut in motion. The momentum of that belief was increased through the rapid dissemination of Bluemel's "primary–secondary" misadventure, which soon became assimilated into Wendell Johnson's widely influential "semantogenic" conjecture. The latter formulation, which carried the development theme in more exaggerated form, was being promulgated and gaining momentum in the middle 1930s. It is particularly noteworthy that during that early period Johnson, the central figure in pressing the claim of stuttering development, was involved in research that revealed the fact, and also the extent, of remission (Johnson, 1934; Milisen & Johnson, 1936).[18] However, those findings remained obscured until very recently (Wingate, 1997).

The belief that stuttering is almost certain to get worse, through the process of reaction and related emotional involvements (the "vicious spiral" notion), engendered many warnings and taboos regarding how to deal with the disorder. Most of these proscriptions were couched in the general injunction to avoid having the child become aware of the stuttering; a goal impossible to achieve.[19] For many years clinicians were afraid to work with stutterers, especially child stutterers, lest they do something that might make the stutter worse. This apprehension was entirely unwarranted (see Wingate, 1971). Although the apprehension may have mitigated in recent times, at least a residual attitude of concern remains among many practitioners (Yaruss, 1999).

The reader will find a considerable range of findings pertinent to the matter of remission in Chapter 5 of *Stuttering: Theory and Treatment* (1976), including a number of formal studies addressed to recovery, extant at that time. The information contained therein remains pertinent, and the reader is encouraged to review that source.

Among the worthwhile findings in the "recovery" studies, one item deserving special attention is the lack of any evidence that the actions of parents cause, or contribute to, the occurrence or uncommon persistence of stuttering. In fact, the pertinent evidence again reveals just the opposite: that parental actions are either benign or helpful (see Wingate, 1976, chap. 5; Nippold & Rudzinski 1995).[20] It is distressing, then, to find in certain current publications, the persisting conviction that some negative parental influence is probable and that evidence for it will yet be found.

Sixty years ago Bryngelson (1938) wrote, in regard to 1492 cases studied, that "forty-eight percent of stuttering children need not worry a clinician, because before the age of eight ... stuttering subsides." Later research has yielded, overall, a general corroboration of these estimates. There is also impressive evidence of major improvement beyond the childhood years, although motivation and action by the individual seems then to be more contributory.[21] Another important dimension of recovery, at any age, is that it happens gradually, and usually more gradually than stuttering onset.

Among the three well-known facts about stuttering emphasized in the first chapter, one was that there is no known cure for stuttering. Standardly, "no known cure" means that no means has been discovered by which one can expect the disorder to be cured, wherein "cure" means elimination—gone, never to return. As in certain other conditions, all attempts at treatment of stuttering have not effected a cure. It is possible that, for certain conditions, some instances of cure may occur spontaneously. However, it is not clear whether stuttering is among them, in view of evidence that recovery is not regularly "full," or complete, even in cases where it may seem to be. About half of the recovered stutterers for whom the pertinent information has been obtained, reported a residual tendency to stutter. The brief, often only momentary, recurrences of stutter are reported to appear unexpectedly, and under casual as well as presumably stressful circumstances. This residual tendency was reported as early as Byrne's (1931) study, and has been recorded many times in later research (Wingate, 1976, chap. 5). Other research has reported findings of related significance—namely, the presence of many very brief silent pauses in the apparently normal speech of acknowledged stutterers. Along similar lines, more recent research has detected various subtle anomalies in the apparently normal speech of persons considered to be recovered stutterers.[22]

Primarily for these reasons, the word "recovered," when used with "stutterer," is routinely written with quotation marks or, when spoken, said with some appropriate qualification. Such special use of "recovered" permits its application to persons who still obviously stutter, but whose speech has improved markedly over a former status. Two such cases are presented as illustration in Chapter 10. These matters, and others that are pertinent to remission and recovery, will be taken up again in Chapter 14.

The fact of stutter remission (instead of exacerbation) in youngsters now seems to have gained some recognition, although hardly general acceptance. However, it is still not understood. At this time prognosis is only actuarial— that is, that by a certain age a certain percentage of young stutterers will no longer be stuttering. The percentage value is not yet very well established, various studies giving values that range from 32 to 79%; an overall approximate figure of 50% seems justifiable (see Bryngelson, above; Wingate, 1976). The percentage remission may well be considerably higher, especially in view of many reports indicating that the prevalence of stuttering among young children is notably higher than the reference figure of 0.7% for "school age children" (see Van Riper, 1971b).

Ironically, now that the fact of stuttering subsidence is acknowledged, sources that concern themselves with stuttering in childhood are not careful to remain cognizant of the fact that, as yet, prognosis has no established foundation or guides. Further, there is scant recognition that remission is most likely to be an expression of neurophysiological maturation. In contrast, one finds, in that literature, assumptions about identifying children who are "at risk" for continuing to stutter. Such assumptions are particularly unwarranted in light of the lack of prognostic indicators. More distressing, however, is the evident readiness to propose, or imply, that certain efforts at "early intervention" underlie the remission reported. There is no evidence at all to justify such suggestions.

PREVALENCE/INCIDENCE‡

The incidence of a condition refers to the frequency of its occurrence over a lengthy time-span (a longitudinal measure). Prevalence refers to the number of instances reported at some particular time. Most reported figures regarding numbers of stutterers are prevalence figures, pertinent to a particular population. The figure may represent occurrence within an age range, a physical locale, a nationality, a culture, etc. In the relevant literature on stuttering published in the United States, the most generally encountered prevalence figure given is roughly 1%. This figure is based on official national surveys of the school-age population (the actual value reported as 0.7%). However, as discussion in the preceding two sections should lead one to expect, this overall value masks considerable variation due to age, which involves the fact of remission. Thus, prevalence figures for younger age levels are considerably higher, and decrease substantially with increasing age.[23]

A REFLECTION

The long-term and widely accepted persuasion regarding the supposed development of stuttering reflects, within the field, the strong inclination to readily accept and adopt some system of belief, and to maintain it in spite of considerable contradictory evidence. This inclination is well represented in the long-standing preoccupation with, and pursuit of, the notion of stuttering as "learned behavior"; it is also evident in other impedimenta to be discussed in the chapters of Part II.

HEREDITY/GENETICS‡

"Heredity" means, properly, the genetic transmission of characteristics from one generation to the next—that is, transmission through the physical substance of an individual's genes. However, "heredity" has been used in a looser sense, to refer simply to the recurrence of certain events in a "family line," with the matter of means of transmission left unclear. A rather formalized use of the term in this way is the reference to "hereditary titles" of a nobility, or the "hereditary home" of some family. Unique to the field of stuttering, a "social heredity" account has been proposed in an effort to explain how this disorder "runs in families" (see below).

Early recorded documentation of the heredity of stuttering appeared in publications by Makuen (1914) and Nadoleczny (1914), and then Bryant (1917). Other reports followed, with fair regularity in the next two decades, becoming most numerous in the late 1930s. Then, inquiry into genetic dimensions of stuttering—and, as well, other physiological aspects of the disorder—were pushed aside by the burgeoning attention to psychological explanation.[24] In fact, early in this expanding new era there appeared a publication that presented a purely psychosocial account of why stuttering "runs in families." This was the "social heredity" contention, proffered by Wendell Johnson through observations made by one of his students (Gray, 1940). That explanation was flawed by many limitations; in addition to not providing a credible fit to the reported data, it also was internally contradictory.[25] In spite of the fact that this account is woefully unrealistic (see Wingate, 1986c), it has been persuasive to many persons in the field, some of whom have continued to believe it well into modern times. It has been recounted favorably in various sources, one of them very recent (Bloodstein, 1993).

Some current sources that address the matter of genetics in stuttering call attention to the fact that the preponderance of human genes is the same in almost all people, and that only a very small number give rise to individual differences. The apparent objective of such notation is to emphasize that stutterers are mostly like everyone else. But it is precisely the, even minimal, difference that concerns us. To make the point clearly, 98% of human genes are shared with the great apes; that 2% is what most concerns us.

In relatively recent times, a return to bona fide genetic inquiry has been led by a highly capable geneticist, K. Kidd. Students seriously interested in acquiring a grasp of genetic study of stuttering should become familiar with his works (Kidd, 1984; Kidd et al., 1981).[26] Current reviews should also be consulted (Andrews et al., 1991; Pauls, 1990; Yairi et al., 1996). It has been known for some time that the pattern of stuttering lineage does not follow the classic Mendelian model. However, in recent times two models under study are compatible with observed familial patterns (Kidd, 1977).

The student is advised to read carefully the article by Gilger (1995) that appeared in the October issue of the *Journal of Speech and Hearing Research*. The author encapsulates, clearly and succinctly, a great deal of fundamental information dealing with genetic principles and concepts that are especially relevant to interests in speech and language. The discussion is developed in reference to several common misconceptions regarding genetic influence, and includes such topics as distal and proximal effects, penetrance, and non-genetic influences. It also contains, as an appendix, a valuable glossary.

It should be recognized that the potential genetic contribution to stuttering is not encompassed within the evidence of hereditary transmission (recurrence in families). The appearance of stuttering in individuals who do not report an extended-family incidence of stuttering does not, *ipso facto*, represent the expression of non-genetic factors. That is, the appearance of stuttering in a person having no stuttering relatives does not rule out a genetic contribution, and thereby imply only an environmental influence. Readers should become aware of the concept of *diathesis*, which refers to a congenital predisposition to develop or acquire certain disorders or diseases.

Some recent discussions regarding the genetic role in stuttering tend to emphasize that environmental factors also play a role. Here a special caveat is in order. Readers should remain aware that, in the context of genetics, "environmental" means "other-than-genetic." Therefore, the term has a very broad meaning: it includes the intrauterine milieu, the circumstances of birth, and subsequent illnesses and trauma of many kinds. To so many persons having a background in a social science, "environment" almost certainly means "psychosocial milieu." This circumstance is especially likely to be true of persons in the field of stuttering, with its long-term immersion in psychological explanations. To encourage an adequate sense of reservation regarding possible influences of the psychosocial environment, the following pithy statement in that regard, made by J. R. Potter (1980 p. 21), is particularly apropos:

> What is there that our environment can influence in us other than what we are endowed with? And what can it activate apart from what is susceptible to activation?

Potter's comment is relevant, in at least certain respects, to one's external physical environment as well; consider, for instance, the matter of allergies.

Another major fact about stuttering, the sex ratio, is somehow involved in the genetics of stuttering, since stuttering is clearly at least sex-modified. However, regardless of the nature of its genetic involvement, the sex ratio is a significant fact in its own right, and will be discussed separately.

Two other items often have been mentioned within the topic of the heredity of stuttering: sinistrality[‡] (left-handedness), and twinning.[‡] These items are presented here as being closer to the tentative level, mentioned earlier, since documentation for them does not match that of items meriting, in this review, the status of fact. However, sufficient support regarding these two items has accumulated that they deserve to be noted at least in the present context.

At one time, earlier in the twentieth century, matters involved in handedness loomed large in discussions of stuttering, especially as related to the concept of cerebral dominance (see later, Chapter 13). Handedness (better, sidedness or laterality) is a difficult matter, primarily in regard to problems of satisfactory measurement (see Springer & Deutsch, 1998). However, laterality continues to arise in study and discussion of stuttering (see Wingate, 1988, 1997).

The second qualified item noted above, twinning, has a somewhat similar status as handedness, with its own complications, and a likely, although unclear, connection with stuttering (see Bloodstein, 1995).

THE SEX RATIO[‡]

The sex ratio in stuttering favors females, because more males than females stutter. The ratios reported, over many sources, range from 2:1 to 7:1, with the generally accepted ratio being close to 4:1. The extent of the ratio is not a critical matter; even 2:1 is a very sizeable difference, adequate to reveal a very important dimension of the nature of stuttering. Still, a larger ratio does make the point more indelibly.

It must be emphasized that the sex differential in stuttering is not a matter of masculine–feminine, which are cultural-behavioral descriptions. Further, efforts to account for the difference in terms of differential cultural treatment of the two sexes have been clearly insupportable.[27] The male:female ratio is a matter of genetic substance, represented fundamentally in whether the individual has two X chromosomes (female) or one X and one Y chromosome (male).

A well-established cultural stereotype identifies females as "the weaker sex." This description is appropriate only in respect to the (average) immediate physical strength of the two sexes. In terms of matters physiological, females are generally the stronger, throughout life. The most readily available attestation of this female organic superiority is clearly revealed in the actuarial tables of any life-insurance company. Those tables, which represent proportional longevity, reveal a clear female advantage. Such casual evidence corroborates many other scientifically based findings of female advantage in physiological strength, such as: endurance, especially under duress; susceptibility to diseases common to both sexes; viability at birth; and vulnerability to many other conditions that either sex may experience.

This physiological superiority of the female is readily explained in terms of the survival of the species: endurance of the female is the more necessary for the succession of generations. It is a fact expressed through every generation.

Another important organismic difference favoring females is that, in general, girls develop and mature earlier than boys. This difference is especially relevant to the higher recovery ratio in females: adult female stutterers are quite rare. Also of special interest relative to the sex ratio, substantial evidence indicates that females are less strongly lateralized than are males (see Geschwind & Galaburda, 1987).

In regard to stuttering, then, the impressive sex ratio carries the clear implication that there is something about the genetic determinants of being a male that renders the individual more vulnerable to the disorder.

MENTAL RETARDATION

Stuttering is found much more often among the mentally retarded. During the first three quarters of this century, data have been gathered on the prevalence of stuttering among more than 13,000 retarded individuals. The extent of prevalence varies among the various reports, but overall the data support an estimate that the average prevalence of stutter in this population is about 8%, clearly considerably larger than in the normal population.

Several subsidiary findings are worth mention. In general, among the retarded, prevalence seems to vary with severity. Nonetheless, prevalence is highest among individuals with Down's Syndrome, in which the stuttering is most often described as simple, that is, consisting predominantly of the essential clonic and tonic markers, with few accessory features.[28] Down's Syndrome is a genetic condition, due to chromosomal aberration. For years prior to discovery of its genetic basis, it was known as Mongolism, principally due to the appearance around the eyes, one readily noticed feature among the many characteristic stigmata of the condition.

It is appropriate to mention here a seemingly unrelated report by Weinberg (1964), which found stuttering to be unexpectedly high among the blind and partially sighted. The relevance of these findings to the present context is that many of these individuals were found to be "neurologically disordered," including mental retardation.

NOT RANDOM

Stutter does not occur randomly in the speech sequence. It is clearly some function of various aspects of word use, including matters of word type (part of speech) and structure. Although this fact regarding linguistic dimensions first became evident later than many of the other facts presented here, it has been well confirmed since that time. This fact, a focal dimension of the disorder, stands as a compelling attestation that stuttering is a disorder of speech. The many aspects of this fact require careful elaboration, and will be considered in essential detail in Chapter 12.

As well as not occurring randomly, neither does stutter occur all the time. Attention to frequency of occurrence has appeared most often in attempts to incorporate frequency into the assessment of stuttering severity. This effort has not been particularly successful, for several reasons, an important one being that the two measures sometimes conflict. Ratings of severity continue to be based principally on the impression gained in observation of the stutter occurrences, essentially in terms of the apparent effort expended in passing beyond the "block." A separate notation of frequency is not often made. Perhaps because most stuttering is reported in the range of mild to moderate,[29] one is more likely to find a frequency notation to accompany a rating of "severe."

In spite of these complications, it is worthwhile to have some reference figure regarding the overall frequency with which stuttering occurs. For some time, an overall figure of 10% frequency has been mentioned in several different sources[30] as though that figure were an established value. The 10% figure cited is almost certainly a value taken from the results of the study by Johnson and Brown (1935) undertaken to search for those speech sounds assumed to be most "difficult" for stutterers. The procedure in that study involved computation of stutter extent in a large corpus of over 300,000 words, which yielded a value of 0.0966, a figure that rounds off to 0.10.

Data regarding stutter frequency have now been reported from a number of other studies, sufficient to warrant attempting to derive an approximate general reference value, one that can be granted at least temporary status as a provisional fact. These data, not previously collated, are presented here as Table 4.1, in which the Johnson and Brown data are entered as the first item. The varying values from subsequent reports are generally within a reasonable range of the percentage yielded in that first report, and would seem to support 10% as an acceptably appropriate figure. It is of special interest that the separate values are based on samples from both spontaneous speech and oral reading and from children as well as adults.

Additional data should be added to this fund to increase its level of stability as a fully credible fact about stuttering. Should further findings corroborate the

TABLE 4.1   Frequency of Stutters Reported in Eleven Studies

Source	Subjects	No. of words	No. of stutters	Percent
Reading				
Johnson/Brown (1935)	32 young adults	311,903	30,131	0.097
Bloodstein (1944)	30 young adults	27,000	3,202	0.0119
Wingate (1959)	18 young adults	4,572	337	0.074
Soderberg (1962)	105 young adults	21,000	2,977	0.141
Spontaneous speech				
Hejna (1963)	18 young adults	248,806	17,143	0.069
Hannah/Gardner (1968)	8 young adults	985	128	0.130
Prins/Beaudet (1980)	16 young adults	( )*	( )*	0.105
Wingate (1988)	20 young adults	4,982	398	0.080
Bloodstein/Gantwerk (1967)	13 children	$(\overline{X})$ 883	$(\overline{X})$ 141	0.160
Wall et al. (1981)	9 children	11,479	958	0.083
Bloodstein/Grossman (1981)	5 children	498	62	0.124

*This report gave only the percentage.

results reported here, they would have considerable import relative to, at least, the facts of remission/recovery and prevalence.

SPEECH DELAY[‡]

Two other speech problems are noted often in young stutterers, or recorded in the development history of older ones: (1) delay in speech onset or progression, and (2) articulation defect. Substantial documentation of these facts is presented by G. Andrews, A. Craig, A.-M. Feyer, S. Hoddinott, P. Howie, and M. Neilson (1983) in their review of a considerable proportion of the numerous pertinent sources contained in the literature, extant at that time. Subsequent sources corroborate those findings (e.g., Wall & Meyers, 1984; Wolk *et al.*, 1990; Gregory & Hill, 1993.)

PERSONALITY

During approximately the first half of the twentieth century, various "theories" of the stutterer's personality were offered in explanation of the disorder. Over many years a considerable amount of research was addressed to investigate these constructions, but the results were quite consistently disappointing for proponents of those offerings.

Reviews of that research are presented in Goodstein (1958), Sheehan (1958b, 1970), Murphy and Fitzsimmons (1960), and Van Riper (1971b). The extensive review provided in these sources, covering over 40 years of pertinent research, included the best available techniques of psychological assessment. Overall, the researches failed to find support for any personality type, or unique personality dynamics, common to stutterers. Clear evidence of individual differences among stutterers, rather than a common theme in their psychological make-up, suggests, further, that the life experiences presumed to be typical for stutterers at least do not appear to have a common effect on the individuals. However, the stereotypes are not relinquished easily (see Horsley and FitzGibbon, 1987).

These findings become especially pertinent to matters of management.

AROUND THE WORLD

Stuttering is known to occur in all the many societies and cultures that have been studied. The prevalence in various societies may vary; however, careful cultural comparisons are limited, in view of the differences in relative population sizes and number of cases discovered. However, relative prevalence is less important than the clear evidence of universal occurrence. From the reasonably adequate basis now compiled, there is no persuasive indication of any special cultural influences, specifically in respect to practices of child-rearing, or in regard to attitudes and practices relating to speech performance. This particular aspect of the fact was well documented years ago (Wingate, 1962a,b,c).

An especially pertinent aspect of the worldwide occurrence of stuttering is that the words for stuttering in the many different languages are quite consistently onomatopoeic—as is the English word "stutter." Moreover, the origins of the words very often reflect the referent descriptively; again like the English word, whose etymological origin also characterizes its sense. A few examples of foreign terms for stutter should suffice here: *hus-sutsuts* (Cowichan, Pacific Northwest Indian); *ankytys* (Finnish); *i'ina* (Hausa, West Africa); *ngak-ngak* (Tabiyang, New Guinea).[31]

IN SUM

Notations of facts about stuttering are scattered throughout the literature of the field, and sometimes are brought into a compilation of sorts. The facts presented in this chapter are a winnowing of those identifiable as most stable because of the extent of their support. Certain sources might contend that there are other dimensions of information about stuttering that possibly merit being listed in this group, by slightly adjusting the criteria for inclusion. However, to my awareness, possible candidates would not add a great deal to, nor detract at all from, what the items presented here have to offer.

The major significance of these facts, as a group, is that they clearly attest to the reality of stuttering and its identity, since stuttering is their common object of reference and source of content. Individually, and in various combinations, these facts shed special light on the nature of the disorder. Although the illumination is not yet as bright as it might be, these facts nonetheless reveal quite a bit about stuttering that is basic to efforts to understand the disorder. They have special relevance for matters to be taken up in the final chapter.

NOTES

1. The basis, and credibility of this claim is reviewed in Wingate (1962b, 1997, pp. 125ff).

2. A criterion of this sort should be required for acceptance as a "fact" about stuttering.

3. General reference sources would include: the three papers addressed to the topic of facts that appeared as pages 226–246 of the August 1983 issue of the *Journal of Speech and Hearing Disorders*, Bloodstein (1997), Travis (1971), and Van Riper (1971). One should consult these sources for the data cited, but be circumspect about accompanying narratives that offer interpretation of the data. There is much in those sources that is like content reviewed in the chapters of Part II of this book.

4. What came to be the American Speech Language Hearing Association. In its early years stuttering was the predominant topic of convention papers and journal articles (see Tables 1.1, 1.2, and 1.3).

5. Quibbling about the identification of stuttering is a relatively recent pursuit, precipitated from some highly questionable issues generated and espoused by Wendell Johnson near mid-century and perpetuated by certain of his followers (see Chapters 2 and 3).

6. Mel Tillis, one of several entertainers who stutter, once told of being awakened one night by noises of someone attempting to break into their hotel room. Unable to speak an alert to his travel-mate, he successfully sang it in a low tone.

7. The early years of the American Speech, Language, Hearing Association.

8. Poems such as Masefield's "The West Wind," Poe's "Annabel Lee," Swinburne's "The Garden of Proserpine," Carroll's "Jabberwocky," and many others. A more recently published source, which contains whimsical poems, many with clear meter, is Silverstein's "Where the Sidewalk Ends."

9. See Wingate (1997, pp. 48ff).

10. In analogy to the visible spectrum, "white" noise contains all frequencies of the audible range. It sounds like rushing air.

11. This attitude continues as a critical problem in the field. For instance, in the effort to substitute "stutter-like disfluencies" or "within-word disfluency" for "stutter." This issue is discussed in Chapter 12.

12. In fact, embraced—to the extent that "feedback" entered the lay vocabulary as an overall substitute for more proper terms, such as "reply," "review," "analysis," etc.

13. This explanation was well addressed in a study by Neelley (1971). However, certain sources persisted in the belief.

14. Although some parents have reported stutter in the single-word stage.

15. What actually grew worse was the propagation and embellishment of this claim.

16. The presentation was published in two professional sources, the same year; see the reference section.

17. The profession's most outstanding figure, especially in the field of stuttering.

18. Also another study, which, although not published until years later (Johnson, 1955), was conducted "between 1934 and 1939."

19. That is, by what means could one expect to *prevent awareness* of stutters, and how could one have any idea whether or not the effort was successful?

20. Corroborated again in a paper addressed to "environmental influence of communication partners" by N. Ratner as part of the program on "Stuttering and the Domain of Language," ASHA Annual Convention, Nov. 16, 2000, Washington, DC.

21. See Wingate (1976) for pertinent data from fifteen studies extant by that date. Subsequent published studies give similar values.

22. Regarding the brief silent pauses, see Watson & Love (1965), Love & Jeffress (1971), Few & Lingwall (1972), and Zerbin (1973). For other anomalies, see van Lieshout *et al.* (1993) and Finn (1997). See also Runyan & Adams (1978, 1979) and Wendahl & Cole (1961).

23. See Bloodstein (1997), Van Riper (1971), and Wingate (1976).

24. See Wingate (1997, chap. 6).

25. For a review and critique of this publication see Wingate (1986c).

26. Other references are Kidd (1977, 1980, 1983) and Kidd *et al.* (1973, 1978).

27. See Wingate (1962b).

28. Once again, "reaction" threatened a confounding. One writer (Cabanas, 1954) proposed that stuttering observed in the speech of Mongoloids was not really stuttering because these individuals did not evidence negative reaction to it!

29. A low-level tentative type fact, but worthy of documentation.

30. Johnson (1948, 1956, 1967), Bloodstein (1969, 1997).

31. The onomatopoeia, and etymology, of "stutter" were discussed in Chapter 3. Other onomatopoeic foreign terms for stutter are presented in Van Riper (1971, pp. 4-5) and Wingate (1976, p. 40).

PART II

Impedimenta

Science is rooted in the will to truth. With the will to truth it stands or falls. Lower the standard even slightly and science becomes diseased to the core.

Max Werthiemer, *Social Research I*

CHAPTER 5

Excess of Testimony

[even] sophisticated people can hardly understand
how vague experience is at bottom, and how truly
that vagueness supports whatever clearness is
afterwards attained.

George Santayana, *Aphorisms, The Life of Reason*

$\mathcal{E}$ xtensive reference to case examples has been a serious impediment to progress in understanding stuttering. Unfortunately, this practice has been a mainstay in the literature of the field.

Case examples always have considerable appeal; they are concrete, personalized, memorable bits of prose that seem to "bring one close to" the disorder. This appeal, of course, is the major part of the problem they present—they bring one too close, where objectivity is easily contaminated or completely lost. One must recognize that case examples, which typically are offered as "representative" examples, are carefully selected and most often presented as support for some particular contention or explanation—which is, of course, what guided their selection. Case examples, though often useful for certain purposes, have a limited range of relevance, and very likely some substantial inherent bias, especially when there is claim or implication of cause and effect.

Even more than the reports of case examples, testimonials from stutterers themselves must be regarded with a highly cautious detachment. Testimonials are simply the personal statements of certain individuals, and any testimony is most relevant to the individual making the statement. Unfortunately, the unspoken, and quite erroneous, implication carried in such testimonials is that they exemplify stuttering in general, or "the stutterer"—which, of course, implies "*all* stutterers." But testimonials from individual stutterers cannot be assumed to represent everyone who stutters. To the contrary, individuals who produce voluntary testimonials should be considered unique in respect to, at least, attitude toward stuttering—and perhaps even in regard to their experiences with stuttering as well. The obvious personal motivation to create an extensive personal statement is itself clear indication of a notable uniqueness, since there are many thousands of stutterers but relatively few testimonials.

The typical case-example reports and testimonials invite criticism not only because they are special instances, but even more because they regularly register or emphasize some negative aspect of stuttering. This common feature constitutes a bias that has no balancing counterpart nor leveling influence. We do not find, in sources prepared by professionals in the field, case examples offered for those stutterers who are casual about their stuttering, or have essentially unremarkable or benign recollections. We also do not find personal testimonials by individuals who are actually indifferent to their stuttering. Many such individuals exist, but their stories remain untold, by themselves or by some professional person. Yet what these individuals have to contribute is at least as important as what one finds in the usual case history found in the literature; such evidence is clearly relevant to a basic understanding of the problem, and it must not continue to be ignored or compromised.

SYMPATHY/EMPATHY

The typical case reports and testimonials are not only misleading in regard to not being representative; they also create a spectrum of insidious influences that plague the effort to understand stuttering objectively and scientifically. Prominent among these collateral influences is what can be called "the sympathy/empathy principle." The personalized statements that appear in the typical case reports and testimonials, usually dramatic in one way or another, readily elicit sympathy and empathy in the person reading (or hearing) the story. Often it is quite clear from the account itself that it is being presented with the intent to elicit the sympathy/empathy effect. However, a biasing and diverting influence of this nature is likely to be active even when not consciously intended. Most people are sensitive to what appears to be the plight of another person. Normally speaking, laypersons, which includes most students of stuttering, are able to appreciate at a personal level the accounts made of, or by, certain stutterers regarding unhappy experiences, and the various feelings of distress they may report, such as embarrassment, apprehension, frustration, and the like. Such reports typically are accompanied by at least the implication of a direct link between the stuttering and the negative feelings reported. Readers of these accounts thus are made vulnerable to explanatory claims that describe stuttering as a psychological problem and, more specifically, to claims that invoke emotion (always negative) as the source, or major dimension, of the disorder.

The sympathy/empathy principle also supports an assumption that is never openly recognized but that is nonetheless pervasive and of fundamental influence in accounts of stuttering. This assumption, arising from implications expressed by at least influential stutterers, is that stutterers are perpetually alert for, and continually aware of, their stutters. There is cogent evidence to the contrary, revealed most impressively in the findings of research addressed to stutterers' awareness of stutter occurrences—a matter addressed later in this chapter.

Sympathy/empathy also has provided leverage to align stutters with "normal nonfluencies." Normal speakers may become aware—more often, are *made* aware by certain writers and practitioners—of some of the irregularities in their own speech, along with certain more memorable circumstances in which these have occurred—for example, speaking to the Highway Patrolman who has just stopped one for speeding. Having one's attention called to such occurrences renders the normal speaker receptive to such homilies as "everybody stutters at some time or other." This remark would be acceptable if it were intended simply as a descriptive simile. However, in its typical casual use it implies a literal identity of stuttering and the irregularities in speaking that are found in some samples of normal speech. In this common connotation, such homilies render the normal speaker vulnerable to the much more unsupportable claim that stuttering and normal irregularities are essentially the same, a claim that cannot sustain objective analysis.

THE PROFESSIONAL TOUCH

Anyone who reads very far into what has been written about stuttering should also remain aware that personal testimonials obtained from case studies of stutterers and published testimonials that appear in books or other media form are not the only sources of information presented by stutterers. A large proportion of the writings about stuttering, including a substantial part of the published research, is written by persons who stutter. In the United States, at least, many stutterers are faculty members in college or university speech pathology programs and therein enjoy the influence and authority common to such positions. Other persons who stutter are to be found in various professional positions within the field, in which settings they have an influence comparable to those in academic positions. Some of these stutterers have attained acceptance as "experts" in the subject.

Personal contributions from stutterers in professional positions have yielded most of the field's evidently appealing, yet faulty and diverting, concepts, beliefs, and explanatory claims. We have already encountered some expressions of such limitations,—for instance, our review of "definitions" of stuttering, in Chapter 2, and the initial analysis of "avoidance," in Chapter 3. Other limitations of this kind will be addressed in directly following chapters. For the present it is important to bring into focus a more immediate dimension of distortion—that which is contained in the personalized information from stutterers.

ALONE AMONG HUMAN DISORDERS

It must be fully appreciated that contributions to explanations of stuttering made by stutterers themselves present a completely unique circumstance in the extensive literature that addresses the wide range of human disorders and diseases. There is no other disorder in which opinion about, investigation of, and explanation for the nature and treatment of the disorder are so extensively contributed by persons afflicted with that disorder, as is the case with stuttering. One will find, of course, that for many other disorders, including some in speech and hearing (e.g., cleft lip and palate, the deaf), patients' relevant attitudes and feelings are sought, and may be given due consideration relative to certain aspects of management. However, for these, and certainly most other human disorders and diseases, patients rarely offer their personal testimonials as cogent information. Most certainly they do not presume to offer their own statements as explanation of the nature of their disorder. Moreover, such statements would not be given serious consideration even if they were offered.

For stuttering, on the other hand, patients' observations and claims are typically accepted when volunteered. Many personal accounts even are invited, and some attain undue persuasive power. Statements from stutterers are treated as veridical data that must not only be incorporated within an account of the disorder but should be given a certain priority.

"ONLY THE STUTTERER KNOWS"

The readiness with which stutterers' reports are assumed to yield especially substantive information reflects the presumption that stutterers have exclusive, privileged knowledge that reaches the interior of the disorder, knowledge that is not accessible except through the agency of stutterers themselves. This presumption is expressed in the claim, made by many stutterers—and many credulous non-stutterers too—that "only the stutterer knows."

Restatement of this frequently expressed, but misguiding, claim continues to appear in the literature. Only a few years ago, Alfonso (1990), contributing to an ASHA publication addressed to research needs in stuttering, expressed a literal current version of the claim that "only the stutterer knows." Surprisingly, the notion surfaced even more recently as a core element in what was presented as a "neuropsycholinguistic theory" of stuttering (Perkins *et al.*, 1991). Personal assertions of the contention recur intermittently: Quesal (1995), in a stutterers' self-help publication, exhorted any stutterer "to remember one thing: he is the world's foremost expert on how he talks." Similarly, Breitenfeldt (1996) stated his "firm belief that we who stutter know more about ourselves and our disorder than people who do not stutter."

Evidence that raises serious question about such claims is reviewed in the next section. In passing, however, one should consider that if stutterers were as knowledgeable about their disorder as is claimed in such assertions, one could expect that at least some stutterers might have pointed out certain important, readily noted aspects of the disorder that have been revealed through (relatively) objective research. For instance, one might have expected reports about matters relative to the various aspects of stuttering to be discussed in Chapter 11—in particular, the critical feature of stutter occurrence in syllable-initial position.[1]

Of course, there are aspects of stutter occurrences to which a stutterer is privy, such as the inner experience of the "block," and what it is like to "know what I want to say but can't say it." There may well be certain other things that "only the stutterer knows"; however, most of what has been recorded is psychosocial in nature, that is, matters regarding their emotional reactions to stutters, and feelings they may have regarding the real, or presumed, actions or views of other people (see the study by Frasier, in a following section). Such knowledge is of limited value for understanding or treating the disorder—unless one is prepared to accept it as explanatory, which too often has been the case.

Personal knowledge of the kind typically reported by stutterers is little different in kind from the unique personal knowledge that might be offered by a patient having some other abnormal condition. One must consider that undoubtedly there is much that is known only to the cerebral palsied individual, to the diabetic, to someone with cleft palate, to the tiqueur, to the alcoholic, and on and on. However, such information is rarely recorded; moreover, even if communicated, it is not incorporated into explanation of those disorders, as is the case in stuttering. In this vein, retrospective accounts of aphasia (Rose, 1948) or even of severe mental illness (Beers, 1945) are neither offered, nor entertained, as significant determinants in, let alone credible explanations of, the disorder.

Similarly, contrary to the regularly implied contention, in some cases openly expressed, what "only the stutterer knows" typically tells us very little about the character of the experience or the nature of the disorder. Most of the testimonies reporting the stutter experience are little more than what is perceivable by an independent observer. For instance, reports of "the block," or "being stopped," or of being "unable to move,"[2] correspond to the observation of *inaction* discussed in Chapter 3 as one of the two cardinal features that mark the stutter *event*. Only rarely does one find an introspective report that reveals something about this experience of stutter that is not discernible to external observation. One especially insightful person, whose stuttering is so improved that occurrences are rare, advised me, "When I'm in a block it doesn't feel like inaction, though it may look like it, or even sound like it. There seems, rather, to be a restraining turbulence, or forceful constriction. My muscles seem anything but inactive." A report of this kind does tell something valuable about the character of the stutter event. Unfortunately, such description is rare.

NOT AS ADVERTISED

The readiness to attribute special authority to stutterers' representations continues in spite of much good evidence that they are not routinely very knowledgeable about their stuttering. A major qualification that limits the value of typical stutterer self-reports derives from the considerable evidence that, on several dimensions, stutterers seem not to know their disorder at all as well as has been claimed, and as has been so widely believed.

THEY KNOW NOT WHAT THEY DO

For some time there has been reason to realize that stutterers are not very conversant with their stuttering—notably, even in regard to what happens during stutter occurrences. An impressively forthright account of this limitation is found in no less a source than Van Riper's (1973) book addressed to the treatment of stuttering.[3] He emphasized that the basic procedure in therapy is to train the stutterer to identify his stutters, pointing out that "he [the stutterer] rarely recognizes what he does" (p. 246). Corroboration of this assessment is found in research such as that reported by Naylor (1953), Cullinan *et al.* (1963), and Aron (1967), which revealed that stutterers underestimate the severity of their stuttering.[4] These findings are supported by occasional testimonies, such as that by David Kehoe, below. The significance of such evidence enlarges when one considers that, in reference to such matters as the anxiety purportedly experienced by stutterers, or such claims as "expectancy," or the assertions regarding struggle and reaction, one would expect the results to have been exactly the opposite.

It is relevant to note here that normal speakers too are unaware of most of the (ordinary) irregularities that occur in their speech, to the extent of being chagrined when confronted with such evidence contained in recordings of their conversational speech (see Wingate, 1988, pp. 47–54). But there is no basis for expecting that normal speakers would be aware of their (ordinary) speech irregularities. In contrast, it is widely believed that stutterers are well aware of all their stutters.

NOR HOW OFTEN THEY DO IT

In addition to the evidence that stutterers are not particularly aware of what occurs during their ongoing stutters, substantial compelling evidence has accumulated revealing that stutterers are not even as aware of the extent of stutter occurrences as has been so long assumed and so sincerely believed. Again, long-term observations made by Van Riper are cogent. In describing the details of his therapy with stutterers he wrote:

> next we ask him [the stutterer] to identify those short, easy stutterings which serve as our temporary primary target and *which already exist unrecognized in his speech.*[5] (1973, p. 249)

My own experience with many stutterers has yielded similar findings. I also am reminded of reflections reported to me by certain respected stutterer colleagues who remarked, in regard to awareness of their own stuttering, that they "undoubtedly miss a lot of the little ones."[6] Occasionally one encounters evidence that some of the "big ones" are missed as well, as supplied recently by David Kehoe (1999), an acknowledged severe stutterer, who wrote that, when an undergraduate at Reed College, he "had no idea of how severely I stuttered."

NOR WHEN THEY DON'T DO IT

A major item in the lore about stuttering, supplied and recited by many stutterers, and echoed by many clinicians, is the claim that they do not stutter when alone. This claim has traditionally been accepted at face value; in fact, it is offered as clear (although inverse) evidence of the deleterious influence of negative emotion; namely, as showing that when a stutterer is not anxious about his speech—because, in speaking when alone, there is no one to hear it—he does not stutter.

This claim, of no stuttering when alone, has been readily accepted because it fits so well into the assumption that stuttering is a psychological problem, based in anxiety and reaction. Largely because of this neat fit, with its apparent support for the belief, exploration of the claim along several potential dimensions of inquiry has not been undertaken. Very worthwhile, pertinent information would be supplied in records of the kinds of things stutterers say when alone, and the manner in which those things are said. Importantly, no one has produced any sort of report on matters of this kind regarding the speech of stutterers when alone. Such matters are very pertinent to the issue, but they have not been investigated. They will be considered in Chapter 12, in discussing the relevance to stuttering of propositionality and, as well, manner of speaking.

However, there is some quantitative evidence pertinent to the issue of no-stuttering-when-alone. This evidence, which has appeared sporadically, is substantial and revealing. Porter (1939) observed 13 stutterers reading aloud when alone, and noted that only two of them did not stutter during that time. Hahn (1940) had 52 stutterers keep a record of their stutters while reading aloud in a situation where they believed themselves to be alone. Unobtrusive observation revealed that all but three of these individuals stuttered during that exercise. Moreover, when the audio recordings of their speech were reviewed with the subjects, it was found that typically they had underestimated the amount of their stuttering—over half of them stuttered from two to eight times as much as they had recorded while speaking. Razdol'skii (1965) compared the solitary and social-situation speech of 125 stutterers ranging in age from 2 years to adulthood. Most of the preschool children stuttered as much when alone as when they spoke in the presence of other people. Most of the school-age children, adolescents, and adults stuttered less when alone. However, only 11 of the 125 subjects did not stutter when speaking in isolation. Later, all subjects who could be expected to answer the question were asked if they had stuttered when talking alone. Initially, most said they did not, but to further questioning many reported "occasional brief lapses" under such circumstances. However, the numbers of "brief lapses" acknowledged were still less than the actual number of stutters that had occurred. Significantly, these studies are routinely ignored in the literature.

THE PERSONAL TOUCH

Findings from another line of research give further reason to be circumspect about contributions from stutterers. Some years ago, Frasier (1955) reported findings that are especially relevant to the criticism that stutterers' personal analyses cannot be accorded a central role in efforts to explain the nature of stuttering. Data obtained by Frasier in individual interviews with 19 adolescent stutterers regarding their "theory" of stuttering revealed that they "tended to stress psychological factors." More importantly,

> The language used by the stutterers was markedly vague, contained a number of relatively or completely unverifiable statements, was relatively lacking in detail, revealed a tendency to overemphasize relatively restricted factors in attempted explanations of causal relationships, and was characterized to a relatively high degree by the seemingly unconscious projection of personal or private evaluations. (p. 333)

The fact that these individuals were adolescents who had done "little or no reading about stuttering" serves to buttress the criticisms leveled here. Having done little or no reading about the disorder, these naive stutterers were not likely to have been influenced by the standard run of material to be found in the literature of stuttering. Significantly, Frasier's summary of these adolescent stutterers' ruminations is just as suitably descriptive of statements made by any number of older, and presumably more sophisticated, stutterers. Moreover, Frasier's summary description of the statements given by those unsophisticated stutterers matches very well the sort of account proffered from within professional ranks, including claims made by "leaders" in the field. One is well reminded here of Jonas' statement, reproduced in Chapter 2, that the accounts of stuttering he had found in his search of the literature were like the "old wives' tales" he had encountered before.

Clearly, stutterers' contributions are an enormously unbalancing consequence for the study of stuttering. Stutterers' personal observations, attitudes and feelings are certainly a source of information that is due some amount of consideration within the broad purview of the disorder—but such consideration must be circumspect, and appropriately qualified. The final limit in attending to these contributions is reached abruptly at the point that they become bent into explanation.

AN UNFAMILIAR PRINCIPLE

Stutterers who proffer their personal experiences, and ideas, as avenues to explanation of the disorder ignore a fundamental principle in science. The

principle is well expressed in the following statement by astronomer Edwin
Hubble (1954):

> The distinction between knowledge and wisdom is fully recognized in our
> time, but it was not always so. Men wanted to explore the universe in all
> its aspects. The attempts began long ago. There was much fumbling; there
> were many false leads and occasional breathtaking achievements. Eventu-
> ally it was realized that only one aspect—the world of positive knowl-
> edge—could be explored with confidence and, moreover, that success in
> the venture was measured in terms of *disinterested curiosity*. Special meth-
> ods for handling the particular kind of subject matter were developed under
> the leadership of Galileo and Newton, and modern science was launched
> upon its extraordinary career.
>
> The requirement of *disinterested curiosity*[7] was never formulated con-
> sciously. Yet it seems to have been the dominant motive in the work of all
> the great men of science. It has inspired the statement that the essential
> characteristic of science is the simple idea of attempting "to ascertain
> objective truth without regard to personal desires."

The serious reservations raised in preceding paragraphs regarding stutterers' biasing influences in the field, particularly an absence of "disinterested
curiosity," do not apply in uniform coverage to all stutterers in the
professional ranks. There are some who give evidence of attempting to
maintain an objective, detached, and rational stance. Many others seem to
convey their biases innocently and to express such influence almost
inadvertently. Still, even such influences are diverting. But the greatest
problem is posed by those stutterers within the profession who continue to
press unsupportable beliefs that either are personally generated or personally
satisfying, and who persistently endeavor to disseminate their biases.

The outstanding case in point is the "evaluational hypothesis" and its
penumbrae, developed by Wendell Johnson in the late 1930s and subsequently
promoted by him and many ardent followers.[8] Its simplicity has accrued an
incredibly wide following over the intervening years, in spite of the fact that,
from the beginning, much of the "evidence" claimed for it, and the interpretations of data based on it, were faulty and incompatible with other sources of
knowledge. Moreover, the formulation is internally inconsistent and contradictory (see, e.g., Wingate, 1962a,b,c, 1986a,b, 1997, chap. 7). The field of stuttering seems now beginning to recover—but slowly, haltingly, and still against
stout and persistent reluctance—from the widespread constraining influence
of this personally based belief system.[9] Still, one finds many sources in which
the essence of Johnson's position is actively pursued. One pervasive manifestation of this condition is the continuing use of the term "disfluency."

The criticism presented here is not limited to certain persons who stutter. There are many non-stutterers in professional positions who, caught up in one or another favored explanation of stuttering, have pressed rationally unsupportable positions as avidly as the more vocal stutterers. Again, the "evaluational hypothesis" provides a pointed illustration. The theme of that position, and certain of its manipulations, continue to recur in many writings, some of which will be noted in Chapters 6 and 7. The most active single proponent has been Oliver Bloodstein, an (evidently) non-stuttering student of Wendell Johnson. The crux of Johnson's theme, with only minimal modification, turns up as Bloodstein's "anticipatory struggle hypothesis." Of course, there are also a number of other stutterers, and non-stutterers, in the profession who actively work at supporting this position and continue to recite its litany. There also are many more who have continued to accept this formulation,[10] which by now should be moribund. The expansive influence of the belief is manifest in a number of other problems in the field, to be reviewed in succeeding chapters.

SUMMARY

The extensive lore of stuttering is based, directly and indirectly, on testimony from stutterers. Testimonies appear frequently in case histories presented as examples in textbooks; many personal statements are reported in organizational publications and pamphlets; a surprising number of lengthy ones have been published as books; and, of course, the lay press and media sporadically feature a "human interest" version.

Testimonies are typically narrow in scope, and emphasize matters that are impressive or have dramatic appeal. However, if details of testimonial reports are reviewed objectively, and further inquiry pursued, much of the appealing surface substance dissolves into inconsistency or contradiction. Unfortunately, these investigative steps have rarely been undertaken in the study of stuttering. Instead, professionals in the field have been ready to accept, and promote, testimonial reports as veridical data. Moreover, the lore from testimonials has been molded into, or served as support for, certain ideas offered as concepts basic to explanation of the disorder.

Actually, so many of the ideas and accounts contributed by stutterers have been misleading in one way or another. Much of this content is the substance of Chapter 6.

NOTES

1. Bluemel (1913) had offered the pithy observation that stutter really involves the following vowel, not the consonant, as routinely claimed. This suggestion was ignored.

2. Of special note in this regard, Van Riper gave the following description in his presentation at a "Recovered Stutterers" Symposium: "that moment in which we cannot make a part of ourselves move the way we want."

3. Van Riper, for many years the foremost clinician in the United States, had worked knowledgeably and successfully with many hundreds of stutterers.

4. A finding that also bears significantly on the issues regarding accessory features.

5. Italics added.

6. In my initial interview with stutterers, of all ages, I first ask what they know about their stuttering, followed later by query as to the frequency, and features, of their stutter during the interview. The results are remarkably like the findings reported here.

7. Italics added.

8. Properly identified as "the Iowa school," an appropriate designation suggested by Hamre (1992).

9. Regarding the personal basis of this formulation, see chapter 7 in Wingate, 1997.

10. St. Louis and Lass (1981) reported that the majority of 1902 university students in 33 states accepted most of Johnson's assumptions.

CHAPTER 6

Deceptive Concepts

Psychologists pay lip service to the scientific
method, and use it whenever it is convenient;
but when it isn't they make wild leaps of their
uncontrolled fancy, and still suppose themselves grounded firmly on objective fact.

Anthony Standen,
Science is a Sacred Cow (1950)

The complaint expressed in the above epigram is true of only some
psychologists. However, it is pertinent to the present context because
it applies particularly well to so many persons in the field of stuttering,
who have had varying degrees of immersion in the subject matter of psychology.

The limitations of extant "theories" of stuttering are best revealed through
a critical analysis of the concepts that, in varying combinations, constitute the
dubious substance of those explanatory attempts. A general, recurring fault in
the concepts around which the theories are entwined is to be found in their
origins in lore—the extensive contributions from case history, patient testimony, and especially personal accounts and affirmations from stutterers who
have entered the field.

A certain number of ideas, advanced as concepts, have attained considerable
explanatory stature in the field. They are properly identified as deceptive
because all except the one to be discussed first (Distraction) have a surface
plausibility that, although it has carried them very far, does not stand up to
critical scrutiny or objective assessment.

This chapter will present seven of these concepts: (1) Distraction, (2) Consonant Versus Vowel, (3) Difficult Sounds or Words, (4) Adaptation, (5) Consistency, (6) Expectancy, and (7) Avoidance. An eighth, Continuity, will be discussed in Chapter 8, within an especially relevant context.

The content of the present chapter follows appropriately that of Chapter 5, because most of these concepts were initiated by stutterers, or have been very actively supported through the testimonies of stutterers. These formulations too have much of the quality of lore about them.

The concepts are interrelated in a number of ways, some having more dimensions in common than others. Traditionally, each has been presented as separate, and so are discussed as such here. The rather lengthy section on Avoidance contains a critical synopsis of learning theory in application to stuttering. Because learning theory can no longer justifiably command as much attention in discussions of stuttering as it has formerly, the consideration it receives in this chapter is essentially the limit of its exposition in this book.

DISTRACTION

There are certain conditions under which a stutterer's production of word sequences does not evidence stutters, such as singing, speaking to rhythm, speaking in chorus, and certain other conditions, the "ameliorative conditions" discussed in Chapter 4; they will be considered again in Chapter 14. At present we are concerned only with the fact that the marked reduction, even elimination, of stuttering that is occasioned by these conditions has regularly been offhandedly dismissed as due to "distraction."

It is not clear when the distraction explanation was first advanced. Although Bertrand (see Klingbeil, 1939) mentioned it early in the nineteenth century; the explanation seems to have surfaced only in rare instances prior to the twentieth century. Unfortunately, relative to the matter of progress in understanding stuttering, the "distraction" account is much more clearly a recourse of modern times, with its focus on psychological interpretation of the disorder. It has been repeated frequently in the extensive literature on stuttering that has accumulated since the time the professional association (ASHA) was established, in the late 1920s. A brief, partial review should note the following entries. Distraction was cited to account for the beneficial effect of rhythm and choral speaking in three of the "Studies in the Psychology of Stuttering" series directed by Wendell Johnson (Barber 1939a,b; Johnson & Rosen, 1937). Much later, Bloodstein (1969) presented it as one of the "Eight General Conditions Under Which Stuttering Varies." Sheehan (1970) listed it as one of "ten things we know about stuttering." Van Riper (1971a,b, 1973) related it to an S–R context, and to fear and expectancy (as did other authors). Most recently, Conture (1990) and Bloodstein (1993, 1995, 1999) continue to treat it as a viable explanation.

The continuing appeal of the distraction account is that it presumably exemplifies the potency of (negative) reaction to stuttering. Proceeding from the assumption that anticipation of (concern about, fear of, preoccupation with) stuttering is what causes stutter to occur, it is further assumed that any conditions that result in minimizing, or eliminating, stutters must then operate through "getting his mind off" stuttering by preoccupying him with something else—namely, the minimizing conditions themselves.

Distraction merits attention among foundation topics in stuttering only because it deserves a sound, clarifying refutation. "Distraction" is undoubtedly the most ingenuous, superficial, and unreflective of the many indefensible explanations that have been offered in regard to stuttering. To accord it any credence whatsoever epitomizes an abysmal lack of basic attributes of a scientific attitude, such as inquiry, circumspection, and rationality. Moreover, its widespread acceptance and recitation by practitioners in the field reflects the catechismal orientation of so many individuals, who nonetheless accept, and repeat, this incredible explanation.

The crucial, absolute fault of the distraction account is that the explanation it intends cannot possibly apply! The meaning of "distraction" is that a person's attention is effectively diverted from that to which he was previously attending. Standard use of the term in respect to stuttering avers, or clearly implies, this meaning. However, in none of the conditions that ameliorate stuttering can the individual be said to no longer have stuttering in mind. In fact, the stutterer himself is well aware that his stuttering has markedly diminished—which means that not only does he have stuttering in mind, but that it is most likely *foremost* in his mind.

It would seem that this flagrant contradiction should have been highly visible at its initial offering. Instead, it has obviously escaped recognition for a very long time. This fact itself stands as additional testimony to the continued complacent superficiality of explanations found so often in the literature of stuttering. The generalized persistence of ideational conviction in faulty concepts about stuttering is well illustrated by finding that distraction is still accepted as a meaningful account in certain contemporary sources (Conture, 1990; Bloodstein, 1993, 1995).

Although it is not clear that "distraction" per se was originally voiced by a stutterer, it is plausible that the term came into use to describe (or interpret) a claim made fairly often by stutterers, although in more ordinary terms. Many stutterers will report that "I don't stutter when I don't think about it." Incredibly, this claim has been accepted at face value among speech pathologists, by whom it is often restated. But this account has its own form of cobweb logic. How can someone report what he does *not* do when he is *not* thinking about it? I trust that, upon reflection, the reader will recognize that this is quite impossible. However, once again the ready, unreflective acceptance of the claim is entwined with the deep conviction that stutters occur as a result of (negative) reaction.

In respect to the stutterer's claim, just noted, it seems quite likely that the actual experience under report is more like the following. In some particular situation, the individual suddenly became aware of stuttering—either from a notable instance of stutter occurrence, or for some other reason being reminded that he stutters. Then, to the best of his recollection, he could not remember having stuttered prior to that time. A statement of recall such as this would be credible, but it is very much different than the report as made, which, as pointed out above, is *not* credible. In considering stutterers' claims, one should keep in mind the well-documented evidence, from studies in psychology, regarding the limitations and errors of personal recollections and report.[1] In particular, one must remain aware of the impressive evidence of fallibility in stutterers' testimony, as presented in Chapter 5.

Much of the lore and myth in the field of stuttering contains certain fragments that may have something of perhaps a superficial plausibility in efforts made at explanation. However, one cannot grant such latitude to the notion of distraction. As invoked relative to stuttering, distraction has none of the partially redeeming features one can find sometimes in lore or myth. In particular, as explanation of any of the ameliorative conditions, "distraction" is not simply a large zero, it is a massive minus. As indicated in the introduction to this chapter, distraction does not have even surface plausibility.

CONSONANT VERSUS VOWEL

The belief that consonants are more difficult for stutterers than are vowels has been a major feature in the lore of stuttering at least since the time, early in the nineteenth century, when an expanding interest in speech encouraged attention to certain dimensions of speech processes. This interest soon extended to speech disorders, of which stuttering has always been the most compelling.

Evidently, belief in the greater difficulty of consonants was an assumption based on observation that stutters more frequently involved consonants—an assumption that undoubtedly was abetted by some stutterers' complaints of stuttering more "on" consonants.

Several challenges to this assumption were made during the nineteenth century, but were ignored, and the idea of consonants being more difficult than vowels persisted as a fact of stutter lore well into the twentieth century.[2] Continued acceptance of the belief received substantial encouragement in the late 1930s from seemingly corroborative findings reported from study addressed specifically to sound difficulties in stuttering. These reports (Johnson & Brown, 1935; Brown, 1938) yielded a rank order of sound difficulty in which consonants clearly filled the higher ranks, and vowels the lowest. Although this gross indication of consonant difficulty helped to perpetuate a misleading concept, certain dimensions of these findings would eventually play a significant role in a linguistic analysis of stuttering. Major features of this analysis will be discussed in Chapter 12.

As mentioned above, the idea that consonants are more difficult than vowels essentially expresses the observation that stutters occur much more often with consonants. Only recently has it been pointed out (Wingate, 1988) that this observed differential is misleading[3]—that it is an artefact undoubtedly occasioned by the structure of words. In fact, analysis of word structure clearly confutes the belief that consonants are more difficult than vowels. First, and particularly important, most words begin with consonants. Significantly, initial position is where stutters occur. Once again, the matter of initial position emerges as critical. Further, another feature of word structure is highly pertinent to the matter of a relationship between consonants and stutter occurrence. As a general rule, word endings contain considerably more consonants than do word beginnings. If stutter occurrence were simply, or even largely, a matter of difficulty with, or fear of, consonants, then one should expect more stutters to occur in final position, since that is where consonants occur most. Several large samples of word composition reveal that well over 60% of consonants occur in final position.[4] This feature can be brought into clear focus with data from the simplest words in the language—words of one syllable. Actually, words of one syllable are additionally valuable for purposes of this illustration, because one-syllable words are also the words most frequently used.

The data in Figure 6.1, based on phonetic analysis of all the one-syllable words of English (Moser et al., 1957), reveal that word-final positions typically contain considerably more consonants than do word-initial positions. If stuttering is some function of difficulty associated with consonants, actual or perceived, or fear of consonants, even particular consonants, then one should expect that the locus of stutters would be, at the very least, more likely and more frequently occurring in word-final positions. Most certainly, this is not what happens; as discussed in Chapter 3, stutters do not occur in word/syllable-final position.

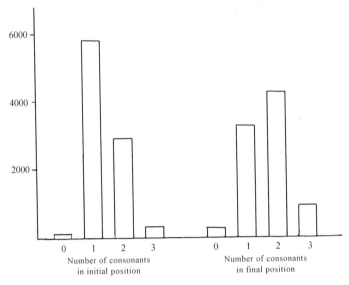

FIGURE 6.1 Frequencies with which 1, 2, or 3 consonants occur in initial and final positions in one-syllable words. Data from Moser *et al.* (1957).

DIFFICULT SOUNDS—DIFFICULT WORDS

The idea that some sounds are relatively more difficult for stutterers has been expressed for a long time. Intermittently during the nineteenth century and into the early twentieth century, various types or classes of sounds (such as "gutturals" or "explosives"), and sometimes lists of individual sounds, were said to present more of a problem than others. However, except for the claim that consonants are more difficult than vowels, there was a notable lack of agreement, among the various sources addressing the issue, regarding which sounds were purported to be difficult. The idea of some differential difficulty among the phones of English received somewhat supportive evidence following upon study addressed to the matter in the 1930s (Johnson & Brown, 1935, 1938, 1939). Although the findings revealed no general factor of phonetic difficulty for all stutterers, that is, no type or groups of phones that were inherently difficult, it did yield a general rank order of apparent phone difficulty—interpreted as such because of the extent to which those phones were associated with stuttering. There were, however, certain other findings from these studies that will concern us in later discussions, especially in Chapter 12.

A different concept of sound difficulty emerged within the developing pre-occupation with psychological factors in stuttering. In this version, the pre-sumed difficulty was not considered to reside in some inherent quality of sounds themselves, but in the individual stutterer's reaction to and belief about certain sounds. In this thema, the difficulty of sounds represented a stutterer's perception and persuasion that certain sounds were his personal nemeses. Such personal beliefs are held to be built upon the individual's recollections of intermittent stutters with certain words or sounds, or the recall of some dramatic stutter instance that involved them. This idea of personalized sound difficulty interlocks with several other beliefs, under review in this chapter and in Chapter 5, that present stuttering as a psychological problem essentially in behaviorist tradition. Before proceeding further with this topic, it is important to emphasize that not all stutterers claim personal difficult sounds, even though they may perceive the disorder in general terms as a problem with sounds.

Most often, a stutterer who spontaneously speaks of "difficult sounds" will make the claim quite straightforwardly, in terms of "trouble with" or "difficulty with" the phone(s) in question. However, literature descriptions of the condi-tion, through the agency of the widespread preoccupation with the purported central role of reaction, have transformed the claim of "difficulty with" into "fear of." Thereby, one will often find this individualized conception of sound difficulty stated in terms of either "difficult sounds" or "feared sounds."

Descriptions of difficult, or feared, sounds are often expressed in terms of difficult or feared *words*. The crux of this equivalence is that, when speaking in respect to words the reference is nonetheless to *sounds*—as, for example, complaint about "s-words" or "l-words" or "m-words" or the like (see case example below). The significance of this equivalence is that, whether expressed in reference to sounds or words, the essential focus is *sounds in initial posi-tion*—which is the actual critical feature that typically is lost in the mist of preoccupation with the sounds themselves. As noted elsewhere in this chapter, and in Chapter 3, the same sounds, when not in initial position, are not "difficult," or "feared"—or stuttered.

The matter of individualized difficult sounds has considerable appeal, espe-cially if one is already persuaded of, or receptive to, psychological accounts of stuttering. The appeal is particularly persuasive when actual stutters involving certain sounds occur in the context of a specific complaint just made about them. In such instances, it seems as though one has immediate, direct confir-mation of the claimed causal connection between the reported sound difficulty and the stutter involving it. However, the listener should be circumspect about the value of such apparent connections—they are misleading by virtue of what might be called perceptual prominence. That is, the concurrences—of com-plaint about a specific sound and stutter with that sound—are impressive, memorable, and persuasive because they often are called to the listener's attention by the stutterer himself. However, one should take care to listen, as well, for recurrences of the same words (with, of course, the same *sounds*) that the individual speaks without stutter. Further, to conduct a full test of claimed sound difficulty, one should also listen for different words that have the same initial phone. These *un*stuttered recurrences of reportedly difficult words or sounds are much less evident and easily go unnoticed, which is one part of the reason this important observation is never undertaken. Another part of the reason is that such analysis is demanding and time-consuming. However, the major part of the reason for not undertaking such logically proper appraisal is that the lore of difficult sounds has been so widely accepted as known fact that both stutterer and clinician are satisfied by an apparent confirmation. Yet attention to *un*stuttered recurrences of "difficult words" is vital information not only of major importance to conceptual matters in stuttering but also of great value in dealing therapeutically with stutterers—especially those who harbor the full belief in the difficult words/difficult sounds notion.

The matter of individualized difficult sounds became elevated quite rapidly from claim into concept largely through an orientation that is based on a persisting set of assumptions and beliefs in which dramatic observations are persuasive and careful objective analysis is discouraged. The matter of difficult sounds has not been studied objectively, and, even in the rare instances in which pertinent data emerge, their significance is unappreciated and ignored. A particular case in point is contained in the report by Brown (1938) that was part of the research addressed to the matter of sound difficulty in stuttering noted earlier. Although Brown reported a "high degree of consistency" of sound difficulty for the subjects as a group, he also acknowledged that "considering the stutterers individually, there is less consistency ... and in some cases there is almost no consistency at all." However, this finding was not considered further, nor mentioned again; yet it stands as the most meaningful result of this, and later, research inasmuch as "consistency" of this phenomenon, or any other, has relevance only in regard to the individual.

The matter of personal sound/word difficulty must undergo objective inquiry before it can be admitted to consideration as bona fide data in the study of stuttering. Appropriate analyses will be time-consuming and require a great deal of care, yet they should be undertaken. The following case (R.S.) is presented as illustration; this particular individual was chosen for example because, in initial interview, he spontaneously claimed having difficult sounds, namely: "s-words, m-words, l-words, and w-words."

Table 6.1 presents the pertinent data provided by R.S., at the time a college junior, age 22. In interview he was pleasant and personable, conversed readily, and was very open about his stuttering, which he reported had been of the

TABLE 6.1 Phones Involved in Stutters in Two Spontaneous Speech Samples of R, S

Phone	Oct. 20			Dec. 6		
	Stutts	# word possi- bilities	%	Stutts	# word possi- bilities	%
s	5	77	6	3	60	5
ʃ	4	11	36			
m	2	30	7	4	31	13
k	2	54	4	2	33	6
d	1	47	2	2	36	5
n	1	37	3	1	31	3
w				2	83	2
θ		22	0	1	18	16
j				1	25	4
f				1	30	3
p	2	32	6			
l	1	15	7			
g	1	26	4			
r	1	24	4			
b	1	40	2			
ð	1	123	*	1	103	*
ɪ	1	100	1			
ʌ	1	71	1			
	24	687	4	18	442	4
Words in sample	1800			1600		
Percentage stutter			1.3			1.0

*Values of less than 1% are omitted.

same nature for as long as he could remember. His stutter, predominantly clonic, was rated as mild.

If "difficult" sounds occur for the reason claimed, they should be evidenced in any speech sample, and therefore more than one sample should be obtained.

Two samples of R.S.'s speech were recorded on separate occasions, 6 weeks apart, under essentially the same conditions. Written transcriptions, including all pauses and irregularities of utterance, were made of each recording. The pairs of transcription and recording were reviewed, and "scored," twice by the same observer.

The data of Table 6.1 are concerned only with instances of stutter. The column at the far left of the table lists the (word-initial) phones involved in stutter in each of these two speech samples. Under each date-heading, the first column records the number of stutters involving each phone; the next column shows the number of words spoken of which that phone was word-initial; the third column shows the percentage of stutter per word for each phone. Thus, on October 20, of 77 words beginning with /s/, R.S. stuttered five, or 6% of them. On December 6, of 60 words beginning with /s/, he stuttered 3 of them, or 5%.

His purported difficulty with /s/ was, as is so often the case, based on ordinary spelling;[5] thereby "sugar" /ʃʊgə/ was for him an "s-word." In fact, he made a point of calling attention to his first stutter on "sugar," identifying it as one of his "s-words." He also made similar casual reference to two other stutters, both of which were true /s/-initial words. In the October 20 sample his percentage stutter with /ʃ/ was substantial; however, not having spoken many words with /ʃ/ in initial position might have inflated this value. Even so, only 36% hardly illustrates persuasively what one should expect of a "difficult sound," especially as typically conceived. Moreover, since he considered such words to be "s-words," from his standpoint words beginning with /ʃ/ and /s/ should be combined in the computations. As such, his overall percentage of stutter with "s-words" was only 8%. Further, his percentage of stutter with true /s/-words is hardly more than his overall percentage of stutter in both speech samples (4%).

Other dimensions of Table 6.1 bear significantly on the matter of "difficult words/sounds," and of "consistency" (see next section). Note the range of sounds involved in stutter, including some that have stutter percentages comparable to that for /s/ but not identified by R.S. as difficult. Note also that stutter involving two sounds, /m/ (claimed to be a difficult sound) and /θ/ (not claimed as difficult) varied notably in the two samples. Note further that the sounds least frequently stuttered are two vowels and the consonant /ð/. These latter findings, and their relevance, will be considered later, in Chapter 12.

The concept of difficult sounds or words is a lore-based and lore-maintained belief in the field of stuttering, couched in a psychological ambience, nurtured by dramatic examples, and supported in default by inadequate inquiry. It is possible that psychological factors may be involved to some degree in certain individualized difficult words/sounds, perhaps even along the lines routinely offered to account for them. Clearly, such account is completely inadequate as a general principle. Conversely, it is abundantly clear that certain factors yet unknown are involved in stutter occurrences—a qualification demanded by the substantial evidence that many sounds claimed to be difficult are not routinely associated with stutters and, to the contrary, that stutters do involve many sounds that are not claimed to be difficult.

THE ADAPTATION AND "CONSISTENCY" EFFECTS

For many years the adaptation and consistency effects were mainstays in interpreting the nature of stuttering. These two phenomena were brought into the literature of stuttering in an article by Johnson and Knott (1937) wherein both phenomena were explained in the stimulus–response (S–R) terms of behaviorism. Both effects were immediately, and for many years thereafter, interpreted in the terms of (behaviorist) learning theory. Over this lengthy period, the adaptation effect was much more often the object of study and analysis than was the consistency effect, evidently because it was amenable to numerical treatment and graphic display

ADAPTATION

The "adaptation effect" refers to the observation that, when stutterers read the same material several times in succession, the frequency of stutter decreases, at first notably and then more gradually. Figure 6.2 shows the typical course of this progression.[6]

In its long-term use, following Johnson and Knott (1937), the designation "adaptation effect" makes improper use of the word "adaptation." Adaptation describes the process in which an individual becomes accustomed to conditions or circumstances. In regard to stuttering, the first, and appropriate, use of the term appeared in the report of a study by Van Riper and Hull (1955),[7] whose research was addressed to the effect of situational influence on stuttering. Finding that stutter decreased in the course of speaking the same material repeatedly, they described the decrease in terms of the stutterer *adapting to the situation*. In this early study, the term "adaptation" was used properly. However, the word was retained in the subsequent extensive exploitation of this particular phenomenon, wherein its correct meaning was supplanted via

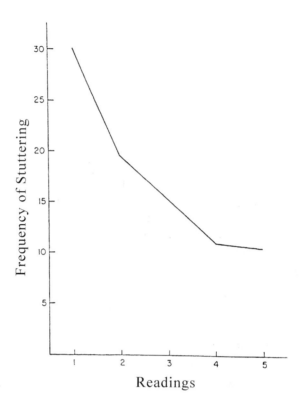

Readings

FIGURE 6.2 Typical curve of stuttering adaptation. Reprinted with permission from
Wingate (1986a).

the assumption that the phenomenon represents "unlearning." Thereby,
through this improper use in regard to stuttering, "adaptation" became an
(unrecognized) misnomer.

Johnson promoted the adaptation effect as representing an unlearning of the
stutter "response," in analogue of experimental extinction, a phenomenon
reported regularly from psychological laboratory studies of animal learning, in
which a learned response "extinguishes" when its reinforcement is withdrawn.
Most likely, Johnson's claim that stuttering adaptation is the analogue of experimental extinction was based on the apparent similarity of the curves that
graphically depict the course of these two phenomena. However, the similarity
is illusory. Stuttering adaptation and experimental extinction are different in
several important ways, a matter eventually brought into focus (Wingate,

1966b,c). Much later, the decrease in stuttering under such circumstances came to be explained, economically and defensibly, as due essentially to rehearsal and practice (Wingate, 1986a,b), in the same way that improvement in any activity follows upon doing it again and again.

CONSISTENCY

The "consistency" effect refers to a tendency for some of the words in the material read, to be stuttered again in one or more of the repeated readings. In contrast to the adaptation effect, the consistency effect—even though actually always more of an incidental finding—was, from the beginning, the phenomenon emphasized for interpretation. This preferential emphasis on the consistency effect was determined by two interrelated preoccupations: (1) stimulus–response (S–R) learning theory, and (2) the claim of difficult (or feared) words (or sounds). In both of these preoccupations, the stutter was purported to be a response, and some feature of the word was held to be the eliciting stimulus. However, from the beginning, both response and stimulus were—and remain—conjectural. Stutter as response exists in name only, that is, simply by affirmation from within a special point of view. There is no credible evidence that stutters are responses. Moreover, careful search of the literature will reveal that no stimulus adequate to elicit a stutter has ever been discovered, let alone demonstrated. From the beginning, use of the word "consistency" has been a presumptuous overstatement. The description of this so-called effect should have emphasized the word "tendency," since the recurrence of stutters did not then, nor in any subsequent research, evidence the regularity implicit in the word "consistent."

In spite of certain seemingly evident gaps in data and reasoning, the phenomena of the adaptation effect and "consistency" effect were for many years widely accepted as research evidence—and thereby scientific evidence—that stuttering is "learned behavior." The term "consistency" continues to appear in the literature, reciting the contention that individual stutterers repeatedly stutter the same words. These repetitions of the claim do not always refer directly to the consistency effect but often imply reference to its purported significance. However, all along the explanations have proceeded more at a level of supposition and conjecture than on a basis of palpable evidence.

INCONSISTENCY AND CONTRADICTION

Serious problems inherent in the adaptation and consistency effects are discussed at length in Wingate (1986a,b); the major faults can be noted here briefly, as follows.

First, the two phenomena represent reciprocal data—an increase in values of one is associated with a decrease in the other. Therefore, both of them cannot independently, or conjointly, represent the same process (learning), as claimed, since the phenomena are contradictory. Second, while the contention that stuttering is learned pertains specifically, and only, to individuals, the data obtained in all these studies have routinely been given for the subjects as a group. Third, values for the consistency effect were based on reversed computation, proceeding from terminal entries to initial ones, rather than vice versa, as actually required by concept, and procedure. Fourth, highly relevant data, contained in stutter recurrences *within* a passage, were never considered. Fifth, attempts to incorporate support for the notion of "continuity" (that stuttering is continuous with normal nonfluency—see Chapter 8) occasioned several *non sequiturs* that contradicted the intended interpretation of both phenomena. Readers interested in a detailed critique of these two phenomena should read Wingate (1986a,b).

RECURRENCE: MORE REALISTIC

The observation that some words are stuttered more than once is more objectively, and properly, described simply as recurrence. Moreover, in assessing recurrence, certain constraints must be incorporated. First, to investigate recurrence objectively the full range of stutter occurrences, and all the words involved, must be included. Second, the observations must be obtained from natural speech samples, not from the highly artificial circumstances of repeated reading of a passage—speaking the same words in the same sequences.

Table 6.2 (see pp. 116–118) presents data regarding stutter recurrence in the spontaneous speech of 20 adult stutterers. The speech samples were recorded as each individual created and told a story about persons in a picture.

The data of the table are separated into two parts. Part A presents data from 12 subjects whose speech samples did contain recurrent stutters, as recorded in the second and third columns. Part B presents data from the remaining 8 subjects, whose samples contained no recurrent stutters.

For both parts of the table, the first column identifies the judged severity level of the individual stutterers, rated on a 7-point scale that is reproduced below Part B. The second column identifies each subject by initials. The third column shows the number of recurrent stutters relative to the frequency with which the stuttered word itself recurred; the fourth column records the actual words involved. For example, the first subject, P.L., said the word "she" nine times, in two instances of which stutter occurred.

Other data directly pertinent to stutter occurrence are presented in the remaining six columns of the table. The fifth column records the number of words spoken only once and stuttered on that single occurrence. The next four columns record words stuttered only once although they were spoken more than once, either before or after the single instance in which the words were stuttered. For example, four words that P.L. stuttered only once were words that, in total, he had spoken 14 times, unstuttered, prior to the single stutter. Similarly, two of the words he stuttered only once were spoken, unstuttered, three times in all, after his only stutter of each of those two words.

Overall, these data reveal that stutter recurrence is a highly individual matter. Further, the extent of recurrence varies considerably among those in whom it occurs. Stutter recurrence as evidenced by J.R. (third subject) and by E.S. (tenth subject), recorded in the third and fourth columns, is indeed impressive. Also, the analogous data for subjects 2, 5, 6, and 7 are notable even though the instances of stutter are few. Such case examples, especially the two former ones, are the kind that attract attention and are the type likely to be given as case illustrations. For someone prepared to find "consistency" in stuttering, cases like these would be cited as illustration. Impressive instances they may be, but representative examples they are not—and it is as representative examples that such cases are typically offered.

The varied, but generally rather impressive, data recorded in the third and fourth columns of Table 6.2A also might serve as reference cases in discussions of stutter "consistency." However, these same data contain grounds for serious qualifications that must be considered. For instance, if a word is stuttered two of the nine times it is spoken, why not *nine* of the nine times, or if three out of four why not *four* of four, (and other instances in column 3)? An S–R account would lead one to expect such result. But the stutter occurrence is not only partial, it is also intermittent. Is it then the "stimulus" or the "response" that is so capricious? Or is it rather that the whole notion is fabrication?

In addition, the kinds of information revealed in columns 6 through 10 are at least as relevant to the notion of consistency. Actually, the extent to which recurring words are stuttered only once places a severe constraint upon attempts to offer anything like "consistency" to explain stutter recurrence, especially for cases in which some recurrence may otherwise be noted. The ultimate contradiction to "consistency" is posed by the frequent occurrence of single stutters of recurring words, that is, *no* stutter recurrence. This finding is particularly damaging to the notion of stutter consistency, with its foundation in S–R rationale and its alignment with the lore of difficult or feared sounds and words.

Further, we have not yet emphasized that 40% of these subjects (in Part B) gave no evidence whatsoever of stutter recurrence. This finding, in itself,

TABLE 6.2   Recurrent Stutters in Spontaneous Speech (20 subjects) — Part A

		Multiple stutters				Single stutter occurrences						
					1. Number of words stuttered on their only occurrence	2. Recurring words stuttered only once					Total number of stutters	Number of words spoken
		Stutters per recurring words		Words restuttered		Number of words & instances of word recurrence before or after single stutter				Total single stutters relative to total word recurrence		
						Before		After				
SEV*	S		Σ			#	inst	#	inst	Σ		
1	P.I.	2/9		she	5	4	14	2	3	6/23	13	230
2	N.H.	2/2		dress; two	22	6	7	3	3	9/19	33	312
2	J.R.	2/2 5/5	7/7	mom; distant Parents	32	7	15	5	20	12/47	51	669
3	R.H.	2/2 3/4 2/7	7/13	come; kind women; looks that	21	5	12	9	15	14/41	42	363
3	B.L.	2/2		married	20	6	14	10	40	16/70	38	241
4	N.W.	2/3		woman	7	1	1	1	1	2/4	11	292
5	T.F.	2/2		girl	13	5	8	2	14	7/29	22	136
5	Ph.S.	2/2 4/10	6/12	such she	7	4	11	2	3	6/20	19	205

Part A, continued

6	R.F.	3/13	who	7	6	11	6	10	12/33	31	162
		5/17	the								
		4/26	is								
		12/56									
6	E.S.	2/2	life; works	37	9	27	11	26	20/73	79	458
		4/4	mother								
		3/4	very								
		6/8	son								
		5/7	daughter								
		2/4	school								
		22/29									
6	J.W.	2/3	woman	15	9	15	5	6	14/35	33	451
		2/4	working								
		4/7									
7	Pl.S.	2/2	works	9	7	18	4	9	11/38	28	146
		3/4	band								
		3/15	girl								
		8/21									

TABLE 6.2 Part B

SEV*	S	Stutters per word	Single stutterer occurrences						Total number of stutters	Number of words spoken
			1. Number of words stuttered on their only occurrence	2. Recurring words stuttered only once						
				Number of words & instances of word recurrence before or after single stutter				Total single stutters relative to total word recurrence Σ		
				Before		After				
				#	inst	#	inst			
1	B.A.	0	1	2	2	2	2	2/2	3	129
1	G.K.	0	2	2	2	0	0	2/2	4	157
1	R.S.	0	1	1	2	0	0	1/2	2	169
1	R.W.	0	0	0	0	2	14	2/14	2	257
2	J.B.	0	0			1	1	1/1	1	264
2	J.C.	0	3	2	5	0	0	2/5	5	121
3	J.B.	0	5	2	4	3	8	5/17	10	108
3	R.L.	0	2	1	1	2	2	3/6	5	124

*Severity ratings: 1 = very mild, 2 = mild, 3 = mild moderate, 4 = moderate, 5 = moderate severe, 6 = severe, 7 = very severe.

certainly weighs heavily against accounts of stuttering that invoke ideas like consistency—or the companion notions of difficult or feared words or sounds, and the claims of expectancy, and of avoidance (covered elsewhere in these chapters).

Another aspect of these data worth noting is that stutter recurrence is more likely to be evidenced by those with severity ratings above the moderate level. At the same time, it is not limited to these subjects, and there is no evidence of a direct relationship between stutter severity and recurrence. This particular finding has been noted previously in other research.

In sum, stutter recurrence is only a partial, varied, highly individualized, occasional phenomenon. It remains an enigma, a phenomenon perhaps worthy of exploration, but it remains tangential to the mainstream of stutter inquiry. It does not come close to corresponding to the meaning of the word "consistency," which therefore is not, by any extent of equivocation, credibly proposed as a principle underlying stutter occurrences. Whatever might underlie the minimal amount of stutter recurrence that has been called "consistency," there is absolutely no evidence, nor even credible rationale, to claim that it represents S–R bonds, or that it reflects apprehension, anticipation, or the like.[8]

EXPECTANCY

"Expectancy" refers to the claim, first made by certain stutterers, that they anticipate stutter occurrence. This anticipation may be expressed as only a vague reference, as a feeling that a stutter is going to occur, or it may be claimed in respect to specific sounds or words. In the latter form it overlaps extensively with the claim of difficult sounds/words, and with the notion of consistency. Not all stutterers claim expectancy, but among the many who do, a seeming majority link their expectancy to specific sounds or words.

Expectancy presents another instance of a claim becoming a concept, the transformation coming about through according the claim a causal role and absorbing it into the reaction-fear explanation of stuttering. As a concept, expectancy is purported to be a reaction to cues associated with previous stutters, cues that the stutterer purportedly recalls at some level of awareness. As such, it is assumed to have a long-term base, founded in and confirmed by previously established associations between certain sounds or words and stutters. These associations, supposedly attached to certain sounds/words, are said to persist over time and to provide the cues that elicit stutters thereafter.

Like the concepts of difficult sounds and consistency, expectancy is also based upon testimony and lore, and maintained by frequent retelling, which has given the notion a status of actuality. There has been very little objective study of the claim; several reports in the late 1930s and a few around the early 1970s. Six of the seven earlier studies were part of the "Studies in the Psychology of Stuttering" series directed by Wendell Johnson; three of the four later ones were reported by disciples of the Iowa school.

Findings from these works give little reason to accept expectancy as a credible concept. Most of the studies were confounded by the method employed, which simply asked subjects to indicate, in the course of reading something, if they expected to stutter on an immediately forthcoming word. This method could, at least, encourage an effect of suggestion. However, the most profound limitation of these studies was their artificiality; they did not in any way approximate the circumstances in which expectancy purportedly occurs. Further, the featured data were group-based values. As pointed out in earlier sections, findings presented as support for explanations based on, and purportedly expressing, individual function must reflect the performance of separate individuals. Even in the studies referenced above, data reflecting individual performance were not supportive of expectancy; they revealed marked individual differences and a generally poor match between expected and actual stutters; typically the agreement was close to only 50%.

A subsequent study (Wingate, 1975) undertook to investigate expectancy in a manner designed to approximate the usual circumstances of expectancy occurrence. At the first of three sessions, each separated by a week, subjects recorded their experience of expectancy and their personal cues of it. Their answers revealed expectancy to be an individual matter: 9 of the 10 of subjects claimed expectancy, 5 of them saying it happened "most of the time." Five (but not the same 5) said their expectancy was based on sounds or words. Later, when asked to indicate, from a list of words, those words on which they would expect to stutter, all subjects identified certain words, and all but one then reported that sounds were the cue. All of the subjects were then given many opportunities to verify their expectancies through readings of various prepared materials presented separately over the 3 weeks.

Overall, the results provided very little support for expectancy, especially as traditionally presented. The subjects varied markedly in confirmation of their stated expectancies, as reflected in the "expectancy ratio," a measure expressing the number of confirmed expectancies relative to unconfirmed expectancies and unexpected stutters. A ratio value of 1.0 would reflect full expectancy-stutter correspondence—what one should find if expectancy is a viable concept; a value of 0.0 would, of course, indicate no correspondence. The expectancy ratios of these subjects ranged from 0.0 (four subjects) to 0.37. These low values clearly contradict the notion of expectancy as a persisting set of associations that determine the occurrence of stutters. These results corroborate the individualized findings of previous work indicating that expectancy is not a long-term process. However, the individual record of the subject receiving the highest expectancy ratio (0.37) yields several features that lead one to propose a plausible account of the expectancy phenomenon.

We begin with the expectancy ratio of 0.37, which, although not in itself particularly remarkable, is truly outstanding in comparison to the other scores, being 22 points above the next highest value. This subject, a female, reported expectancy only "sometimes." Significantly, she did not link expectancy to identifiable sounds or words; instead, she described her cues as "throat tightens," and "oral postures for sounds"—in essence, kinesthetic or somatosensory cues. It is pertinent to recall here Van Riper's (1937b) description that expectancy "consists of tiny rehearsal movements and increases in tonus of the musculature."

These findings suggest that expectancy is basically a short-term happening, a kind of prescience, a marginal awareness of impending difficulty, based on subtle sensations.[9] The experience of the stutter, involving a particular word or sound, becomes associated with that word or sound in immediate awareness, and in short-term recollection, which, for some instances, may be remembered over a longer period of time. Once again, the conditions suggest that registry of the event is occasioned by perceptual prominence, akin to circumstances that underlie the claims for "difficult words or sounds."

AVOIDANCE

In application to stuttering, avoidance was expressed initially in terms of a wish to avoid stuttering. From such a humble—and more importantly, credible—origin the term came to be invested with more elaborate and specialized meanings. Within the brief span of a few years, through interrelated sets of testimony, reflections and assumptions that yielded a sequence of non sequiturs, the term came to represent a concept, and ultimately a principle, in an attempted explanation of stuttering.

Along the way to its elevated explanatory role, the wish to avoid stuttering (a general objective) came to be stated in reference to instances of stutter, namely, as an intent to avoid specific occurrences of stutter. Within this context, the broad notion of avoidance incorporated the satellite features of difficult words/sounds and expectancy. At this level it also took on a cause-and-effect character, accruing support from certain other claims, such as, that unless a particular word were avoided it definitely would be stuttered. It was in the context of this line of thinking that the accessory features came to be identified—inexplicably—as "avoidances." This condition set the stage for the final step in the aggrandizement of avoidance—to the level of explanatory principle. With the melding of stutters (the speech features) and the accessory features as all being "symptoms" of stuttering (covered in Chapter 3), the way was open to contend that all features are avoidance. Thereby, stuttering itself could be construed as avoidance.

This contention, first formulated in 1936 (Johnson & Knott, 1936), was subsequently presented many times, often embellished in the form of a slogan-like expression—"stuttering is what the stutterer does trying not to stutter again" (see Johnson, 1946; Johnson & Moeller, 1948, 1956, 1967). The elevation of avoidance to the levels of concept and then principle was essentially the work of Wendell Johnson, the major figure in promoting the belief that stuttering is "learned behavior" based in emotional reaction, principally fear. Johnson wanted stuttering to be conceived as something the stutterer *does*, not, as traditionally accepted, something that *happens*, for reasons unknown. The notion of avoidance—understandably something that someone does, and based in reaction—fit his preconceptions well. The contention that stuttering was itself avoidance neatly encapsulated the range of his view.

The claim that "stuttering is the effort to avoid stuttering" is patently a paradox,[10] and on those grounds alone it should have been received as little more than a whimsical remark. To the contrary, however, it was clearly appealing and persuasive, as attested by its wide acceptance and perpetuation. Accepted as an account having substance, it was enhanced by the effort to fit it to learning theory. This effort was first published in an article by Wischner (1950) that was based on his doctoral dissertation, completed three years earlier at the University of Iowa[11] under the direction of Wendell Johnson.

Further discussion of avoidance in stuttering will be more readily understood if a brief review of learning theory paradigms is presented here.

LEARNING THEORY PARADIGMS

In psychological laboratories addressed to the study of how organisms learn, the basic process is referred to as "conditioning," of which there are two major types: classical conditioning, and instrumental conditioning.

CLASSICAL CONDITIONING

In classical conditioning, so called because it replicates the original procedure reported by Pavlov, there is an unconditioned stimulus (UcS), which is necessary and adequate to elicit a response (R). If another, originally neutral, stimulus is associated sufficiently often with the adequate stimulus, the former will, in due time, become able to elicit the response. Now being able to elicit the response, the originally neutral stimulus will then be called the conditioned stimulus (CS); the response has now become a conditioned response (CR), "conditioned" to that specific CS. The hallmark of classical conditioning is that the occurrence of the response does not influence the circumstances of the process.[12]

INSTRUMENTAL CONDITIONING

Instrumental conditioning bears this name because what the organism does (the R) is *instrumental* in the occurrence of the reinforcement (of that R). There are several types of instrumental conditioning:

1. Instrumental Reward

Some act of the organism results in immediate positive reinforcement whenever that act is performed. The reference example is the delivery of a food pellet when a bar is pressed. There are two forms of this type:

    a. Respondent. This form incorporates a stimulus (S), which, though initially inadequate, comes to elicit the act (R) through its repeated association with the reward, whereby the stimulus becomes adequate to elicit the act and is then a conditioned stimulus (CS).

    b. Operant. This form omits mention of any stimulus that elicits the act. The act is simply considered from the time it occurs—is "emitted." It too is said to be acquired via the effect of a reward that is contingent upon its occurrence. In repeated concurrences of the act, a reward and some "cue," the act will become linked to the "cue."

2. Instrumental Escape

Some act (R) of the organism terminates or substantially reduces an existing, or developing, noxious circumstance (UcS). The reference example is that pressing a bar turns off the increasing electrification of the floor on which the animal is situated.

3. Instrumental Avoidance

Some act (R) of the organism, performed in response to a signal (S), enables it to avoid a noxious condition (UcS). The reference example is that by pressing a bar when a buzzer sounds, the animal avoids delivery of an electric shock.

STUTTERING IN LEARNING THEORY FORMAT

The proposal that stuttering is learned, couched in the terms of behaviorism, was broached by Johnson in interpreting findings of the first study in his "Studies in the Psychology of Stuttering" series (Johnson & Knott 1937).[13] In this interpretation, and in many subsequent statements, Johnson did not invoke any particular model of learning theory but spoke only in general terms of "stimulus" and "response," in which stutters were said to be the response. Stimuli were not specified but were assumed to be embodied in words or their sounds. In later statements, the range of assumed stimuli was extended considerably, but they continued to remain conjectural. The formulation presented in the Wischner report (see above) was generated with a view to explaining stuttering in the terms of formal learning theory, aligning the effort with achievements in the psychological laboratory.

Among the models available for casting stuttering in a learning theory mold, the escape learning paradigm would seem most suited to the supposed circumstances of stutter occurrence. That is, in the instrumental escape paradigm an organism acquires a "behavior" that has relieved it (the organism) from an unpleasant state.

THE FAVORITE BY NAME

Although the escape learning model has a certain plausibility for an account of stuttering, the avoidance learning paradigm was the one selected and pursued by the proponents of a learning theory explanation. Almost certainly, preference for the avoidance model was influenced by the word "avoidance" and pursued in literal association to Johnson's claim that stuttering is "an avoidant response."

However, the avoidance learning account soon faced a serious dilemma, in the general form of no clear agreement as to what it is that the stutterer is supposedly trying to avoid. The dilemma was revealed early in Wishner's presentation, in a section titled "What is the Stutterer Attempting to Avoid?"[14] The crux of Johnson's explanation—that stuttering is the effort to avoid stuttering—could not be applied literally because it provides no explanation for the *first* stutter, the presumably original "noxious stimulus," and how it arose. So, it was necessary to find something else that could be fit into the "noxious stimulus" slot. Prominent among the alternative agents that have been suggested for filling this purported stimulus role of "what the stutterer is attempting to avoid" have been: (a) the "label" (the word "stuttering"), (b) nonfluency, (c) disapproval of nonfluency, (d) the original (parental) disapproval, (e) specific words, (f) specific sounds, and (g) perhaps any or all of the foregoing.

Wischner chose "the original parental disapproval of nonfluent behavior," citing the rationale presented in Johnson's *People in Quandaries*. At the same time, he revealed that stutterers give "only vague answers, if any" when asked about what they are avoiding.[15] Vagueness continued to be a feature of avoidance formulations. In effect, then and in subsequent elaborations, the instrumental avoidance learning paradigm provides no more lucid an account of stuttering than does Johnson's paradoxical claim,[16] which was its forerunner.

It is critical to note that all of the events suggested for "what the stutterer is attempting to avoid" are mounted from the assumption that the stutterer *must be* attempting to avoid *something*—an assumption based entirely in conjecture.

There should have been at least some occasional uneasiness among proponents of the S–R account of stuttering, since all the conjectured parts do not fit quite as they should. In fact, it has not even been very clear what all of the parts are. First of all, stuttering was only *assumed* to be a response (R). Second, no necessary and adequate stimulus (S) for the assumed response has ever been isolated or demonstrated, although routinely claimed retrospectively. Third, no credible supposed reinforcement of stuttering-as-response has come into clear view either. Reinforcement has remained a particularly vague assertion, ventured simply because there is a part like that in the model.

So, with S–R formulations facing such evident limitations, considerable relief attended the introduction of the "operant" learning concept, through which at least one of the two missing links could be dismissed.

AN APPEALING MIRAGE

In the operant framework there is no need to specify an eliciting stimulus; "operant behaviors" are said to be "emitted." However, according to the operant paradigm such behaviors are stabilized (acquired, learned) through some reinforcement that is contingent upon their occurrence. So here too, then, one of the missing links—the reinforcement assumption—still remains in limbo. But then, it is easier to explain away one missing link than to somehow have to account for two undiscernibles.

The operant concept, which permitted evasion of the serious missing-stimulus problem, was actively embraced and vigorously pursued in a new generation of explaining stuttering as "learned behavior." However, the deliverance from dilemma seemingly provided by the operant concept was only apparent. Those who gladly embraced the operant notion did not confront certain basic problems faced by the effort to invoke this seemingly "better" learning theory account.

Advocacy of the operant learning account of stuttering has failed to recognize the essential requirements for utilizing this model. If stuttering is to be credibly explained as an operant, then its occurrence must fit the sequence of events that characterize "operant behavior." According to the operant learning formulation, operants are acts ("behaviors") that occur initially under some unspecified circumstances, and very likely at random. Operants become stabilized (acquired, learned) if they are attended by fortuitous reinforcement of their occurrence. Also, standardly, operants are acquired by being *rewarded*, that is, *positively* reinforced. In addition, they are best stabilized if the reinforcement is intermittent and if it is "delivered" considerably less frequently than 100% of the time. This means that: (1) the behavior (operant, act) is not always reinforced, and (2) the behavior (operant, act) occurs much more often than it is reinforced.

So, for stuttering to be veridically explained as an "operant behavior," it must originally have been *emitted*, not elicited—that is, it must have occurred as a *de novo* act of the individual, *before* it could then be reinforced. Further, the stutter would have to have occurred many times without being reinforced. That is, for stuttering to be subject to reinforcement, quite a few instances of this unique "emitted behavior" must have occurred, during only some proportion of which occurrences it was reinforced.

Now, the foregoing description does not at all match the conditions and events by which stuttering is supposedly learned as an operant. In all accounts invoking learning theory, the question of the initial stutter(s) has remained unaddressed. More important, in direct contrast to the critical role of positive reinforcement in the operant paradigm, the efforts to explain stuttering as "learned behavior" have, throughout, assigned the prominent role for its acquisition to some form of *punishment*, not reward. Moreover, this punishment is assumed to be steadily present, affecting each instance of stutter. So, the observations and the data relative to stuttering do not fit the operant model either. Stuttering is no more credibly explained as "operant behavior" than as "avoidant behavior."

ENTER: COGNITION

It has been something of an irony that the rush to employ "operant technology" in the treatment of stuttering has called for the use of *negative* reinforcement of the stuttering "behavior" to cause it to be "unlearned." Such procedure also contravenes the long-term, paramount proscription regarding how stuttering should be managed. The standard proscriptive "rule" in dealing with stuttering, basic to the formulation pressed by Johnson and his followers, is that this "behavior" should not be disapproved (punished), even at the level of calling attention to it.

Somewhat surprisingly, then, operant approaches to stuttering therapy (using presumably negative reinforcement, such as calling attention to it) have been associated with a certain amount of success. However, there is good reason to believe that whatever results have been achieved in such programs have had only a peripheral connection to the learning theory model proposed to account for them. To the contrary, it seems clear that the successes actually have been a function of two circumstances that typically have not been recognized, or at least acknowledged, by the practitioners. First, these treatment "programs" (or pertinent studies) have regularly made use of some fluency-inducing procedure to "instate" fluency. Second, the real substance of any of the "contingent reinforcement" utilized is to be found in its cognitive aspect. Regarding the latter, there is good evidence from the relevant research that even little children quickly discern what is going on in the supposed reinforcement schemes. Also, they perform appropriately whether the supposed reinforcement is describable as positive, negative, or neutral. Moreover, they do even better if given initial instructions, that is, if they "know the rules" of the procedure beforehand rather than having to discover the connection as the procedure unfolds. In other words, even children catch on to the scheme, which indicates that their "behavior" is based principally in a cognitive function rather than being "controlled" by some schedule of reinforcement manipulated by an experimenter or therapist.

In closing this section on behaviorist efforts to explain stuttering, the following quotation from Miller *et al.* (1960) is especially germane.

> It is so reasonable to insert between the stimulus and response a little wisdom. And there is no particular need to apologize for putting it there, because it was already there before psychology arrived. (p. 2)

"DYNAMIC" AVOIDANCE

Explanatory efforts that have attempted to combine ideas from psychody-namics and learning theory are exemplified in the "conflict theory of stuttering" proposed by Sheehan (1953), another stutterer with a background in psychology. Sheehan's creation is appropriately introduced here because it pivots on the notion of avoidance.

Being familiar with the literature of clinical psychology, Sheehan found "avoidance" in another area of psychological specialty. His account was constructed on the schema of the "double approach–avoidance conflict," one of the motivational conflict paradigms described by Neal Miller (1944). It also incorporated contributions from Freud's writings on anxiety (Freud, 1936), the "two-factor theory of learning" proposed by O. H. Mowrer (1956), and Sheehan's own personal experiences and reflections. The crucial, although unrecognized, fault of this construction was that it could not logically be fitted to the hypothetical model on which it was based.

In Neal Miller's paradigm, the organism, initially in a neutral circumstance, becomes motivated to move toward either of two "goals," both of which have attracting and repelling "valences." The attracting dimensions of either goal are initially the more potent, eliciting approach. But as the goal is neared, its repelling features become more potent than its attraction, causing the organism to then move toward the other goal. However, upon approaching the second goal, the events that transpired relative to the first goal recur, and the organism is then caught in a vacillation between the two alternatives. In Sheehan's use of this paradigm, stuttering is explained as representing a vacillation between the opposing "goals" of *speech* and *silence*. However, this intended application of Neal Miller's paradigm contains a critical hiatus not recognized by its author or by many others who have accepted this account. The critical, nullifying element in this transposition is that, in contrast to the model on which it is based, there is no neutral starting point from which to move toward either presumed goal—of speaking or of being silent. There is no separate, neutral, initial condition from which an individual proceeds to begin speaking or to begin being silent. One is either silent, or speaking!

This serious discrepancy did not, however, limit the range of speculation and interpretation through which the "conflict theory" formulation was spelled out. In fact, it should be noted in passing that this construction also contained certain other damaging limitations, in the form of various assumptions and inconsistencies. Beyond these, the overall nature of the formulation is well reflected in the treatment of several instances of paradox that arise. Here, as in the Iowa school "evaluation" theme, paradox was not only tolerated but presented as explanatory. The most flagrant of the paradoxes in the "conflict theory" account is the following. As a summary statement of a section that purports to explain how his "fear-reduction hypothesis" clarifies "a number of relationships," Sheehan writes, "Hence we have a paradoxical relation—the stuttering produces the fluency and the fluency produces the stuttering" (1958a, p. 133).

Thus, both of these major attempts to explain stuttering in terms of avoidance (learning theory and conflict theory) center in paradox. Thereby, both accounts at least lack scientific merit; the rational and scientific treatment of paradoxes endeavors to resolve them, not to offer them as explanation.

Other accounts of stuttering that contain some mixture of personality variables and learning principles do not attempt so formal a structure as does the preceding account. In these less formalized views, ideas from the two conceptual sources are casually intermingled and not differentiated. As could be expected, their presumably relevant treatment approaches incorporate some mix of counseling and instruction.

It should be understood that these less formal accounts are no more tenable or supportable than the formal efforts reviewed above. In fact, because they have little formal structure, the lack of "wisdom" noted by Miller, Galanter, and Pribram (see above) is the more difficult to assess.

AVOIDANCE: EPILOGUE

The point of this brief section is to direct attention to the fact that there are many individuals, having normal speech, whose apprehension about speaking is at least as intense as that so often claimed for stutterers. These individuals, identified as "reticents," report, and manifest, various levels of personal distress about speaking to others, even though their speech itself contains no notable anomalies. This condition was first reported in publication by Phillips (1968)[17] and has since been studied extensively under the general rubric of "communication-avoidance" (see Ayres & Hopf, 1993; Daly et al., 1997).

The levels of communication-avoidance extend over a broad range, from a poignant aversion to speaking in public to an apprehensiveness about conversing with other individuals. The various expressions of this condition involve thousands of individuals, and treatment programs have been developed to deal with their unique problems. The use of "avoidance" in this context is considerably more appropriate and realistic than its use in stuttering, simply because of what these affected persons tell, and what they do—which is in marked contrast to what is found among stutterers.

It is important to recognize that none of the affected persons express concern about the quality of their speech, or of any unique features of it. Of particular significance for our purposes—especially in view of certain claims made in some of the literature of stuttering—there is no evidence in the extensive literature on communication-avoidance of any person with normal speech expressing a concern about fluency. Rather, the apprehension of individuals affected with communication-avoidance has to do with some dimension(s) of personal image and identity, often not recognized.

The student of stuttering should be encouraged to become familiar with the literature of communication-avoidance and to have at least a general knowledge of it as a worthwhile reference. Even a minimal awareness of its content should serve as a valuable antidote to certain unfortunately influential dimensions of the lore of stuttering.

SYNOPSIS

This chapter is addressed to several foci in the lore of stuttering that have been considered, rather inappropriately, as concepts. They have been accepted widely and have had extensive influence in efforts to explain the disorder. Directly or indirectly, they are contributions from stutterers, based principally on personal accounts and recollections. A few of them are partially credible if one is satisfied to take them at face value, which may account for their unwarranted acceptance and longevity. At the same time, the one in existence the longest (Distraction) is, and always has been, logically indefensible. Moreover, the one that has received the greatest amount of attention and has been most widely deployed (Avoidance) began as a paradox and has, throughout, maintained that essential character in its several applications.

The heavy absorption in testimony, reviewed in Chapter 5, emerges clearly in the most prevalent concepts of present day accounts of stuttering, reviewed in this chapter. Because of its heavy immersion in lore, the study of stuttering openly loses whatever claims to scientific status have been made for it.

The remaining notion that is properly included in this group of ideas, Continuity, is considered in Chapter 8, in an especially pertinent context.

NOTES

1. Reports and examples will be found in many good introductory psychology texts.
2. See Wingate (1997), especially chapter 5.
3. And, to careful analysis of stutters, fundamentally in error. This matter is covered in Chapter 12.
4. See Wingate (1988, chap. 5).
5. See discussion in Chapter 9 regarding the effect of literacy that establishes the primacy of spelling.
6. It was soon recognized that five readings were adequate to reveal the effect.
7. This research was done in 1934 but not published until 1955.
8. The kind of rationale offered in support of "consistency" is exemplified in the following excerpt from Bloodstein (1984, p. 177), repeated in Bloodstein (1997, p. 173). He asks a rhetorical question as to whether a stutterer would stutter again on a name recently stuttered in the same social context. His answer: "the *theory* says he will be more likely to block again." Followed immediately with another rhetorical question: "What are the facts?" He then gives, as the *facts*, that "Among *stutterers* and *their clinicians*, the prevailing *impression appears to be* that the prediction is correct" (italics added).
9. One might offer, in analogy, the (variably detectable) sensation that sometimes precurses a sneeze.
10. And was recognized as such. Moeller (1975, p. 76) cited Knott as referring to "that well-known paradox."
11. G. J. Wischner, *Stuttering Behavior and Learning: A Program of Research* (1947).
12. This learning theory paradigm shows up in only one account of stuttering, and then as only part of the explanation (Brutten & Shumaker, 1967).
13. The source of the adaptation and consistency effects.
14. Note the assumption that the stutterer *is* attempting to avoid something, indicating that (from this position) avoidance has therefore been accepted as an established principle.
15. Suggesting that the question was not meaningful to the stutterers.
16. That "stuttering is the effort to avoid stuttering."
17. They were described originally by Muir (1964).

CHAPTER 7

A Matter of Words

And therefore the ill and unfit choice of words
wonderfully obstructs the understanding. Nor
do the definitions or explanations, wherewith
in some things learned men are wont to guard
and defend themselves, by any means set the
matter right. But words plainly force and overrule the understanding, and throw all into
confusion, and lead men away into numberless
empty controversies and idle fancies.

Francis Bacon, *Essays* (1612)

*W*ords are basic tools of science. They are central to the structure of an
orientation; they shape the way problems are approached; they underlie concepts and influence collection of data, and the interpretations
mounted from data. Words are the means of implementing careful inquiry, and
scientific analysis. They must be used with great care.

There is much in the literature of stuttering that is aptly described in the
above quotation from Sir Francis Bacon. The "ill and unfit choice of words" is
the most insidious of the influences confounding the study of the disorder.
Largely a modern-day problem, it is an influence that is active in many sources
and contexts. It is one good reason that the literature of stuttering must be
read critically.

This chapter addresses a most profound influence of this kind, namely, the
improper use of certain terms that are basic to both description and concept.
Many of the verbal distortions that confound the subject of stuttering arise
circumstantially; others are true dissemblances. Whatever their origin, the

continued use of terms that should be brought to careful scrutiny and revision, but are not, remains a persisting major fault in the literature regarding this disorder.

USE OF GENERIC TERMS

A fundamental requirement of any inquiry and study presumed to have a scientific orientation is that its terms be as accurate and precise as possible. This requirement has been ignored in the literature of stuttering for many years, especially in the repeated use of certain words that represent a *class* of features instead of employing subordinate terms of the classes, terms that express important distinctions within each class.

There are four generic terms that are used in the improper manner noted above: *repetitions, hesitations, interjections,* and *disfluency.* Unfortunately, there is substantial reason to believe that the improper use of these four terms has been in large measure intentional, the objective being to support efforts to align stuttering within the range of normal speech, a matter to be addressed in Chapter 8. However, whether due to intention or carelessness, the continued use of these four generic terms, in circumstances that call for more careful and explicit reference, represents the unscientific quality of much of the literature of stuttering.

Of these four improperly used class terms, the two used most often are *repetitions* and *hesitations.* Frequently they have appeared as a presumably descriptive pair—in fact, almost as a refrain, as in such frequently encountered broad-spectrum claims as "the repetitions and hesitations known to be characteristic of the speech of normal young children." The word "repetitions" often appears singly, in equally sweeping contentions, such as "repetition is a normal characteristic of speech from the beginning." This indefensible practice is like a forester blandly talking about "trees" when the topic calls for differentiating conifers from deciduous trees, or palmaceous, or other special types— and, as well, noting variants within those classes.

ORDINARY WORDS

It seems likely that the first three of these words—repetitions, hesitations, interjections—were readily accepted and used because they are quite ordinary words, familiar to everyone and thereby easily applied, unreflectively, in special contexts. However, scientifically oriented word use would require that the generic nature of these words be recognized, and that efforts be made to identify distinctions within each class, and to use these distinctions carefully.

REPETITIONS

The class of "repetitions" contains subordinate distinctions simply in terms of length, ranging from repetition of the simplest element, sounds (phones) to repetition of words, phrases, sentences, and so on. These distinctions should be obvious; moreover, they surface repeatedly in the literature of stuttering, even though they are seldom specified. In other words, despite their disuse, these subordinate types should be well known to anyone having even minimal sophistication in the topic.

As discussed and illustrated in Chapter 3, the smallest repetitions—those of less than a completed syllable—are the hallmarks of stutter, even though repetitions of longer lengths (words, phrases) may sometimes appear in their vicinity. Moreover, research comparing stuttered to normal speech, of both children and adults, has consistently shown that these "part-word" repetitions[1] characterize stuttered speech. These partial repetitions contrast with repetitions involving full syllables, that is, repetitions of monosyllabic words, polysyllabic words, and phrases. Repetitions of these longer lengths are not distinctive of any certain kind of speech; they occur in the speech of all speakers. In passing, it should be noted that in the occasional instance when someone is said to be "repetitious," the reference is to a frequent restatement of certain ideas or issues, not to features of the speech sequence per se—such as individual words, of any length.

The contrast between the repetition types just noted is considered further in Chapter 10. The occurrence of the longer repetitions as ordinary aspects of speaking is discussed at length in Chapter 11.

HESITATIONS

Essentially, "hesitation" signifies inaction, so when used descriptively in respect to the speech sequence it should mean simply "a silent interval." However, in many ordinary contexts of its use the word also carries the implication of concurrent uncertainty or indecision. Unfortunately, this qualitative, subjective penumbra has characterized usage of the word in respect to stuttering—epitomized in such catchy, but misleading, expressions as "the stutterer hesitates to hesitate." Primarily for this reason, the word "hesitation" should be supplanted by the use of "pause" in references to silent intervals in speech. The word "pause," established in the psycholinguistics literature concerned with analyzing the speech sequence, is more objective, having none of the surplus meanings or implications of "hesitation." It is also more comprehensive, including different types and lengths of pause. To be explicit, in the Pause classification, "hesitations" would be equivalent to a subcategory limited by two qualifiers: *silent*, and *non-grammatical*.[2] Some elucidation of this matter will emerge in following paragraphs of this section; however, the important subject of Pause is deferred to extended discussion in the early chapters of Part III.

In the literature of stuttering, "hesitations" has been used casually in its full generic sense to refer to all noticeable silent intervals. The reader should make careful note of the qualifying word *noticeable* because, as will be discussed at some length later (especially Chapter 10), many silent intervals in speech are not readily discerned, because (a) they are very brief, and (b) most important, they are integral with the message.

These most frequently occurring, typically brief silent intervals in connected speech are the *juncture pauses*. They are also known as *grammatical pauses*, because they are part of the structure of the spoken message. These frequent little silent intervals are not identified in any writings as "hesitations," because "hesitation" refers to silent intervals that are noticeable. They are noticeable silent intervals primarily because of their length, although other features contribute, as discussed below.

The term "hesitations" is not suitable as a category of speech phenomena because, in addition to the implication of indecision it carries, it is also an overly inclusive class term. As such, and as typically used, the term "hesitations" disregards several differences in kind that can be readily discerned among these noticeable silent intervals in speech. Noting such differences is important for an accurate record of connected speech.

Noticeable Silent Intervals

Four subclasses of such intervals have been described. These distinctions, although largely qualitative, are pertinent to any effort to differentiate ordinary forms of noticeable silent intervals in speech from ones that are not a normal part of the speech sequence. Originally presented as necessary refinements of the category of "hesitations" (Wingate 1976),[3] the distinctions are equally pertinent to their better identification as *non-grammatical silent pause* in the Silent Pause classification, to be presented and discussed in Chapter 10. Consequently, the word "pause" is used here in each description of the distinctions.

a. *Voluntary Pause*. One may intentionally stop speaking at any time, for various reasons. A common form of voluntary pause is the *rhetorical* pause, which the speaker uses for effect, often with the objective of emphasis. Such pauses vary in length depending upon the speaker's intent.

b. *Meditative Pause*. Many silent pauses are of this kind, reflecting a condition when one stops speaking momentarily to search for a particular word or phrase, or to reflect briefly on what to say next, or just how to say it.

c. *Circumstantial Pause*. This frequently occurring kind of silent interval is occasioned by some external or internal event that distracts the speaker from what he was about to say. The kinds of potential distracting events are legion.

d. *Involuntary Pause*. For each of the three kinds of silent interval just described, some features of the verbal or situational context in which it occurs provide a circumstantial "justification" or "account" for its occurrence. In contrast, there is a kind of silent interval for which there is no evident contextual justification and which, moreover, often occurs at an unexpected locus in the speech sequence. Such intervals are not readily accountable as being one of the first three described. Largely because instances of the fourth type are thereby not "justified," they have a quality of being unusual, anomalous. They are the kind most readily noticed in a speech sample.

Lacking a discernible justification, they are likely to be considered unintended, therefore most likely viewed as involuntary. Especially if they occur more than occasionally, silences like this soon raise the suspicion that they reflect transient inability to continue speaking—a "block." This suspicion is often aided by other cues, of an accessory nature, that many times are very minimal, such as eye-blink (see Chapter 3).

The qualitative dimensions of silent intervals pose some amount of problem to their use in stutter identification. In fact, some stutterers are able to camouflage at least some of their involuntary instances as being one of the other three kinds described above. These, and other matters relevant to pause are deferred until the extended discussions of pause presented later (Chapters 10, 11, and 12). The principal concern in this chapter, regarding the issue of silent intervals in speech, is largely to emphasize that: (a) silent intervals are not all of a kind, in anyone's speech, and (b) that the practice of using a term like "hesitations" gives inadequate and misdirecting information.

INTERJECTIONS

The word "interjection" means simply, and literally, "to throw in between." The word occurs in lay usage with this literal meaning, for instance, when someone speaks of "interjecting a personal anecdote," or "interjecting a question." In many lay writings, and in much ordinary spoken use, "interjection" has the limited meaning of "exclamation," since exclamations are the more dramatic kinds of expressions "thrown into" what is being said.

In writings and discourse addressed to description and study of speech, the term is used in its generalized literal sense, wherein it refers to anything verbal or quasi-verbal (unintelligible or meaningless speech-like sounds) that are not intrinsic to the intended message. "Interjections," then, is another broadly inclusive *class* term that has several variant meanings. For instance, when referring to an exclamation it carries an emotive significance; in many instances it means an off-hand remark; in other cases it refers to a lengthy statement, carefully formulated, and so on. However, the most common use in ordinary description is in reference to the use of so-called "pet phrases" such as "y'know," or "I mean," and the like.[4]

In the literature of stuttering, "interjections" has been another class term used with an impropriety equal to the use of "repetitions" and "hesitations," although not as frequently or imposingly. In actual use in this literature, interjections refers most often to audible versions of "hesitations." As such, one can identify distinctions among interjections that are direct counterparts of those under hesitations—namely, voluntary, meditative, circumstantial, and involuntary. Discussion of these subtypes will be deferred to Chapter 10.

For purposes of this chapter, the particular issue being drawn regarding "interjections" is that it is another class term whose improper use obscures important distinctions that are necessary for careful study of the disorder. In the more objective and suitably descriptive Pause classification arising from psycholinguistic research, the vernacular category of "interjections" is sub-sumed under the category of Filled Pause. This term is appropriately descriptive of what is observable, in contrast to "interjections," which carries surplus meaning, as noted above. Filled Pause is considered in detail in later chapters, especially Chapter 10.

DISFLUENCY

This is the grandest class term of them all in that, being a most general referent, it encompasses *all* kinds of phenomena considered to be irregularities of fluency, the large variety acknowledged to be normal and, as well, the ones conceded to be abnormal. As should become evident in the following para-graphs, this term truly does epitomize the role featured in this chapter's epi-gram, in which words "force and overrule the understanding, and throw all into confusion."

Words containing "dis" as a prefix are most comprehensive referents. The prefix "dis" signifies a contrast with whatever the suffix may be—it denotes separation, negation, or reversal; the core reference is "apart," the simplest equivalent is "not." Thus, "disfluency" means "speech that does not have fluency" and, as routinely used, refers to all irregularities in the apparent "flow" of words, that is, words in continuous, uninterrupted sequence. However, such reference is a notable departure from the standard, and realistic, meaning of "fluency," which incorporates more than words. This important matter is taken up at length in Chapter 10.

There are two issues that bear critically on the meaning and use of the word "fluency." First, fluency refers fundamentally, and almost exclusively, to speech—*as ordinarily spoken and heard.*[5] Second, a clear appreciation of the meaning of "fluency" catches the use of "disfluency" in a remarkable irony— namely, that many irregularities in the sequences of connected speech—the so-called "normal nonfluencies"[6]—are standardly accepted as aspects of ordi- nary (normal) fluency. So, actual "disfluencies" are quite rare. These issues, although highly pertinent to the present context, are mentioned here only briefly because they are discussed at length in Chapter 10. For purposes of the present chapter, our interest is in the problems created by "disfluency," which, as another class term improperly used, has injected extended confusion into the literature of stuttering.

Unlike the other three class terms discussed in this chapter, the word "disfluency" is a true oddity that will not be found in any standard diction- ary[7]—including the ultimate lexicon, the 12-volume *Oxford English Dictionary*, which contains a great number of "dis-" words, including many that are remarkably special and esoteric. "Disfluency" is a rare word, promoted specially by Wendell Johnson for use in talking about stuttering.[8]

The character of the word, and its use in the field of stuttering, compel one to deduce that it was inserted into this literature, and also is otherwise widely employed in the field, to serve a salient role in the effort to meld stuttering with normal speech. The word first appeared in the 1961 report by W. Johnson, to be discussed in Chapter 8, in which the clear objective was to intertwine seeming irregularities of fluency in normal speech with those anomalies char- acteristic of stuttering. This matter too will be covered at some length in Chapter 10.

By using "disfluency" in a seemingly appropriate[9] way as an all-encompass- ing term, it then became possible to speak of stutters and "normal nonfluen- cies" together, in composite, as forms of "disfluency" and, moreover, with the clear implication—in many instances, the forthright contention—that the two phenomena are essentially of the same substance. Under this obscuring canopy a number of confusions have appeared, sometimes from naivete or insouciance, at other times from evident intent. Gradually "disfluency" has come to be used when the actual reference is "stuttering." In some instances, such substitution has resulted from ignorance or carelessness, less frequently as apparent euphemism. However, the major thrust of this substitution is the intent to have "disfluency," the broadly encompassing *class* term, *replace* "stuttering," a specific limiting term (see, as exemplary of this effort, Silverman & Williams, 1967). This bold, incredible venture is like attempting to substitute the word "animal" for "cattle," or some (any) other distinctive animal form.

DYSFLUENCY

A general basis for the confusion introduced through "disfluency" resides in the fact that *disfluency* is a homophone of *dysfluency*. This phonetic artefact has led particularly to a generalized uncertainty about the latter term, evidently because so many persons seem not to recognize its distinctive meaning. As noted above, the prefix *dis* is a broadly comprehensive, umbrella notation. In full contrast, the prefix *dys* is a special notation having a specific meaning: it signifies "abnormal." The prefix *dys* is most widely used in medical sources, where it denotes various anomalies, or departures from normal, for example, dysostosis, dyspepsia, dysplasia, and dystrophy. However, use of the prefix is not exclusive to medical literature. In particular, anyone presumed to be knowledgeable in speech pathology should know its meaning well, since there are abnormalities of speech function that are properly identified by the prefix *dys*, in which it signals "abnormal" or "defective," such as dysarthria, dyslalia, dysphasia, and dysphonia.

Within the context of drawing attention to extant *dys-* words in speech pathology, students of stuttering should be made aware that, in the early years of the developing profession, West (1943) proposed a classification of speech anomalies under the rubric "dysphemia." This proposal, which evidently arose largely from West's interest in anomalies of fluency, received very little attention. Most likely, disinterest in the proposal was due to the foment surrounding explanation of stuttering as a psychological problem, which was at that time well under way.[10]

Although confusion of *dys-* with *dis-* references might be excused in careless lay usage, the confusion should not occur in professional use. Actually, any good standard desk dictionary will identify the difference in meaning between words beginning with *dis* from those beginning with *dys*. It is of particular interest, then, that a dictionary compiled especially for use by speech pathologists (Nicolosi *et al.*, 1978) equates *dysfluency* with *disfluency* by cross-referencing the two words and, moreover, by stating that the two words are alternate spellings.

A more frequently occurring example of this particular dimension of the "disfluency" confusion is found in the remarkably self-contradictory description "normal *dys*fluency." This error has surfaced, over many years, in a number of sources in the literature of stuttering.[11] An especially notable example appears in an illustration to be discussed in Chapter 8 (Table 8.1). These instances of word usage error are not simply spelling errors; they are ideational errors that pointedly reflect the confusion being discussed here.

The extent of conceptual confusion embodied in the foregoing errors is well reflected in the many sources that write (and speak) of dealing with "the disfluent child." Here one finds both inconsistency and contradiction. Since it is often stated (in many of these same sources), and also widely accepted, that all children are disfluent, does working with "the disfluent child" mean that *all* children are being treated (or somehow managed)? It should be obvious that this is not what is meant. Rather, it must be that only certain selected children are the objects of such special attention. But then, as seems clear, if only certain children are the objects of attention, how is "the disfluent child" identified, since all children are claimed to be disfluent?

The answer must be that the youngsters selected for this special attention are ones who evidence *dys*fluencies—which have to have been discriminated out of all the purported *dis*fluencies the children must evidence. I should hasten to remind the reader of the true meaning of *dis*fluency, discussed earlier in this chapter, and that in its widespread use in the literature of stuttering the term is, in several ways, the grandest impropriety.

SPECIAL VERBAL DIVERSIONS

The problems of word usage addressed in this section have not arisen in isolation since, as will become evident, they have a lineage to matters discussed above, especially "disfluency." In some respects, there is direct lineage to the word "disfluency" itself, and certainly to the underlying construction which that word represents.

EUPHEMISM AND TABOO

Euphemism refers to expressing something through use of a word or phrase that is more acceptable, or less unpleasant, than the one it replaces. A common example of a euphemism is to say that someone "passed away," rather than having died. Sometimes a euphemism becomes so soundly established that the word it replaces becomes taboo, a phenomenon that reflects the potential power of euphemistic intent.[12] A good illustration of euphemism eventually leading to taboo is provided by the sequential changes in acceptable reference to limited mental ability. Even into the twentieth century, persons identified as being not of normal mental capacity were referred to as "feeble-minded." This term became increasingly objectionable, especially to many families of those affected, and by mid-century the term came to be supplanted by "mentally retarded," and then by simply "retarded." Although the latter terms are still in use today, certain sources have attempted further replacements, such as "developmentally disabled" or "the special child." The term "feeble-minded" has been taboo for some time.

Euphemism has played a considerable role in beliefs about stuttering. As in the case of using more acceptable words for subnormal mental ability, the objection to the word "stutter" (and derivatives) emerges from among those close to the disorder. Actually, the original repudiation of "stuttering" quickly reached the level of taboo. Prompted by his immersion in general semantics, Wendell Johnson arrived at the position that stuttering is just a word—moreover, a bad one. According to the "semantogenic" or "evaluational" conjecture he constructed, Johnson claimed that stuttering resulted because ordinary irregularities of speech were "mislabeled" as stuttering. According to this contention, there is no such thing as stuttering; it is just a damaging word mistakenly applied to certain occurrences in normal speech. Purportedly, "the problem called stuttering"[13] lay in the overly critical evaluation of normal nonfluencies and then "labeling" them with an incorrect term. From this position, parents and others concerned with the welfare of children were enjoined not to use the word "stutter" and its derivative forms—especially, it seems, "stutterer." Johnson's persistence in expounding this contention was persuasive and, with the aid of numerous followers, was widely disseminated, especially in the United States.[14]

The taboo against use of stutter words is not now as wide ranging or as potent as it was some years ago, yet the ambience generated by Johnson's contention is still active in the field, as revealed in the survey by St. Louis and Lass (1981), and in certain writings that still state the Johnson position verbatim (for instance, Selmar, 1991). However, the most pervasive expression of its influence is in use of the word "disfluency" and related euphemisms.

At base, euphemism represents an effort at denial; it expresses an attempt to at least mitigate reality through the use of words. One should recognize, as well, its connection to sympathy/empathy, discussed in Chapter 5. "Disfluency" is not only a major euphemism; it embodies other attractions for those who do not want stuttering to be viewed as something abnormal. The euphemism of "disfluency" is entwined with an intent to meld stuttering into normal speech. As noted earlier, both aspects are evident in such references as "the disfluent child."

Other current efforts at euphemism relative to stuttering appear in the use of "children who stutter" in place of "child stutterers" (also "adults who stutter" rather than "adult stutterers"). Also, one finds objection to use of "stutterer," evidently because "er" is thought to carry the implication of an inherent condition.[15] Actually, "er" is simply an agentive suffix, having a variety of uses. In cases like "stutterer" it is comparable to hunter, rider, singer, farmer, etc., and means only "someone who..." (hunts, rides, sings, farms, etc.). Although the suffix may convey the meaning "characteristic of," it does not imply anything about the reason for the activity, nor that the person does it all the time. And it has none of the penumbra of implication associated with certain other words with the "er" suffix, such as "drinker."

BANNING THE WORD "STUTTER"

Motivations underlying the appeal and use of "disfluency" in reference to stuttering reach their zenith of expression in the endeavor to eliminate the word stutter itself. Quite recently Yairi (1996) mentioned a current search for "better labels," an effort that involves "attempting to avoid the word 'stuttering.'" He added that a substitute for stuttering had already been suggested, namely, "replongations." The strength of the motive to get rid of "stuttering" is well revealed in this willingness to consider, as replacement, such a cumbersome neologism as "replongations." The reader will no doubt recognize that this construction is a compounding of "repetitions" and "prolongations." If the field of stuttering were reduced to using a neologistic substitute for stuttering, "blocketitions," the converse though equally clumsy term, would at least contain the critical reference—"block."

However, the whole matter is folly. It seems clear that the urge to jettison "stutter" is simply continuation of the effort at denial pressed by Wendell Johnson. If clarification of nomenclature were the objective of this concern about "labels," then something should be done about "disfluency," the most confounding label in the field. Any effort to supplant "stutter" (and derivatives) with a "better" word is not justifiable on either descriptive, professional, rational, or semantic grounds. As discussed earlier in this book (Chapter 3), the word "stutter" is, from all relevant dimensions, the ideal word to signify its referent.

SHAPING BY CLASSIFICATION

In recent years, two schemes for classifying "disfluencies" have been proposed: (1) "Within-Word Disfluencies vs. Between-Word Disfluencies" and (2) "Stutter-Like Disfluencies." Both of these proposals embody the spirit of euphemism and, as well, the motivation to erase, or at least smudge, the border between stutters and normal irregularities of speech. Their common flaw is that both are built with the sand of disfluency. However, each also has additional limitations.

BETWEEN AND WITHIN

Conture (1990) repeated a classification scheme he had proposed almost a decade earlier in which the various apparent irregularities in the speech sequence—that is, departures from a literal smooth continuity of words—are separated into two broad subclasses: "Between-Word Disfluencies" and "Within-Word Disfluencies."[16] In this scheme, the former category includes what ordinarily are called "normal nonfluencies"; the latter category is presented as the equivalent of stuttering.

This classification scheme finally aroused complaint, which was directed essentially at the within-word category. Cordes and Ingham (1995) pointed out that not all within-word disfluencies are necessarily stutters. Yairi (1996) expressed concern about "the vague and inconsistent treatment of monosyllabic word repetition," noting that Conture (Conture, 1990, and elsewhere) lists some monosyllable words as within-word disfluency and some as between-word disfluency. Such inconsistency itself reveals that the scheme has real limitations.

Issues regarding single-syllable words are a matter deserving separate attention, to be addressed shortly. However, at this point, attention should be directed to the overarching fault in Conture's classification scheme—namely, that *both* the "between" and the "within" categories are vague and over-inclusive; they force unnatural and erroneous differentiation.

A scientific objective of classification is to clarify. Both of these categories lead in the opposite direction—they obscure. In this respect, they are true extensions of their base word, "disfluency." Both dimensions of this classification scheme are expansive glosses that reflect either unawareness of, or indifference to, some fundamental psycholinguistic research that bears particularly on matters of fluency (to be discussed in Chapter 10).

The Between-Word Category

"Between-word" obscures the important differences among items that would be appropriately placed in this category. There are many types of occurrences between words in connected speech that have various special significance to the psycholinguistic analysis of an utterance—a matter discussed at length in Chapter 10. Most of these occurrences are demonstrably a significant aspect of connected utterance, that is, of ordinary fluent speech. It is for this reason, in particular, that "disfluency" is itself a contradictory misnomer, and thereby a profoundly confounding term. Psycholinguistic research of normal speech has revealed that many "between-word" phenomena are an integral part of ordinary *fluency*—among which, most notably, are grammatical pauses, rhetorical pauses, and several kinds of repetition as well. It is, therefore, contradictory and incorrect to refer to them as being *any* kind of "*dis*fluency."[17] Most sources in the field of stuttering evidently continue to assume that fluency means *verbal* continuity—that is, that "fluency" equals "words in uninterrupted sequence." It is an orientation that reveals insulation from an adequate awareness of the nature of normal fluency. As noted above, fully fluent utterances include much more than the word sequences within them. Fluent speech is not the acoustic version of a written prose narrative.[18] "Between-Word Disfluencies" is an expansive generalization—imprecise, incorrect, and misdirecting.

The Within-Word Category

"Within-Word Disfluencies" has its own unique and critical limitations, of which the most serious is that it is by no means a substitute for "stuttering." It too is a generalization that obscures or ignores several important distinctions within it—distinctions that are readily evident.

For instance, what sort of "disfluencies" might occur within the word "stuttering"? Among many potential "disfluencies" that might occur within that word, only a certain kind would be recognized as "stuttering." Putting the matter simply via illustration, "stuttering" means occurrences like /st..st..st..stʌtərɪŋ/, or /stə..stə..stə..stʌtərɪŋ/, or /stəəəəʌtərɪŋ/. It does not mean /stʌt.. tə.. tə.. tə.. rɪŋ/, nor does it mean /stʌtə.. rɪŋ rɪŋ rɪŋ/, nor /stʌtə_ rɪŋ/, nor /stʌtərɪŋ..ŋ..ŋ./, nor other possible variations.

The foregoing illustrations point up the critical feature of *locus*. It is axiomatic that stutters do not occur in word-final position. Even more fundamental: stutters do not occur in *syllable*-final position. Stutters might more properly be called a within-*syllable* anomaly, but even that would be imprecise. Stutters involve syllable-*initial* position. Although this fact is extensively documented, it is, surprisingly, so frequently omitted or ignored!

STUTTER-LIKE DISFLUENCIES

This classification was introduced by Yairi and Ambrose (1992), and used by other coworkers, as a designation to replace "stuttering." This scheme, which violates ordinary reasoning as well as scientific principle, is thoroughly unacceptable; the critical fault in the scheme is the word "like," which, in this common usage, means "resembles." Briefly stated, "stutter-like" is not stutter, nor in any substantial way equivalent to stutter.[19] Even without knowing what might be encompassed within "Stutter-Like Disfluencies," the intended substitution of this term in place of "stutter" must be rejected.

As noted in regard to the "between–within" scheme, the objective of classification is to clarify, through organization and, particularly, specification. But "Stutter-Like Disfluencies" (SLDs), even more than the "between–within" scheme, leads in the opposite direction; it confounds. Especially in undertakings purporting a scientific orientation, it is not justifiable to incorporate into the study of a phenomenon some other phenomenon that might resemble it. In contrast to bunching resemblances into a common amalgamation, a scientific orientation seeks to carefully distinguish among phenomena within which there may be some resemblance, and to just as carefully identify the differences to be found among them.

The invalidity of "SLD" is revealed in results reported in a recent article (Watkins *et al.*, 1999) in which SLD was the substitute, and the criterion, for "stuttering." The authors reported that the (so-called) stutterers "consistently demonstrated expressive language abilities well above expectation." This finding is opposite to those reported in much previous research; in fact, any time the matter arises. Delay in speech acquisition has been found so often that it has been featured in several lists of facts about stuttering, the most recent one published in 1983 (Andrews *et al.*). When findings of a study are so clearly contrary to previously accumulated evidence, it could mean a grand revelation, or that something is grandly wrong in the method. In the present instance, it must be the latter, especially since the flaw is so obvious.

It is now relevant to note the composition of "Stutter-Like Disfluencies." This classification includes "part-word repetition, monosyllabic word repetition, and dysrhythmic phonation" (Yairi & Ambrose, 1992). Traditionally, the first and third items[20] have been identified in the field as characteristic of stuttering. In marked contrast, monosyllabic word repetitions have not been so identified. Monosyllabic word repetitions are by no means unique to, and are certainly not criterial of, stuttering. In fact, it is well documented that monosyllabic word repetitions occur in the speech of everyone, a fact revealed through extensive research with normally speaking children and adults. Even if such repetitions were found to occur more frequently in the speech of stutterers, that would be no justification for conglomerating them with stutters. It would be a matter worth investigating, but that is all.

MONOSYLLABIC WORD REPETITIONS

The speech-irregularities categories of word repetitions and interjections have been the greatest source of confusion and equivocation in the identification of stuttering, a matter considered as part of the analyses presented in Chapter 10. However, certain issues concerning word repetitions need to be addressed here because monosyllabic word repetitions have figured so prominently in the two classification schemes under review.

Typically, writings that list types of speech irregularities[21] have contained word repetitions as a category, without specifications of length. However, relative to the preponderance with which single-syllable words occur in general usage,[22] it seems quite certain that most word repetitions in speaking are monosyllabic.

Both the "between–within" and the "stutter-like disfluency" classification schemes, whose substance spirals around the issue of monosyllabic word repetitions, epitomize the word-borne anomalies in the literature of stuttering. The anomalies found in the treatment of monosyllabic word repetitions can best be brought into relief by first setting forth fundamental considerations regarding these phenomena, as follows: (1) monosyllabic word repetitions occur in the speech of all speakers; (2) many monosyllabic word repetitions are found as ordinary occurrences in the speech of normal speakers; (3) monosyllabic word repetitions also occur in the speech of stutterers, and there is no reason to assume that those repetitions, as such, are inherently different from ones in the speech of normal speakers. In essence, any monosyllabic word repetition claimed to be other than normal in character must be identified as intrinsically different from ordinary occurrences.

SIMILARITY AND IDENTITY

The narratives of both classification schemes manifest a failure to distinguish similarity from identity, a matter that has clouded discussions of stuttering for many years. Similarity does not indicate, nor even imply, identity. Many things that are quite similar in appearance are significantly different, in important ways. Iron and steel provide a pertinent illustration. The two metals are in most instances indistinguishable to unsophisticated scrutiny. Moreover, they are of almost identical origin and substance. However, there are significant differences between them, in properties and in function; adequate discrimination between them requires knowing the unique properties of each. In analogy, single-syllable word repetitions are clearly repetitions of short entities. But, in addition to being not as short as are the repetitions of stutter, there are other intrinsic structural differences that should quickly come into focus in even minimally sophisticated observation.

Several dimensions of difference should be illuminated. Throughout, keep in mind that monosyllabic words, although properly called "words" are, fundamentally, syllables.

A fundamental problem in the effort to claim monosyllabic word repetitions as equivalent to stutter is the failure to consider the production of such words in reference to proper criteria. There is an important difference between (a) monosyllabic word repetitions and (b) stuttered monosyllabic words. The reader should take careful note of the difference between "a" and "b." The distinction between the two should be mounted in regard to the salient features of normal versus abnormal *syllables*. The core of the issue is the failure to recognize—or acknowledge—that the syllable involved in stutter, whether in a polysyllabic word *or* as a monosyllabic word, is in some extent incomplete. Normal syllables, in contrast, are completed, whether in a polysyllabic word *or* as a monosyllabic word. It follows that the principal criterion for distinction should be whether or not the syllable is completed, as ordinarily spoken. Briefly put, the essential characterization is this: single-syllable word repetitions are repetitions of a complete unit; they have a linguistic, and an expressive "coherence." In contrast, stutters are incomplete; they are only some fraction of a linguistic "integer," in structure and in expression.

Whether or not a monosyllabic word is completed should ordinarily not be a particularly demanding discrimination. For "bounded" syllables, essentially those having a *terminal* boundary (CVC, or VC), the distinction should be made readily. For example, there is a clear difference between /k...k...k... kæn/ or /kə.. kə.. kə... kæn/ and, in contrast, /kæn...kæn...kæn/. Ordinarily, the word "and" may be pronounced fully (/ænd/) or, very often as /æn/ or even as syllabic /n/. Repetition of each of the three versions is discriminably different from /æ..æ..æ..æn/ (or /æ..æ..æ..ænd/). For monosyllabic words without a terminal consonant, like "see," there should also be no problem of discriminating /sə.. sə.. sə... si/ or /s.. s.. s.. si/ or /sssssi/ from /si.. si.. si.../. For the latter repetition to be viewed as suspect, one would need to consider other, attendant, cues that aid the discrimination. Such cues have been elaborated in Chapter 3, in the discussion of accessory features

THE CATEGORICAL REQUIREMENT

The matter of considering other cues to aid identification raises the other major problem in the struggle over the status of monosyllabic words. Ironically, in spite of the position which claims that stutters are not reliably discriminated from "normal nonfluencies," there is nonetheless a clearly expressed requirement that a differentiation be made. As a major feature of this requirement, there has been a clearly evident unwillingness to consider use of an "Uncertain" category. The study of stuttering is not so well developed or so finely tuned that unquestionable differentiation should be routinely required, or even necessarily sought. The apparent yearning for perfection, expressed by certain sources, has plagued the issue of identification for decades. Recurring assertions regarding the claimed inadequacy of stutter identification have been mounted simply on grounds that agreements about all instances are not absolute. The reservations that are then routinely expressed are presented as being of grand import for understanding the disorder, and for efforts to manage it. However, the reality of the situation is that neither therapies, nor worthwhile research endeavors, are in any important way constrained by such imperfection as is purportedly revealed in the "lack of agreement" so often emphasized by certain sources. Moreover, in view of repeated findings of high levels of even inter-judge agreements,[23] the matter of agreement is hardly the issue some sources persist in claiming. In large measure, continued recitation regarding the lack of complete agreements in stutter identification serves to perseverate the aspiration to deny the reality of stuttering.

CUES UNEXPLORED

In addition to accessory features, there are aspects of monosyllabic words themselves, contextual and physical, that may be found useful in differentiation. The most evident dimensions are such aspects as word type and use-frequency. Also, certain intrinsic features of words may contribute importantly. For instance, Throneberg and Yairi (1994) reported finding that *some* monosyllabic word repetitions of stuttering youngsters showed certain physical differences from those of nonstuttering children "in terms of internal segment duration properties." The authors did not describe the character of these properties. However, simply having found certain differences between the single-syllable words of the two groups should, alone, militate against including monosyllabic words indiscriminately as stutters. Further, even if all of the monosyllabic words in the stutterers' samples showed those certain physical differences from ones in samples from normal speakers, this still would only be grounds for further careful study. To find that some of the monosyllabic repetitions of young stutterers show certain physical differences from those observed in samples of normal speech might suggest one lead for possible evidence of an aberration in the speech production capability of stutterers. However, this only suggests inquiry that might lead to a bona fide objective basis for differentiating certain monosyllabic word repetitions in stuttered speech from those in normal speech samples, but it is little more than an intriguing partial finding. It does not corroborate anything, and especially it does not call for such a sweeping generalization as proposing that (all) monosyllabic word repetitions should be classed as stutter, a matter discussed below.

Classification Logic

Inscrutable

As noted earlier, Yairi (1996) criticized the "vague and inconsistent treatment of monosyllabic word repetition" evident in Conture's application of his between–within scheme of classification. Those documented limitations alone reveal illogic in Conture's classification scheme. Yairi, in turn, contended that, unless a separate class of disfluency were established, "plain logic" would call for monosyllabic word repetitions to be classed as within-word disfluency.

How can a *word* be a *within*-word event? The rationale for contending that anything should be classified within itself is indeed obscure. Whatever logic underlies such a position, it is certainly not plain.

Unsupportable

Yairi (1996) claimed that monosyllabic word repetitions occur more frequently in the speech of young child stutterers, citing findings reported in some of his earlier work (Hubbard & Yairi, 1988; Yairi & Lewis, 1984). On the basis of those reports he suggested that, *therefore*, monosyllabic word repetitions should be classed as stutters. This position has faulty logic, on several counts. First, just because something is observed more frequently in group "A" than in group "B" does not give reason to claim that it embodies the unique characteristics of, or even is equivalent to, members of group "A." In this particular instance, the clear dissimilarity is why monosyllabic word repetitions have always been distinguished from stutters. Second, on a practical level the position would, by decree, extend stuttering to all children—in fact, to everyone, since these speech features are common to all speakers. Beyond these reservations, the claim is a distortion. Many studies[24] have shown that all kinds of "nonfluencies" occur more frequently in the speech of stutterers, of all ages. Moreover, this same finding was clear in the data of the two studies cited by Yairi in support of his claim. To have singled out monosyllabic word repetitions from those reports, as support for his contention, was a clear instance of bias. In addition, even if monosyllabic word repetitions actually had been the only other nonfluency found by Yairi and his coworkers, those repetitions had already been distinguished from stutters. How, then, can they be claimed to be the same?

Tangential

Another error in logic within this context involves previous report that the perception of "stuttering" in a speech sample is enhanced by the occurrence of multiple repetitions per instance. Yairi (1996) cites the work of Sander (1963) in this respect. However, Sander's findings are not relevant to the issue regarding monosyllabic word repetitions. Sander employed specially created speech samples in which alterations of repetition extent involved incomplete word-initial syllables of polysyllabic words—a mimic of stutter. Nonetheless, even if multiple monosyllabic word repetitions, occurring in a sample of stuttered speech, enhance the judgment of stuttering, this finding does not support a position that the two phenomena (monosyllabic word repetitions and stutters) are therefore the same—or even similar. It indicates only that the impression of "stuttering" is enhanced. In this respect, however, it tells a lot about what listeners understand stuttering to sound like. One can appreciate how the impression of stuttering might be enhanced by multiple-unit repetitions of these brief entities—it might suggest *iteration*, one of the two compelling hallmarks of "stutter." But suggestion is not equivalence, much less identity.

Overall, illogic underlies the whole effort to construe monosyllabic word repetition as stutter. One should recall the well-recognized fact that stutters do not involve word-final position, a fact that is disregarded in this effort. Repetition of a monosyllabic word is repetition of a complete word, which includes, of course, its word-final position. The effort to have monosyllabic word repetition be classed as stutter thus contains an inherent contradiction.

CLASSIFICATION AS CIRCUMLOCUTION

The two classification schemes reviewed above are the latest examples in the literature of stuttering to represent the "empty controversies and idle fancies" mentioned in the epigram for this chapter. The evident theme underlying both schemes, couched in words of explanation that "force and overrule the under-standing" is to talk around the reality of stuttering. The "classes," or categories, that are generated therein (Between–Within Disfluencies and Stutter-like Dis-fluencies) are verbal constructions that distract the reader's attention to chimera clothed in faulty logic. Throughout, word choice and word use are the means to circumlocute what is meant by "stutter."[25]

It should be recognized, too, that these classifications represent implicit definitions, a basic problem in the field, discussed in Chapter 2. In one classi-fication, stutter is "within-word disfluency"; in the other, stutter is "stutter-like disfluency." Criticism of both claims is contained in the preceding pages. Other pertinent criticisms are presented in Wingate (2001).

IGNORING THE CRITICAL

In none of the work under review here is there evident recognition that *stutter* refers to unique fluency anomalies of which the most typical, most widely recognized, and perhaps the most frequent is *iteration of less than a complete syllable*. In the sources reviewed here, and in many others, much is said about all kinds of "disfluency." However, although frequent references are made to "stutterers" and "non-stutterers" (or normal speakers), there is no acknow-ledgment of the very criteria by which those two groups are differentiated. Clearly, the two groups are not distinguished in terms of monosyllabic word repetitions, or any of the other similar types of "disfluency" typically men-tioned, since these phenomena are the object of argument. The regularly omitted, but critical, criterion for the differentiation is *stutter*, which is mani-fested in the iteration or protraction of syllable constituents—that is, something less than a full syllable. This criterion has been repeatedly confirmed over many years and in many ways. It continues to stand as the essential reference; even though so often ignored and evaded, it is always at least implied.

This essential criterion cannot be supplanted by constructions like "Within-Word Disfluencies," or "Stuttering-Like Disfluencies," or any other formula-tions created to sidestep a clear recognition of the objective realities of stutter.

SYNOPSIS

Improper word use is a major, but unacknowledged, problem in the literature of stuttering. It constitutes a serious impediment to implementing a rational, scientifically oriented study of the disorder. The range of misuse is wide, extending from unsophistication, to carelessness and indifference, to intentional misconstructions. Much of the erroneous usage may be carried forward in relative innocence by the rank and file of the profession, by repeating what has been uncritically accepted.

The literature contains an excess of contributions that mislead, not simply through undisciplined word use but, as well, from casual shufflings of word references and meanings. The major theme underlying these verbal anomalies is the intent to have stuttering construed as within the purview of normal speech.

The evident professional tolerance, even indulgence, of so much cavalier dealing with words has characterized the literature in stuttering for many years. Representative writings in the field bespeak its distance from the scientific model, which calls for rational, objective inquiry and careful, coherent analyses. The quotation from psychologist Max Wertheimer, entered on the introductory page of this Part II, is appropriately recalled here: "Science is rooted in the will to truth. With the will to truth it stands or falls. Lower the standard even slightly and science becomes diseased to the core."

NOTES

1. As described here, repetitions of less than a completed syllable.
2. Ironically, via terminological limitations, they would also be identified as one kind of "hesitation phenomena." This anomaly should become understandable from later discussions addressed to the analysis of fluency, especially in Chapter 10.
3. However, these distinctions have been ignored routinely in the literature of stuttering.
4. I have observed some quite unusual ones in normal speakers, for example: "On it." and " 'N everything 'n all that." However, both of these occurred only at a terminal juncture.
5. Although infrequently applied to certain other phenomena (e.g., fluency of ideas), speech remains the ultimate reference.
6. Called "hesitation phenomena" in the original psycholinguistic research.
7. Major, frequently available unabridged sources consulted include: *Funk and Wagnalls Standard Dictionary of the English Language* (1963), *Random House Dictionary of the English Language* (1973), *Webster's Third New International Dictionary of the English Language* (1981). Example esoteric "dis-" words: "disrudder" and "dispauper." It is of note that Van Riper (1992) reported having told Johnson that disfluency is "a garbage can word."
8. See discussions in Wingate (1997).

9. But see pertinent discussion in Chapter 10.

10. Of special interest here is that one of the four classes of dysphemia proposed by West is "spasmophemia" (stuttering). However, with the word "spasm" being effectively expunged from the literature by Wendell Johnson, during his tenure as editor of the *Journal of Speech and Hearing Disorders* (1943–48), spasmophemia was certain to have a short life. For a rather brief period, West, and a few others, used "dysphemia" to refer to a hypothesized underlying, organismic condition of which stuttering is the outward manifestation (symptom). Another category in West's proposed system is "tachy-phemia" (cluttering), a term that captures the major feature of cluttering: rapid rate. West's proposal was quickly submerged by the expanding absorption with explaining stuttering as a psychological problem.

11. For a more detailed review of this problem see Wingate (1984a).

12. Some English words that are now taboo were at one time not offensive.

13. A favorite Johnson reference, encapsulating his contention that there is no condition, or reality, of stuttering; it is just a "problem" of misevaluation and mislabeling.

14. A review of this phenomenon is presented in Wingate (1988, chaps. 7 and 8).

15. Several citations are referenced in Wingate (1997, p. 160).

16. Also found in Bloodstein (1987).

17. And certainly not *dysfluency*—see later.

18. See discussions in Chapter 8.

19. A daily-life analogy might make the point clearly. Suppose a young bachelor were to vacillate about accepting a party invitation, and then is pressed by the hostess, who says, "Do come. We already have you all set up with a very nice female-like person."

20. These items are taken from the Johnson list of "disfluencies." See Chapter 10.

21. See Wingate (1988, chap. 2).

22. See Wingate (1988, fig. 5.2).

23. Correlation values in the high 80s and above. In*tra*-judge agreements are typically higher.

24. See Wingate (1988, chap. 2).

25. It is pertinent to note, at this point particularly, the very likely rationale behind Yairi's persisting concern with the categorization of monosyllabic word repetitions—it is central to the classification scheme he has contrived.

CHAPTER 8

Two Faces of Normal

It is the common wonder of all men, how among
so many millions of faces, there should be none alike.

Sir Thomas Browne, *Religio Medici* (1662)

he above quotation speaks to the long-recognized reality of individual differences, ultimately identifiable in many respects: external and internal structures; capacities, capabilities and processes; from DNA to how one speaks. Yet within all this variation there is a persuasive "sameness," stabilized in perception through our casual, and predominantly superficial, observations of others that support a basic orientation to similarities. This "leveling" in regard to individual differences is abetted by the concept of "normal," which allows a range of variation to be accommodated to the perception of sameness. However, the range of variation itself varies considerably in extent, depending upon the variable (feature, characteristic, etc.) that is in focus.

"Normal," like the word "speech," is another term with more than one meaning that also has engendered problems in the study of stuttering. Within the principal reference supplied in a dictionary definition of the word,[1] one can identify two major uses of "normal," which, although overlapping in a general way, have considerably different implications. "Normal" is used in what may be called the Natural (or Observational) sense, and also in a Statistical (or Probabilities) sense. Each form has a special significance. The unique substance of each sense must be fully appreciated and the distinction kept in mind in discussions wherein the concept of normal is in focus. Unfortunately, the distinction is not clear in the literature of stuttering. This chapter will present discussion of these two schemas of normal, and their relevance to the study of stuttering.

NATURAL NORMAL

"Natural" conveys what is intended in a number of other words having similar meanings, such as "usual," "typical," "regular," "standard," "ordinary," and "expected." Importantly, all of these terms carry, as well, the implication of their opposite, or contrast, namely: "natural–unnatural," "usual–unusual," "typical–atypical," and "regular–irregular." All of these pairs are subsumed under the general encompassing reference: "Normal–Not Normal," or "Normal–Abnormal." A defining feature of the natural sense of normal is this implicit distinction of a contrasting condition.

This sense of normal is the original, age-long, and still the ultimate reference for what is meant by "normal." It is based in observation and experience of the real world and reflects all kinds of observations—everyday commonplace ones and careful scientific observations. It represents an observational structure for events and conditions of a physical or material nature, such as the climate, or weather, the status of a river, and the longevity of an automobile. It reflects matters having to do with plants and nonhuman animals, such as the emergence of leaves, and the migratory patterns of birds. It expresses the reference for the wide range of human attributes, including many physical aspects of size and appearance and, as well, matters of personality, conduct, attitudes, beliefs, etc. In some of these areas, there may be a relatively broad range to what is accepted as being normal, sometimes expressed as being "within normal limits." In some areas the limits may not be particularly well-defined. Nonetheless, themas of what is normal in any of these areas contain certain criteria, often not formalized, for what is to be accepted as normal, and that serve to identify what is considered to be not-normal. Furthermore, many areas have criteria that are very specific and rigorous. The human form provides the most relevant example. Thus, the normal human has two eyes, two ears, one nose, one mouth, all of which are arranged in a normal pattern on one head. Every normal individual also has two arms, each with a hand that has five fingers (no more, no less), all arranged in a normal pattern. The list could easily be extended, and include internal body structures as well. Such a standard (usual, regular, etc.) set of features is normal; any departure from this standard set is not normal. There is no range of variation—that is, one head, no more; two eyes, no more, no less; etc. These, and related observations of human functions, have long served as the foundation of medical diagnosis—to identify what is normal and what is not normal.

As noted above, normal in the natural sense contains implicit reference to not-normal. It is of particular interest that this implication is often expressed in the opposite direction; that is, many things identifiable as not-normal are sufficiently unique as to be given a pertinent name, for which there will be no specific contrasting term for a normal counterpart—the implied contrast to normal being adequate. If a specification of contrast is for some reason necessary, the word "no" or "not" will suffice. For example, there is no specific contrast term for "shivering," or "glaucoma," or many other descriptions. The same is true for "stuttering."

Many variables in the areas noted above are amenable to measurement, and each of them may then be cast, independently, in numerical terms (see especially the remarks on anthropometry in the next section). However, such treatment does not transform, nor in any significant way modify, the role and status of variables identified as normal, and not normal, in the natural sense of the term.

STATISTICAL NORMAL

The statistical sense of normal has a considerably different connotation than the natural sense of the term. Statistical normal is based in mathematics and carries the meaning of quantification and measurement, of numerical gradation and continuity. Importantly, within this schema there is no inherent normal/not-normal contrast. In fact, not-normal raises a complicating issue, which will be brought into focus later in this chapter.

Statistical normal seems generally to be viewed as more scientific than natural normal, largely because it is grounded and expressible in numbers and computations, has numerical reference tables, etc. However, statistical normal is not an alternative to natural normal, nor necessarily an improvement on it. Statistical normal does not discover, identify, or create variables; rather, it is a means of applying quantification to many variables identified through (natural) observation. By means of measurement, whatever frequency and extent of variation occurs in that variable can be represented concretely. Such data are often visualized graphically via histograms (see Figure 8.1), for which standard procedure registers the number of instances (cases, etc.) on the vertical axis and the variation in extent (amount) of the variable is registered on the horizontal axis. The "amount" dimension represents a continuous, graded scale of values.

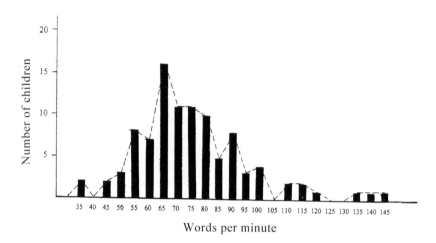

FIGURE 8.1 Bar graph and resulting "curve." Data from Voelker (1938). Speech rates of 98 deaf children.

Histograms are readily transposed as curves by connecting the topmost points of each bar. Some histograms—those based on substantial numbers of instances—may have a pattern of distribution whose fitted curve approximates the idealized "curve of normal distribution" (Figure 8.2), often called simply "the normal curve." This curve is the reference—most often implicit—whenever the statistical sense of normal in intended. Unfortunately, statistical normal and natural normal are often confused, in fact, not even differentiated. Further,

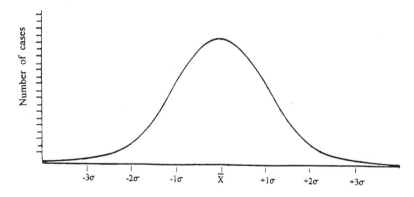

FIGURE 8.2 The ideal curve of normal distribution.

the "curve of normal distribution" has become such a common image and reference that it has essentially usurped an overall meaning of "normal."

It is difficult to characterize the level of sophistication, in respect to the statistical schema of normal, of persons who come to the study of stuttering. It seems safe to say, however, that the reference for "normal" that is usually, and implicitly, held in mind is the image of the idealized "curve of normal distribution." It is a memorable figure with (1) its neatly symmetrical dispersion around the actual mean (average) value, and (2) the wide overall range, with, in particular, its broad central area that speaks of considerable latitude in regard to what is to be considered as "average." Further, there is (3) the clear indication of gradation and continuity on the horizontal axis that represents the extent, or amount, of the variable being described. These aspects of gradation and continuity have had critical appeal for certain contentions about stuttering, to be addressed later in this chapter.

THE NORMAL CURVE

A brief review of the origins and employments of the statistical schema should help the student to appreciate its nature, conditions of its proper use, and the problems it presents.

The curve of "normal distribution" emerged from interests in the field of mathematics. It is a *probabilities* distribution, first derived in the mid-eighteenth century as a convenient approximation to the binomial distribution.[2] In the early nineteenth century it was accepted as the basis of much practical statistical work, particularly in astronomy. It then came to be applied in a variety of special interests. Karl Frederick Gauss (1777–1855), one of the greatest mathematicians of all time, and Pierre Simon de Laplace (1749–1827), a famous astronomer and mathematician, applied the relevant mathematical principles to data, such as the spread of hits around the center of a target, and runs of luck at games of chance. Quetelet (1796–1874), a noted Belgian astronomer and mathematician, made the same kind of analysis of data he had obtained for chest sizes of a large number of Scottish soldiers, and heights of French soldiers. Plots of these measurements showed a pattern of distribution similar[3] to ones for the data analyzed by Gauss and Laplace, which suggested that variation in at least certain dimensions of human physique was distributed in a manner comparable to certain other living and nonliving phenomena. Francis Galton (1822–1911) extended this line of investigation; initially to a variety of human physical dimensions, an area of study known as anthropometry, and eventually to measurements of certain psychological functions, particularly in his *Inquiries into Human Faculty and Its Development* (Galton, 1883).

Plots of the data gathered in these inquiries showed patterns of distribution that were similar to those found in the preceding work reported by Gauss, Laplace, and Quetelet. These, and later, studies in anthropometry laid the basis for the assumption that many other kinds of human qualities, physical and mental,[4] occur in the pattern of variation reflected in the "curve of normal distribution." It is well to keep in mind that this remains an assumption.

It is important to first emphasize a point that is crucial to a proper appreciation of the basis for applying the statistical schema of "normal" to human characteristics and functions. The human measurements that yielded the data plots recorded by Quetelet and by Galton—and later, others—were obtained from individuals who, to begin with, fit the "natural" criterion of normal. That is, we can be sure that among the Scottish and French troops who were the source of Quetelet's data there were no midgets, dwarfs, or giants; no individuals with missing or stunted arms or legs, and so on for many other human features and functions. In brief, they were all physically normal—in the "natural" sense of the term. Similarly, the physical measurements obtained by Galton also were obtained from individuals already accepted as being normal in the natural sense. Importantly, so were the measures of various psychological functions he obtained. The crucial point here is that, in regard to whatever variations have been obtained in the "normal" distributions of anthropometry, the variation represents differences among individuals who have already been identified as within normal range, in the fundamental and original sense of the term—natural normal. That variation also excludes data from individuals identified, on similar grounds, as being abnormal, in regard to the variable(s) being assessed. Here "normal" has a double meaning: (a) the dispersion of numerical values yields a (statistical) normal distribution that represents data obtained from (b) measurements of (natural) normal individuals. In such instances, there is a *statistical* normal distribution of some measurable feature of each person in a group of *natural* normal individuals.

In instances such as the foregoing, the two references of "normal" coincide. However, this coincidence does not occur regularly. It is important to remember that the idealized reference curve shown in Figure 8.2 is a statistical representation, and is fundamentally mathematical. Data yielding a curve of this approximate form may be, and often are, obtained from many different kinds of events and observations for which there is no *natural* normal reference. A clear example is found in the pattern of hits (range of scores) on a dart board. The "normal" distribution refers simply to the frequency with which the various scores were obtained; it means *statistical* normal, which refers to the pattern of hits as determined by probabilities to be expected under "normal" conditions, that is, conditions not influenced by non-chance factors. Confusion arises from the fact that a similar curve may, in certain other instances, represent the distribution of some feature in a large group of individuals who meet certain criteria of normal in the ordinary, basic sense—identified here as *natural* normal. However, there are certain measurable variables in a population of (natural) normal individuals for which the distribution of measurements does not approximate the (statistical) normal curve. For the moment it is necessary to point out that the two senses of "normal" are not equivalent, nor are they interchangeable. Unfortunately, the difference between these two meanings of "normal" is not recognized in many sources, especially in the literature of stuttering.[5]

OUT OF PSYCHOLOGY

Most likely the majority of persons in speech pathology have become familiar with the curve of normal distribution through acquaintance with its prominence in the psychological literature, or in sources that have borrowed from that literature, especially in reference to psychological tests. In such contexts the image of the idealized curve is offered as representing how some measured psychological variable is distributed in the population under study. However, students in speech and hearing science seem unlikely to be aware of certain major qualifications that must be kept in mind about this apparently stable reference.

First of all, it seems to be regularly overlooked that actual, real-data distributions often depart from this idealized form, a matter that importantly qualifies many of the implications of the idealized curve. Many data plots yield curves that are considerably narrower, as in Figure 8.3, which indicate a rather restricted range of what is within the extent of "normal." Even more important,

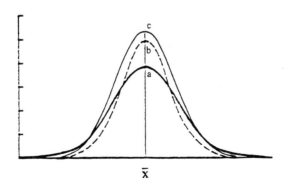

FIGURE 8.3 Normal curves: "a" is the standard normal curve; "b" and "c" have narrower ranges of values.

a goodly number of data plots yield curves that are skewed, in varying degrees, as represented in Figure 8.4. A feature that is described by the latter type of curve is not "normally" distributed, in the sense implied by the idealized curve. Neither of the curves in Figure 8.4 has those comparable departures (to the left and right) from the "average" that are seen in the standard "normal" curve, derived from mathematics. Nonetheless, each of these non-idealized curves, and other variations of graphically portrayed distributions, do accurately reflect data obtained from many (natural) normal populations. Many physiologic functions provide excellent examples of "natural normal" distributions that do not conform to the idealized curve; body temperature is a classic instance.[6]

Data from two relevant sources, addressed to several dimensions of verbal expression, illustrate the potential variety in distributions that represent naturally occurring phenomena. Goldman-Eisler (1968) recorded the variation in rate of the many utterances spoken by each of four individuals as

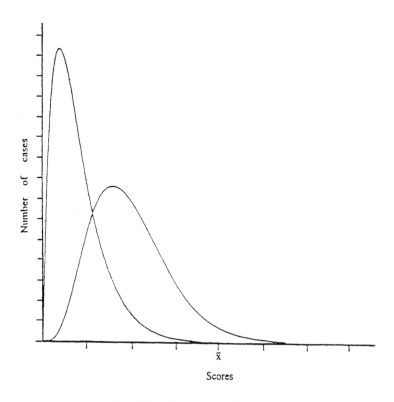

FIGURE 8.4 Two curves with marked skew.

each participated in a two-person conversation. Graphic plots of these data, for each individual, yielded an approximate "normal curve," as in Figure 8.2, although the pattern for each speaker varied somewhat, as suggested in Figure 8.3.

In contrast, data representing word lengths, and lengths of sentences, have consistently yielded distributions with marked skew. For instance. Kucera and Francis (1967) analyzed the lengths of words and of sentences in 15 different "genres" (various content areas) that contained well over a million words, in over 52,000 sentences. For each genre, and for the corpus as a whole, graphic plots of the data, for both words and sentences, yielded curves very much like the two skewed curves in Figure 8.4.[7]

Especially pertinent to our interest: data representing fluency variables typically yield skewed distributions, which is well represented by the data obtained in each of the two studies of "disfluencies" to be discussed later. Note that the data from both studies yielded distribution curves (Figures 8.6 and 8.7) that have the same extent of skew as in the more extreme curve of Figure 8.4. Simply put, these are marked departures from the "normal curve."

There are a number of other problems inherent in application of the normal curve that require attention. The construction of psychological tests provides illustration of such problems. Many issues regarding test construction cannot, and need not, be addressed here. However, the critical matter of concern to us has to do with the assumption, noted earlier, that human capabilities, including intelligence, are distributed in the population in a manner represented by the statistical normal curve. In most sources that mention or discuss psychological testing in one way or another, one will find that the normal curve is either displayed, or stands as the clear reference in the discussion. However, the pertinent assumption regarding the normality of distribution, just noted again, is most often not mentioned; certainly it is not called to attention. The impression typically rendered is that the distribution represented in the idealized normal curve represents reality, revealed graphically. Failure to qualify that assumption leads to further assumptions, which are likely to be grossly misleading.

MAKING IT FIT

Except for certain literature dealing directly with psychological test construction, I have found no mention of the fact that the reason the curve showing the distribution of psychological test scores matches the idealized curve of normal distribution is because the tests are so constructed as to yield such a curve. That is, the representation that intelligence, and other measurable psychological functions, are "normally distributed," in the form represented by the idealized statistical curve, is a contrived representation, not one that was discovered. This essentially force-fit procedure is assumption-driven: by the long-held assumption derived from certain findings in anthropometry, as mentioned above. This force-fit procedure has been standard practice since the time, early in this century, that formal tests of mental ability have been constructed. The rationale for the procedure has been that, since many measurable physical characteristics of humans seem to vary in a manner reasonably comparable to the normal curve, it seems likely that intelligence and other psychological functions are probably spread around in a similar configuration. The only defensible justification for such procedure is that there is no other plausible recourse.

The rationale for constructing intelligence tests so that results will produce conformity to the mathematical curve of normal distribution involves two further assumptions. First, that intelligence occurs in varying degrees, or gradable levels, in the general population. Second, that this assumed graded variation is truly represented by the idealized curve of normal distribution—that is, in a continuity from "least" to "most," with the large majority falling in the middle and fewer and fewer toward the extremes. These assumptions too are founded on the works in anthropometry and their extensions.

However, as acknowledged by early leaders in the development of mental measurement, these assumptions may not be correct. Terman and Merrill (1937) noted that there are biological characteristics that are not distributed in the statistically ideal form,[8] and pointed out that intelligence may be one of them. Those authors acknowledged that the effort to measure intelligence was "in the unfortunate position of having to assume the answer in advance in order to derive the equal-unit scale" (p. 25). Without an equal-unit scale of measurement it is not possible to determine the actual distribution of such a variable, and the only methods for obtaining equal units, in these areas, is to assume that the variable is normally distributed—a circular dilemma.

For physical features (e.g., height and weight), standard (equal-unit) scales of measurement are available—such as inches, centimeters, etc., and pounds, kilograms, stones, etc.—from which a distribution can be plotted. For intelligence, and other psychological functions, there is no evident scale, and therefore it was necessary to create one having features that correspond to the physical model. Although the end result of these manipulations has turned out to have utility in practical application, one must remember that their base lies in assumptions, and that what they represent may not reflect reality as it seems to be represented in the data distributions derived from readily measurable physical attributes.

A CLOSER LOOK

The curve of normal distribution for intelligence provides an especially clear illustration of the difference between natural normal and statistical normal. The curve of Figure 8.5 depicts the standard (statistical) distribution of intelligence as measured. The extent (degree) of intelligence, registered on the horizontal axis, ranges in graded continuity from lowest (left) to highest (right).

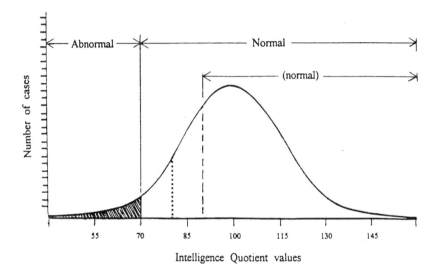

FIGURE 8.5   The normal curve with reference intelligence levels indicated (see text).

It is sufficient for our purposes to identify only major categories of classification.[9] IQ values below 70 are classed as Mental Deficient, between 70 and 80 as Borderline, and between 80 and 90 as Dull Normal. The mean, or average IQ value is 100. However, the classification "Average" extends between 90 and 110. The several classifications for values above 110 (Bright Normal, Superior, Very Superior) are relevant here in only a general sense.

   The crux of this illustration is that statistical normal—the "normal curve" distribution—encompasses the natural categories of normal *and* abnormal intelligence. This is because, in a broad, *unselected*, population one would expect that all levels, from most to least, would be included. (Recall that the soldier "populations" of Quetelet, and Galton's samples, were *selected* "populations" from which the abnormal were excluded.) Now, for practical purposes, there are just two major categories of mental capacity: Normal and Abnormal. The criteria for inclusion in either category lie in evidence of being either not mentally retarded, or being mentally retarded; these criteria are based ultimately on observation and experience, and supported by measures developed to assess mental capacity.[10] Note that, by intelligence test scores (a statistically based distribution), the bulk of the population is identified as Normal, and that this designation includes a wide range of values. In fact, the category of Normal includes two classifications of intelligence level that fall below the level of Average. The statistical normal is based on test scores, which overlap with and have a substantial level of correspondence to, practical criteria. However, among those who are not (either practically, or by test) mentally retarded, there is considerable range in mental ability.

Lay judgments of mental capability, of course, are made directly from observation of the individual, without reference to intelligence test scores. The general distinction between normal and abnormal is made from the same basis as the formal diagnostic designations of Normal and Abnormal, wherein the reference of normal is in the natural, or empirical sense of the term. Certain finer differentiations, all of which fall within the broad range of Normal, also are frequently made in lay terms, many of them expressed in words such as "slow," "very bright," etc. At the same time, in much lay usage the terms "normal" and "average" are not very well differentiated: in fact, they are often used as though synonymous. Still, in certain contexts "average" is used to refer to the base category in normal, as when average is contrasted to "well-above-average." This frequently expressed, but unacknowledged, differential in the use of "normal" and "average" is represented in Figure 8.5 by the added entry of "normal" in parentheses. Similarly, in a common lay expression, "below the norm," the norm may refer to either "average" or "average-and-above." However, in "above the norm," the reference must be to "average" or the average range. The essential point being made, however, is that, in spite of such descriptive vagaries, the judgments, extending from the basic distinction between normal and abnormal, are made in reference to relevant observations of individual function. The descriptions are imprecise because the available descriptive terms are themselves vague. It seems pertinent to mention again, in the present context, that what is considered to be "normal" in respect to mental ability is founded on observation, and that this assessment may be aided, but not supplanted, by test measurement.

NORMAL AND STUTTERING

For centuries, and still today, stuttering has been acknowledged in reference to normal in the natural sense, in regard to which stuttering has occupied the status of *ab*normal. However, in the latter half of this century efforts have been made to dissolve this age-long distinction and to claim that stuttering is simply a marked degree of "normal nonfluency."[11] A review of these efforts will reveal that, in the final analysis, they all fail by reason of one or another important fault in conception or argument. Yet they continue to be expounded and, surprisingly, accepted in many sources as credible. The claim of "continuity" between stutter and normal speech exemplifies this condition.

"CONTINUITY"

The foundation of the effort to meld stuttering with normal speech lies in the contention, originally posed by Wendell Johnson, that stuttering arises from "normal nonfluency." The endeavor to normalize stuttering almost certainly arose through reference to the curve of normal distribution (statistical normal), especially from its appealing assumptions of gradation and continuity that encompass a range of ability. Johnson's contention, and the image of the normal curve, are cardinal features of the claim that stuttering is continuous with normal nonfluency. The claim that stuttering and normal speech are on a continuum is frequently cited as though it were actuality; in fact, the claim is frequently restated simply as "Continuity." The reader should recognize this assumption as the remaining Deceptive Concept, among the several identified in Chapter 6.[12]

The Original Assertion

The initial statement expressing the claim of continuity between stuttering and normal speech (through "normal nonfluency") appears in *The Onset of Stuttering* (Johnson & Associates, 1959), in which the author writes

> There are no "natural" lines of demarcation between "normal" and "abnormal" degrees of non-fluency. (p. 205)

The statement is a cleverly presumptuous set of contentions. Note that it speaks of *degrees* of nonfluency. Other than in literature sources reflecting similar presumption, stuttering is not, and had not previously been, identified as a *degree* of nonfluency but, rather, a difference in *kind*—a notable anomaly in the speech sequence, a departure from *any* degree of nonfluency. By speaking of *degrees of nonfluency*, Johnson implicitly contends that all irregularities of speech are simply variations, presumably in amount. Further, the contended "no natural lines of demarcation" purports that one cannot distinguish among the presumed degrees. Thereby, stuttering is just one expression of variable occurrences of "nonfluency" that occur in normal speech.

Efforts to support the claim of stuttering as an extension of normal nonfluency have been expressed along both purely descriptive lines, and in reference to what is presented as quantitative support. At the same time, the claim has often simply been stated as such, with no attempt to justify the contention (e.g., see Brutten & Shoemaker, 1967, p. 31). Descriptive attempts have tried to link stutters to certain kinds of ordinary (normal) nonfluency (for example, Bloodstein, 1970; see also Table 8.1, below.). Quantitative attempts have compared various measures of the extent of "disfluency" in speech samples obtained from stutterers with those from individuals having normal speech, hoping to show some kind of continuity.

The initial, major quantification effort of this type was mounted by Johnson (1961) in a study whose primary stated objective was to analyze speech samples from stutterers and from normal speakers "with respect to discernible varieties of speech disfluency."[13] An unspecified objective of the study—to obtain support for the claim that stuttering is a *degree* of nonfluency—was revealed in Johnson's disclosure that

> The design of the study serves to place in focus particularly the question of *the referential equivalence* of the terms "stuttering" and "disfluency." (p. 1, italics added)

It was also intended that the study should yield "normative" as well as comparative data, based on a frequency count of each of the "varieties of disfluency." These data were expressed in decile format, rather than in the standard computations regarding dispersion of data. Still, it is clear that none of the distributions could have approached a (statistically) normal form. The data afford no support for the contention of gradation or continuity *over* the two sample populations—that is, the findings contradict the contention that "disfluency" is normally distributed in the population at large. The stutterers' samples contain more of all "disfluency" types. For both subject groups the dispersions for most types were markedly skewed, especially those for the stutterers. As could be expected, marked skew was especially pronounced in stutterers' samples for those features that are the hallmarks of stutter—sound and syllable repetitions—as revealed in Figure 8.6.

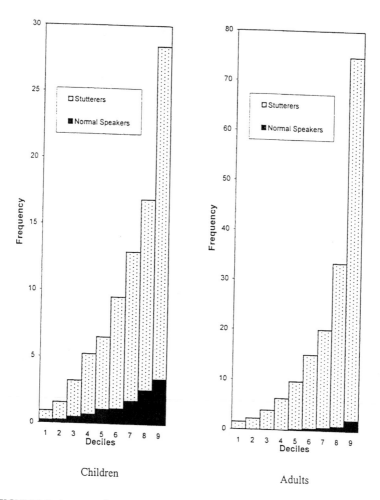

FIGURE 8.6 Amounts of sound and syllable repetitions in spontaneous speech samples from 136 children and 200 adults. Data from Johnson & Associates (1959) and Johnson (1961).

A Clear Difference

Figure 8.6 reproduces in graphic form the data for sound and syllable repetitions recorded from the speech of 68 child stutterers and matched normally speaking controls (Johnson & Associates, 1959), and similar data recorded for 100 adult stutterers and matched normal speakers (Johnson, 1961). Each display reveals the dramatic differences in frequency of sound and syllable repetitions observed in the speech of stutterers in contrast to the speech of normal speakers; the extent of skew emphasizes this uniqueness. It is of particular interest that the extent of stuttering among the children is clearly greater than in the adults, corroboration of other evidence that stuttering is principally a disorder of childhood. This finding is particularly pertinent to the matter of remission, one of the important facts about stuttering reviewed in Chapter 4.

The Issue of "Overlap"

In spite of the evidence in the foregoing two studies that clearly revealed marked differences between the stutterer and normal speech samples, the findings were nonetheless claimed by Johnson, and others, to portray stuttering as simply a degree of nonfluency. This interpretation was mounted on grounds of a claimed "overlap" in the frequency with which certain nonfluency types occurred in the speech samples of the groups being compared. The essential irrelevance of this finding, however, was that the only "overlap" noted for the 1961 study was evident for just one type of nonfluency—revisions, which are hesitation phenomena found routinely in anyone's speech.[14]

This claim of "overlap," which is based on the minimal sharing of only one (normal) category, should be recognized as a desperate attempt to salvage the contention that stuttering is an aspect of normal speech. One's ordinary experience is replete with perceivably different things for which comparison will show many more features of "overlap" than in this claim. The issue of overlap, in this context, is hollow; the error it represents should be obvious. It is then surprising that the notion still is recited by certain individuals within the profession; evidently persons who need to cling to the contention of "continuity" of stuttered and normal speech.

"Normative" Distorted

In the two works discussed above, no attempt was made at application of, or direct reference to, the (statistical) normal curve, and none of the significant procedures in those studies were consistent with its employment. At the same time, the image of the normal distribution was steadily implied by incorporating, as one *stated* objective, the gathering of *normative data*. However, the meaning of "normative" was thoroughly confounded by combining comparative and supposedly normative approaches. The stated objective of obtaining normative data was vitiated by the following critical circumstance: half of the individuals in this purportedly normative population sample were selected in reference to the major variable of the study, *stuttering*, the criterion on which this half *differed* from the other half of subjects. Thereby, fully half of the subjects participating in the study were individuals who could be expected to produce certain "discernible varieties of nonfluency" that are not normal, kinds that were not likely to occur in the speech samples of the other half of the subjects. In this way, the procedure was inherently biased in favor of the unspecified objective noted above—namely, gathering stutters and normal nonfluencies into a common pool.

Normative data regarding any particular variable should be obtained from an unselected population. The only concession that might be made in this matter would be to collect data from a subject sample defensibly representative of the population at large, the approach used by Wechsler in developing his intelligence test. As applied to stuttering, 0.7% of the participating subjects could have been stutterers (also to be chosen randomly), since this value is an arguably reasonable estimate of stuttering prevalence among individuals of the age-level serving as subjects in that study.

The two publications considered so far in this section (Johnson & Associates, 1959; Johnson, 1961) have had extensive and profound influence in the field of stuttering. The continuing reference to the purported "normative data" in both of these studies (as, for example, in Bloodstein, 1984, 1997) has itself been a steady detriment to understanding stuttering. However, the most stultifying influence has been the continuing use of the list of "disfluencies" created through this work.[15] For well over 30 years, this list has been the standard source in many studies of stuttering vis-à-vis normal fluency, and cited in many other publications. However, it is inadequate for meaningful use, for it is incomplete, inaccurate, and imprecise. This matter will be discussed at some length in Chapter 10.

OTHER NORMALIZING EFFORTS

The Disfluency Index

The next publication seen as relevant to the issue of continuity of stuttering with normal nonfluency was pursued in terms of a "disfluency index" (Minifie & Cooker, 1964). The index was based on what were presented as "two basic types of fluency interruption": one called "disfluencies of syllable insertion," the other called "disfluencies of deliberation." Each of these types were aggregates of the nonfluency varieties in the list created by Johnson (1961). Importantly, both types in the Minifie and Cooker index were hybrids that included a mixture of items, some of which are identifiable descriptively as stutters, but others that are clearly normal kinds of "nonfluency." The hybridization, which obscured important distinctions, created *de facto* "overlap," which confounds the issue.

Although the findings of this study are, as in the Johnson study, contaminated by the mixing, the data plots representing them are of great interest. Figure 8.7 is reproduced from Minifie and Cooker. The values for the plotted distributions are the "disfluency scores" for individuals, computed as a ratio of the total number of syllables uttered (S) divided by the words per minute spoken (W/M). A marked difference between the two distributions is clear. The data for the normal speakers show essentially a modal score with a remarkably minimal range of scores; there is hardly any "distribution." The data for the stutterers are a marked contrast. These data do not yield a normal distribution form; the wide range of scores is markedly skewed. Notably, the amount of skew is similar to the skew present in Johnson's 1959 and 1961 data, as presented earlier in the chapter (Figure 8.6). Clearly, the data for the stutterer samples do not constitute a normal distribution. It is equally noteworthy that the data for the normal samples show such minimal dispersion, evidence that the distribution of fluency is not accurately represented by the standard normal curve.

Descriptive Gradation

Attempts to effect a union between stutter and normal nonfluency via description are also without real substance. Arguments claiming "continuity" ignore the realities of objective analysis—realities that nonetheless emerge routinely.

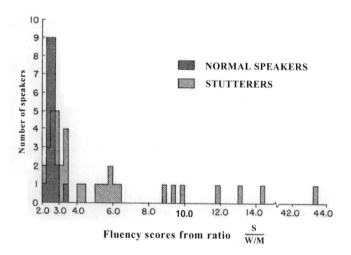

FIGURE 8.7   Distributions of "fluency scores" for 37 stutterers and 22 normal speakers. Reprinted with permission from Minifie & Cooker (1964).

An especially relevant illustration is presented in a publication by Diehl (1968). Table 8.1, reproduced from that source, represents an effort to portray stuttering as continuous with normal nonfluency by employing qualitative descriptors arranged on a continuum; the bottom horizontal line evidently is intended to suggest the gradation and continuity typical of the curve of normal distribution. One might note, first, the technical error of arranging qualitative descriptions on a quantitative framework; there is no progression of measurable values. However, a more important error of this display is the erroneous use of *dysfluency* with *normal*. "Normal dysfluency" is an inherent contradiction, since the prefix *dys* means *ab*normal. The error derives from: (a) the fact that *dys*fluency is homophonous with *dis*fluency, and (b) a lack of adequate sophistication in the use of the two terms. This error is found in other literature sources in the field, in fact, much too often. It appears even in a dictionary devised especially for the field (Nicolosi *et al.*, 1978), in which, moreover, the two terms are cross-referenced as equivalent.

The descriptors used for the several different types in the sequence of Table 8.1 are of particular interest in that they contradict the implication of continuity, and are instead consistent with the long-established differentiation of stuttering from normal speech. Types I through IV evidently represent normal speech, since the remaining types are identified as "Stuttering Behavior."[16] The latter types, notably, emphasize matters other than speech. It is particularly significant that the descriptors in Types IV and V reveal a line of distinction in regard to the all-important speech features. In Type IV (normal speech) one finds "repetitions of monosyllabic words and phrases," whereas in Type V (stuttering) the features are "hard contacts on sounds by prolongation or repetition." These contrasting descriptors are clearly consistent with the differentiations emphasized in Chapter 3.[17]

Nonetheless, continuing efforts are made to obscure the distinctiveness of stuttering and to bring it into the range of normal. As reviewed in Chapter 7, a current maneuver is to construe monosyllabic word repetitions to be the same as stutters. The whole matter of fluency, its dimensions and departures therefrom, has not been approached from a scientific orientation. Necessary considerations for such endeavor are presented in Chapters 10 and 12.

Normal Curve Failure

Efforts to meld stuttering with "normal nonfluency" by reference to the curve of normal distribution are not viable. As a general referent, "disfluency," no matter how structured, is a hodgepodge of variables, most of them clearly normal in nature but certain others long recognized as not normal. In view of this variety in composition alone, "disfluency" cannot, in any meaningful way,

TABLE 8.1 An Attempt to Portray Stuttering As Continuous With Normal Nonfluency (Diehl, 1968)

Fluency–stuttering categories

Type I	Type II	Type III	Type IV	Type V	Type VI	Type VII	Type VIII
Superior fluency (skilled speaker).	Normal dysfluency (average speaker).	Excessive dysfluency (hesitant speaker). Not considered defective. Variety of dysfluencies. Seeming lack of facility with words.	Excessive dysfluency. Considered stuttering by some listeners. Occasional, inconsistent repetitions of monosyllable words & phrases. Prevalent at 2½ & 3½ years. Usually lasts only 3–6 months.	Dysfluency with persistent hard contacts on sounds by prolongation of repetition. Consistency appears related to overt or subliminal apprehension. Some minimal struggle usually noticeable.	Dysfluency with occasional acute, bizarre, struggle-type associated symptoms, especially when excited. Apprehension but no withdrawal.	Dysfluency with consistent, bizarre, struggle-type associated symptoms. Anger and irritation at self. No withdrawal. Apprehension but no avoidance of self-expression orally.	Dysfluency with consistent, concealed, fearful, interiorized, socially withdrawn, non-vocalized behavior. Occasional catastrophic, struggle-type bizarre associated symptoms. Consistency effect. Severe apprehension.
				Primary Stuttering (Bluemel). Phase I (Bloodstein). First Stage (Van Riper).	Transitional stuttering (Van Riper). Phase II (Bloodstein). Second Stage (Van Riper).	Secondary stuttering (Van Riper). Phase III (Bloodstein). Exteriorized: Vocalized (Douglass-Quarrington). Third Stage (Van Riper).	Secondary stuttering (Bluemel). Phase IV (Bloodstein). Interiorized: Non-vocalized (Douglass-Quarrington). Fourth Stage (Van Riper). *Inneres stottern* (Freund).

⟵——————— Stuttering behavior ———————⟶

⟵——————— Speech behavior (fluency variable) ———————⟶

Fluency: a facility to communicate orally without blockings, interruptions, repetitions, interjections, or hesitations.
Stuttering: dysfluency with associated symptoms.

be said to vary simply in degree or amount. By the same token it has no natural equal units of measurement, nor is it amenable to a devised equal-unit scale. Categories of "disfluency," most unlike the categories of intelligence, cannot be fit under a common rubric.

A Different Tack

In the final decade of the twentieth century, a new effort to align stuttering with normal irregularities in speech appeared in the form of the "covert repair hypothesis." In this construction, stuttering is rationalized as simply one form of disfluency that results from the effort to "repair" an impending speech error. As stated by its authors (see Postma & Kolk, 1993), the formulation, like the Johnson endeavor, is "intended as a global frame of explanation for all types of speech interruptions." The central contention of this notion is that all disfluencies are byproducts of internal (therefore "covert") attempts to "repair" potential speech errors detected prior to overt expression. Stutters are claimed to be one kind of byproduct; normal nonfluencies are presented as other disfluency forms that reflect the same effort.

The notion of "covert repairs" in the speech process is extracted from Levelt's (1989) complicated and involved effort to explain normal speech production. A substantial dimension of this endeavor centers on literature concerned with speech errors, and in this context Levelt assigns a prominent explanatory role to "internal monitoring" of speech. Levelt's formulation itself contains some questionable assumptions, as well as certain evident faults and inconsistencies. Overall, there is good reason to entertain reservations about an explanatory conception based on speech errors, phenomena that occur relatively infrequently. One especially pertinent lacuna deserves mention: the concept of an internal monitor is weak. Many errors in ordinary speech go uncorrected, which reveals that, at least then, no monitoring is active. Further, Levelt acknowledges that the "internal monitor" is not on duty full-time. However, the overall proposal is too complex to attempt an adequate review here. Rather, our interest is principally in the derivative scheme conjectured for stuttering—the "covert repair hypothesis."

There are several ways in which reality considerations reduce "covert repair" to contrivance, rather than hypothesis. First, Levelt himself gave such possibility little consideration. He ignored the 25% of repairs in his corpus that were of this kind, which he called covert "because we don't know what was being repaired" (p. 478). Second, if, as claimed in the covert repair hypothesis, normal nonfluencies and stutters are both byproducts of repair effort, why should stutters take the form they do, rather than the form of normal nonfluencies, which are claimed to reflect the same "repair" effort?

There are several important descriptive differences between stutters and the supposed "repair" of ordinary errors—differences that Postma and Kolk do not recognize, although evidently aware of them since they (Postma and Kolk) distinguish between the two phenomena. The most obvious difference is that, in an ordinary error "repair," the intended objective supplants the error, as correction of—and *different from*—the error. In stutter, the error persists; there is no correction. Fifth, as documented in Chapters 3 and 5, stutterers are not aware of many of their stutters, especially "the little ones." In other words, these occurrences are not sensed by the individual who produced them, so how could they result from some repair effort, which purportedly follows from some very careful monitoring? Sixth, in any stutter occurrence, whether or not recognized by the stutterer, it is difficult to discern how the stutter represents an effort at "repair." Seventh, stutterers are said to be, and many stutterers claim to be, on the alert for difficult words or sounds. If so, then they should be well prepared in their internal planning-ahead and thereby be able to avoid potential errors.[18]

The aspect of the "covert repair" scheme that turns normal nonfluencies into simply the wreckage of attempts to "repair" potential speech error reveals the contrivance of the entire conjecture. The attempt to explain disfluency of any kind, especially normal nonfluencies, as the byproduct of error contains the implicit assumption that normal speech should be smoothly continuous—that is, an error-free sequence of *words*! This assumption represents a long-standing misunderstanding of "fluency," a matter to be discussed at length in Chapter 10. At the moment it must suffice to point out that fluent speech contains much more than words; it includes varying numbers of various non-verbal phenomena. The extensive research concerned with "hesitation phenomena" has yielded sensible and credible accounts of the occurrence and functions of these nonverbal features in normal (normally fluent) speech. Significantly, this important area of research is not considered by Levelt, nor by the authors of the derivative "covert repair" account nor, unfortunately, by the large majority of sources within the field of stuttering.

IN BRIEF

The word "normal" is regularly used very loosely, most often without adequate sophistication regarding its several meanings. Ordinary usage reflects a traditional lay generalization that is based largely in common casual observation and experience. A specialized, and separate, meaning of normal, mathematically derived, is statistical in nature. These two meanings of normal are not equivalent, although they overlap to some extent—a circumstance that underlies an evident confusion in some of their intended application.

Statistical normal does not provide a means of changing the form or character of observational normal. However, the assumption that this can be done is an evident misunderstanding in the attempt to apply statistical normal to stuttering. Certain nonverbal phenomena in speech, referred to as "normal nonfluencies," have been erroneously so labeled, because they are "nonfluencies" only from a constricted and artificial understanding of fluency. In the literature of stuttering, the concept of "fluency" continues to carry the meaning expressed in unsophisticated lay usage, namely, "words in continuous sequence." From such reference, common irregularities occurring in connected speech are thereby identified as "normal *nonfluencies.*"

Although there is continuing effort to normalize stuttering through attempts to align stuttering descriptively with what have been called "normal nonfluencies," these efforts nonetheless continue to reveal the unavoidable differentiations that exist between "normal nonfluencies" and stutters. A persisting effort to achieve this goal is mounted through use of the term "disfluency."

Overall, the various efforts to meld stuttering with normal nonfluency have clearly come to naught. The open failure of this endeavor serves to confirm the long-recognized uniqueness of stuttering.

Notes

1. *Webster's New World Dictionary of the American Language*: "conforming with or constituting an accepted standard, model, or pattern; especially, corresponding to the median or average of a large group in type, appearance, achievement, function, development, etc.; natural, standard, regular."

2. Actually, the curve for the binomial expansion $[(a + b)^n]$ is narrower than curve "b" in Figure 8.3.

3. It is well to keep in mind that "similar," in these contexts (as in so many others), does not mean "identical." In so many instances it means simply "reminiscent of."

4. Unfortunately, easily extrapolated to *all* human characteristics and functions.

5. Of stuttering, certainly; but of other disciplines as well.

6. For other examples see sources such as Bennett & Plum (1996), Ganong (1997), or Wallach (1992).

7. See Kucera & Francis (1967, p. 367, pp. 397–405). For the approximate normal curves in Goldman-Eisler (1968), see her pp. 19–22.

8. As noted earlier in regard to body temperature, etc. See also footnote 5.

9. The classifications here reflect deviation IQs based on a standard deviation of 15. The numerical limits of classifications vary slightly for various tests, but remain essentially equivalent.

10. Edgar Doll (1953) criticized the use of intelligence test scores to identify mental deficiency, pointing out that social competencies are the essential criteria, for which test scores are *ex post facto*.

11. Discussed elsewhere in previous chapters, especially Chapters 2, 6, and 7.

12. It continues to be championed especially by Bloodstein (1970, 1984, 1997).

13. The "disfluencies" identified in this study will be a subject of Chapter 10.

14. The same method, procedures, contentions, and interpretation are found in the parallel study involving young children (Johnson & Associates, 1959).

15. The list was developed in the study reported in 1961, which actually preceded the work reported in 1959, where the list was first used.

16. The superfluous use of "behavior" is a hallmark of the era caught up in learning theory, Behaviorism's core.

17. Note also the discussion in Chapter 7.

18. Comparison of stutters and true speech errors is considered in Chapter 12.

CHAPTER 9

Speech Minimized

We meet Thee, like a pleasant thought,
when such are wanted... Thou unassuming
commonplace of Nature.

    William Wordsworth, *To the Daisy* (1798)

*S*everal times in preceding chapters the point has been made that, at least in this century, concurrent with the persuasion that stuttering is a psychological problem, attention to speech has been largely incidental—in spite of the fact that stuttering is manifestly disordered speech. All of the psychologically oriented accounts of stuttering are forced to deal in some way with at least certain aspects of speech, simply because stuttering is so patently an anomaly in speaking. However, interest in speech processes has been largely peripheral.

This relative indifference toward speech, which deals with it as more or less of subsidiary concern, is founded in several insidious and seldom recognized, yet potent influences: (1) the ubiquity of speech, (2) vagaries in use of the word "speech," and (3) the matter of general literacy. We will consider these influences in that order.

EVERYBODY DOES IT

Throughout the long formative years of reaching adulthood, most people have very little if any awareness of, let alone experience with, humans who cannot talk. For most individuals, everyone with whom they come in contact not only talks, but talks quite well, and seemingly effortlessly. Add to this the fact that, if one were to reflect on his or her own fuzzy awareness of one's self speaking, it seems to be little more than a matter of "have thought, open mouth." At times, such as when needing to search for a word, there may be a brief perplexity about the process, and at some of these times one may even become aware of using certain techniques to search for the word. However, on the whole, speaking seems to occur without any particular effort, or even attention to the process. Further, this comfortable, casual, essentially indifferent attitude toward speech is stabilized through the assumption that the capability for speech and the process of speaking are the same for everybody.[1]

As a result of these several happenstances, there seems to exist, in the mind of most persons, an underlying, unverbalized, most likely non-conscious assumption that speech is an ordinary, unremarkable accomplishment. Even in those instances in which speaking might receive special appreciation, such as in the discourse of an articulate, practiced, verbally capable speaker, it is the particular style and proficiency of performance that is admired, not the function itself. Speech, therefore, is taken for granted; acknowledged, if much at all, with an offhand attitude.[2]

PROFESSIONALS TOO

Interestingly, but unfortunately, this cavalier attitude toward speech, established over long years of everyday immersion and experience with it during the course of growing up, does not seem to undergo any substantial modification for many people in certain areas of the behavioral sciences who have a special interest in speech, and who presumably study it—namely, persons in some areas within psychology, and especially individuals in speech pathology. A major, and most regrettable, dimension of this casual orientation is the belief that ordinary speech is automatic. This understandable but unsupportable assumption is at least a major contribution to, if not the source of, certain conceptual misadventures in psychology and speech pathology, especially in the area of stuttering. This issue, of speech as automatic, will receive attention in Chapter 11.

Evidence that speech is so routinely taken for granted will be found in many places, for example, in professional as well as lay sources that speak of children "learning to walk and talk," as though the two achievements were of similar quality. Actually, neither function develops in the way "learning" is usually understood, such as learning to read, to write, to play tennis, or to drive an automobile. Even so, talking is exquisitely more complex a process than is walking—as well as any other skill that actually is learned. But the most distressing reflections of naivete regarding, or indifference toward, the marvel of speech are found in "theoretical" formulations that treat speech simplistically. Most notable among such attempts are efforts to invoke the tenets of learning theory, especially behaviorism, which received its principal exposition in B. F. Skinner's *Verbal Behavior*, published in 1957.

While Skinner's literary effort was under way, other comparable statements from the behaviorism orientation surfaced. One account of this sort, which has had considerable appeal in speech pathology, is the effort to explain speech in the terms of operant learning principles, using the example of "talking" birds. This account, called the "autism theory" of speech development, was first presented as part of a Symposium on Speech Development of the Young Child in the 1951 national convention of the American Speech and Hearing Association. The following year it appeared as an article in the *Journal of Speech and Hearing Disorders*, becoming then a reference for many years. Subsequently, in 1980, the article was reprinted in a book titled *Psychology of Language and Learning* (see Mowrer, 1952).

The sweeping appeal of behaviorism overwhelmed not simply scientific attitude, but common sense as well. Many persons exposed to the autism theory of speech acquisition found revelation in it; many others either accepted it or found no grounds for objection. Clearly, those who found the account persuasive overlooked what should have been obvious—that the only parallel between a child's words and the croakings of a bird was a very superficial, approximate similarity of sounds. The intended isomorphism with speech was hollow, in which regard it is pertinent to mention that Chrysippus, the third century BCE Stoic, noted that some animals, especially parrots, "utter something which is like speech, but it is not."[3] There is an extensive literature concerned with the complex vocal communication of birds, some aspects of which have interesting relevance for certain dimensions of human speech, but not in terms of equivalence nor of conditioning principles. For a recent excellent review, see Ball and Hulse (1998).

Attempts to explain speech or its acquisition within a framework based on stimulus and response can only be undertaken by proceeding from a most superficial and limited awareness of the nature of speech processes. At base, learning theory deals with speech in units that can be cast in the roles of stimulus, or response, or both. Rather than attempt any further criticism here, I will refer the reader to an appropriate authoritative source. Chomsky (1957), in his careful review of Skinner's book, described it as a *"reductio ad absurdum* of behavioral assertions" that is based in what is largely "a mythology whose widespread acceptance is not the result of empirical support, persuasive reasoning, or the absence of a plausible alternative." Chomsky's criticism was clearly not very persuasive to the audience most deserving of it. The need for a second attack on the Skinner ideology was given expression 13 years later (Chomsky, 1970). Still, the appeal of behaviorism has persisted, and many of its adherents continued to cling to their views. At the present time, in linguistic circles at least, behaviorism has come to be viewed as an outmoded brand of psychology (Harris, 1993). Nonetheless, behavioristic notions have been long-lived, as reflected in the time required for a change in the title of a psychology journal that has focused on language content. The *Journal of Verbal Learning and Verbal Behavior*, established in 1962, continued with that title until 1985, at which time it became, mercifully, the *Journal of Memory and Language*.

LOOKING ELSEWHERE

One might expect that individuals who are presumed to know something about speech should not so readily accept, and avidly repeat, simplistic fabrications. Yet psychological conceptualizing has long been attractive to many speech pathologists, who have sought to imitate certain preoccupations found within psychological disciplines. Some individuals were attracted to the proposals of dynamic psychology—the discipline concerned with personal problems believed to reflect inner turmoil, conflicts, and hidden motivations that are expressed in convoluted symptomatology. However, the learning theory framework of behaviorism was more readily understood and by far the more appealing. The behaviorism movement was well established, broadly supported, and vigorous by the time speech pathology was beginning to assume a professional status. It also had a substantial academic base. It is of particular note that the academic source contributing most heavily to development of the profession of speech pathology—in this country at least, the University of Iowa—included a heavy emphasis on coursework in psychology.[4] Further, the emphasis there centered on learning theory, with its focus on the instrumentality of conditioning principles, whether expressed in the clearly reductionist concepts of stimulus and response, or the comparably mechanistic tenets of the operant viewpoint.

For many years, the strength of psychology at Iowa lay in learning theory, and, during that long period preparation in speech pathology was heavily invested with behaviorist concepts, principally through the efforts of Wendell Johnson, who employed these concepts particularly in his interpretation of stuttering.

A substantive theme of this chapter is that most persons are only vaguely aware of their own speech, and are essentially indifferent to its properties except for sporadic awareness of the words they speak, and to some extent the sounds of their words. Understandably, in lay conception, most persons also readily accept that speech is learned. These circumstances support a point of view that renders speech amenable to a variety of simplistic explanations, especially the view that the evident aspects of speech—sounds, words, *and* anomalies thereof—are all "learned behaviors." Only an ingenuous view of speech could support attempts to account for it in S–R terms. Speech is not a function to be treated casually, regardless of how many people do it so well and so effortlessly. Edwin Newman, in his book *Strictly Speaking*, complains about the hackneyed, improper overuse of certain words, and offers the word "wonderful" in example. "Wonderful," he says, means "to excite wonder." He goes on to point out that there are actually few things or events we experience that can be said to be truly "wonderful," and he gives several illustrations from the physical world. To those persons who can overcome their lay ingenuousness about speech, and move beyond such simple notions as stimulus and response to gain some familiarity with the intricate processes involved, speech becomes revealed as something that fully merits description as "wonderful."

We are still a long way from understanding how speech is accomplished (despite presumption to the contrary in certain sources), but even considering what is now known about all that must happen, and so rapidly, in order to (in lay conception) transduce "thoughts" into acoustic signals having an exquisite range of meanings, one can only appreciate speech to be—to use another good word appropriately—marvelous! We will consider important dimensions of this marvel in Chapter 11.

SPEECH CONFOUNDED

Traditionally—that is, for centuries—"speech" has referred to the human capacity to convey meanings by creating patterns of unique vocal sounds. The word "speech" has had a comprehensive reference, one that incorporates all aspects of the process, from intended meaning to phonetic execution. The word continues to be used in this inclusive, comprehensive sense.

Over this long span of time, the most common use of the word "language" was in reference to the differing speech of various nationalities. When appearing as a generalized term, "language" was used principally as equivalent to "speech," although sometimes it was used to analogize methods of expressing meaning other than with words—such as "sign language," "the language of bees," and "the language of love." However, the common reference of speech and language has always been assumed,[5] as reflected in the fact that the grammatical classes of words long have been known as "the parts of speech." Also relevant are the discussions of "inner speech," and the long-used references to "speech areas" in the brain. Typically, speech has been contrasted only with writing, which is recognized as the graphic representation of speaking.

However, early in the twentieth century the two words came to receive differential treatment within two separate areas of study: (1) the established discipline of linguistics, and (2) the newly developing interest in speech correction. In linguistics, language came to be used as a generic term, having a reference quite removed from speech. A formal statement of differentiation was presented in de Saussure's (1915) contrast of *parole* and *langue*, which evolved essentially from linguists' interest in the structure of a language. *Parole* referred principally to the observable aspects of verbal expression (what can be recorded—in other words, speaking); *langue* referred to a system hypothesized as underlying this external expression. In this conception, language was assumed to be a system that has an internal consistency quite apart from real-life verbal expression.[6] In the middle years of the twentieth century, this view was cast into more literal form in the position developed by Chomsky (1957, 1965). Chomsky pressed the evident fact that humans have a *capacity to acquire* language into the contention that language is a special mental "organ," created through the human genetic program—in a word, an instinct (see *The Language Instinct*, Pinker, 1994).

The foregoing concepts from linguistics are not simply of historical and background interest, but have had a substantial influence in the field of speech disorders. They affected especially the attitude regarding language, through which the differentiation of speech and language, already under way within the field, was encouraged.

Chomsky's concepts did not themselves specify a differentiation of speech and language, but, understandably, his writings were addressed exclusively to verbal formulation and structure—essentially, grammar—which in theoretical linguistics is the substance of "language." His extensive discussions of language, the elaboration of its inferred properties, and its reification as innate, gave the concept of language a stature and aura that eclipsed the then seemingly mundane matter of speaking. Also, a speech–language differentiation is at least implied in other linguistics literature. For instance, in a book whose title, *The Role of Speech in Language* (Kavanagh & Cutting, 1975) implies the differentiation, a statement in the Introduction proposes "speech to comprise the part of language that extends from the phonetic message to the sound."

The speech–language differentiation of special concern in the context of this book came about initially as an artefact of the speech correction movement. Since the major activities of speech correction traditionally have been addressed to some aspect of pronunciation, it followed that the principal focus of interest was directed to the production of speech sounds, which in turn meant special attention to the motor functions by which speech sounds are produced. Thereby, in the field of speech and hearing disorders, "speech" came to be used very often in this special limiting sense. Although the word continued to be used with its age-old significance in certain generalized references, it also became more widely employed in its special sense of signifying essentially motor performance. From this orientation, speech, as sound-makings, is quite separable from language, conceived as an amorphous entity or process somewhere in the central nervous system that comprises the truly verbal functions—the "rules" by which words are related to each other to convey messages.

One effect of this speech–language distinction is well reflected in the sequential name changes of the professional association. At its inception in 1925 it was called the *American Academy of Speech Correction*, in which its foundation interest was stated directly. In 1947, acknowledging attention to the other major dimension involved in oral communication—hearing—the name was changed to the *American Speech and Hearing Association*. Eventually, in 1979, the implicit speech–language distinction was installed into the organization's title through insertion of the word "language"; thenceforth the *American Speech–Language–Hearing Association*.[7]

In certain respects the reification of language leaps beyond some important realities. Language lacks certain features characteristic of instincts, and although it is properly conceived as based upon certain neuronal systems in the brain, one must recognize that language could only have arisen through, and represents, speech. Briefly stated, "the role of speech in language" is as its source and essence. Language is not defensibly conceived as something bigger, better, and more profound than speech. Even in contexts limited to a focus on verbal formulation and arrangements, "language" is essentially a synonym for "speech" in which attention to the acoustic aspect is reduced. Although, for certain purposes, use of one or the other term may seem preferable, the two words have a common referent.

THE LITERACY COMPLICATION

The vast majority of individuals in western cultures are literate, that is, able to read and write. The ability to read and write is not a native capacity like speech, which, as noted earlier, is not learned in the usual sense of learning. Reading and writing are skills that must be learned; in fact, a great deal of time, considerable teaching, and much application are required to learn to do either.

The acquisition of literacy typically begins quite early in life. Most children have had informal instruction in at least reading well before entrance into a formal school program, which usually commences at about 5 years of age. Thus, familiarity with the printed page is almost as extensive as is one's experience with speech; moreover, it is much more memorable due to its visual representation. This long-term familiarity with writing—more accurately, printing—is particularly pertinent to the typical insouciant, casual attitude toward speech. It underlies an assumption that spoken and written expression are isomorphic; that the two are essentially equivalent forms expressed in different media. The resulting orientation leads to a concreteness in the conception of speech; in particular, in the view that the sounds of speech are matched in the letters of print. This orientation must be recognized, and rectified.

NOT EQUIVALENT FORMS

Fundamentally, writing is the graphic record of speech. However, in all but highly specialized, esoteric forms of transcription, the written record is an incomplete, inadequate, and in certain important ways inaccurate version of the utterances it is intended to reproduce. Much of the information, and most of the complexity, embodied in the spoken message is left out of the standard printed version. The omission is especially marked in respect to prosodic features, for which conventions of punctuation are a limited compromise. However, other significant dimensions of the speech signal, pertinent to words, and phones themselves, are also omitted in transcription. We will presently note some effects of these differences that are relevant to the topic of this chapter.

Although printing is a shadow version of speaking, there are some ways in which a written record refines the spoken version. Ong's book on orality and literacy (Ong, 1982) contains a chapter titled "Writing Restructures Consciousness," in which the author describes a number of advantages to writing that inhere in its differences from speech. Many of the interesting, substantial, and important differences between speaking and writing need not concern us here, but one clear difference between them is of particular significance to the present analysis.

The printed word is a physical entity: concrete, objective, stable, permanent, ever reviewable. It is variably composed of little marks, called letters, that have the same characteristics as the printed words they constitute, that is, they are concrete, permanent, reviewable, etc. In marked contrast, speech is ephemeral and evanescent. However, in being equated with the little marks of print, the sounds of speech are vested with the impression of concrete physical reality. Significantly, the words people think and say are thus, to them, words as known from the printed page. The literate speaker, through his longstanding immersion in both speech and writing, assumes an isomorphism between what is spoken and what is written. Ong put the matter this way:

> For most literates, to think of words as totally dissociated from writing is simply too arduous a task to undertake.... The words keep coming to you in [the form of] writing, no matter what you do. (p. 14)

An especially pertinent illustration of this phenomenon is represented in the extent to which reversion to ordinary spelling routinely plagues individuals learning to transcribe speech in IPA[8] symbols. For example, learners frequently ask, during practice transcription of unfamiliar words from dictation, "How do you spell it?" Sometimes the standard printed form of a word is especially difficult to abandon; for instance, more than once a student has complained that "There is no "ing" (meaning /ŋ/) in [the word] ink!"—or some similar evidence of the power of print. Of special relevance are examples that show up frequently in the literature of stuttering in regard to claims of difficult sounds or words. For instance, the stutterer noted in Chapter 6 who, in his claim of difficulty with "s-words," listed among his examples the words "sugar" and "sure." The initial *letter* of these two words is "s" but the initial *phone* is /ʃ/. This phone is clearly differentiated from /s/ by almost any speaker—including this particular subject when it was brought to his attention. However, the print representation was his spontaneous (and incorrect) reference.

Similar examples will be found in many literature sources wherein the purportedly difficult sounds are expressed as letters.[9] In this regard, it is of note that, in the "language factors" research extending from the Johnson and Brown (1939) search for difficult sounds, word length was measured by counting the number of *letters* (not phones) and syllables (initiated by Brown & Moren, 1942).

SPEECH AS PRINTING

This common, and commonplace, orientation to speech conceives it as though it were in printed form. The sounds of speech become the letters of print, and vice versa. Thereby, spoken words become sound sequences in printed-letter format, wherein sounds, implicitly identified with the independent, separate letters of the printed version, are thought of as beads on a string that, moreover, are ever the same wherever they occur.

But the sounds of a spoken word are not separate unchanging entities, nor do they have little spaces between them. Unlike words in print, spoken words are not like beads on a string; they do not consist of parts that can be moved about, interchanged, and remain the same wherever they appear. This difference is well illustrated with examples of palindromes, in which words that are spelled exactly in reverse are also real words, although they differ in meaning—and also differ in sound! Clear differences between letters and sounds are obvious with palindromes such as "yard" and "dray," and "laid" and "dial." The differences may not be so evident in a pair like "stop" and "pots" since the vowels and their letter representations in both words seem the same and the consonants, in isolation, have some letter–sound correspondence. However, there are two very important differences between the printed and spoken versions of each of these two words: (1) in respect to the essential differences between phones (speech sounds) and letters representing them, and (2) the even more critical differences relating to the sequences of phones as compared to sequences of letters, that is, in their relationships to each other. In print form, the difference between "st" and "ts" is simply a matter of which letter appears first. In each word, each letter, "s" or "t" is the same letter regardless of where it appears, and each has no influence on the other, nor on what precedes or follows. In contrast, it should be clear, for example, that pronunciation of /st/ is considerably different than speaking /ts/.[10] Moreover, the difference is enhanced by whether the combination follows or precedes some particular vowel. Similarly, the letter "p" is the same regardless of where it appears; but the sound /p/ varies depending on its phonetic context. Although the /p/ is not part of a consonant combination, it too differs in production when in syllable-initial as compared to syllable-final position, via coarticulatory influences. The reader might then deduce, correctly, that the "same" printed vowel in "pots" and "stop" also are not identical when spoken, but are influenced by what precedes and what follows.

The foregoing analysis of "stop" and "pots" is equally applicable to even simpler palindromes such as "mad" and "dam." The crux of the matter is that the nature of speech sounds is not adequately reflected in their printed representations. In addition, other important speech variables are represented in these examples, and have been suggested in preceding content of this chapter. Discussion of them is appropriately deferred to Chapters 10 to 12.

One major effect of literacy has been to give speech a visualizable physical reality wherein words are accepted as being made up of interchangeable parts. Underlying this orientation to speech lies the image of the printed page, with its words lined up in left-to-right sequences. The activity of speaking thus becomes viewed as, in essence, a kind of reading from script.[11]

An especially relevant illustration of this image, one especially pertinent to the interests of this book, is represented in the claim that stutterers "look ahead" for difficult words.[12] Testimony of this sort has come largely from circumstances involving oral reading; nonetheless, it also has been stated in regard to spontaneous speech. The substance of this claim suggests that the words to be said are all lined up in script form ready to be rendered audible.

Literacy, through its influence in concretizing the sounds of speech, has had several effects significant to our interests. (1) It has helped to render speech—and especially stuttering, with its focus on sound making—amenable to mechanistic explanation, especially behavioristic accounts. (2) It has abetted the literal speech–language distinction. (3) It has enhanced the belief that, in stuttering, some influence external to speech intervenes to impede the rendition of the speech script, which, it is further presumed, ordinarily occurs automatically. The latter issue is addressed in Chapter 11.

These views derive from another effect associated with literacy, namely, the impressiveness of the printed page. Things that are written, largely because they exist as a physical, visible reality, take on an aura of special value and credibility. In certain important respects, the effect is much like other forms of visual record—statues and pictures, physical realities that have permanence. People tend to be unduly impressed by what is recorded in print which, as Ong (1982) pointed out, may last forever, continuing to influence indefinitely.[13]

In spite of the fact that most people speak much more extensively than they read and write, the literate person seems bonded to the written version of what is said. To illustrate, if you ask someone "What does the word 'city' begin with?" almost invariably the reply will be "c." If the same question is then asked about the word "country," again the answer will be "c." If you then go on to ask "What *sound* does each word begin with?" most often the person is a bit perplexed—and some people clearly need a little time to figure it out. This little quiz becomes more illustrative if one adds, in the sequence, the same questions about words like "this" and "who." Even though the latter words are used with great frequency, the task becomes noticeably more demanding. I have found that these questions are dealt with in much the same way among speech professionals as they are by laypersons.

SUMMARY

Speech, unquestionably the most remarkable of all the amazing functions observable among the wide range of earth's animals, is a capacity unique to humans. Because this capacity finds expression naturally in almost every individual from a very early age, it is ordinarily so taken for granted that the uniqueness and wonder of speech go unrecognized and unappreciated, and its marvelous processes are trivialized in premature explanations of it.

A second mundane influence is occasioned by the average person's long-term familiarity with the printed page as the graphic transcription of speech. This influence has not only encouraged the attitude of indifference about speech but also has contributed substantially to a reductionist, mechanistic view of speech processes.

In the twentieth century, the original and traditional meaning of speech—"man talking"—has been split into two references: (1) speech as equivalent to the entire process (the traditional meaning), and (2) speech as referring to the external effects. In this latter sense, "speech" is juxtaposed to "language," which, in many contexts, refers to an amorphous source conceived as underlying what the literal acts of "speech" make audible. However, in many other contexts the word "language" is used as interchangeable with "speech" in the general, traditional meaning of the word.

The word *speech*, in its general reference, is still widely used, most notably in lay sources. The use of speech in its most limited sense, and contrastive to language, is found regularly in speech pathology. This limited meaning of the word, through its focus on literal acts, has made speech, in its traditional sense, vulnerable to efforts at explanation in mechanistic terms.

A superficial, insouciant conception of speech generated and maintained by the circumstances reviewed above is especially evident in much of the literature of stuttering. In the chapters of Part III, the word "speech" will be used in its traditional, comprehensive sense, except in circumstances where citations from other sources force use of the word "language."

NOTES

1. This routine assumption remains untested. There are reasons to consider it fallible.
2. A more realistic appreciation of speech is the subject of Chapter 12.
3. Cited in O'Neill (1980, pp. 49–50).
4. See Wingate (1997, pt. III).
5. The reader is advised to inspect the entries for "speech" and "language" in any good dictionary.
6. de Saussure's writing, considered by many to be the most influential work in linguistics of the twentieth century, contained other dichotomies. His formulations reveal the extent to which some linguistics is largely philosophy. de Saussure's juxtapositions seem to reflect the influence of dialectics, which was "in the air" philosophically during that era, especially from the writings of Hegel and Marx.
7. The resolution advocating the addition of "Language" (ASHA, LC 22-78) cited, in the rationale for the name change, the "historical involvement" of the association

"in the study and management of language disorders" and, as well, the prior endorsement of an official title of "speech–language pathologist" for qualified members of the association. It seems pertinent to ask how "language disorders" differ from "disorders of speech," and what a "speech–language pathologist" does that a "speech pathologist" does not, or cannot do. As implied in the final sentence of the next narrative paragraph, lacking objective differentiation, "speech–language" is redundant.

8. The International Phonetic Association.

9. Although most often presented therein as example of reaction.

10. In fact, /ts/ in initial position is a difficult combination for native speakers of English to master.

11. A conception possibly enhanced in recent years by awareness that many statements on television are read from well positioned cue cards.

12. I recall having heard Van Riper, in a convention address, tell of being able to "see that word coming." This description suggests analogue to the printed page; however, it also could represent the matter of speech planning, a major focus of Chapter 12.

13. Epitomized by the Bible-thumping preacher. In a lighter note, as remarked by comedian Carol Burnett, "Words, once they're printed, have a life of their own" (Reader's Digest, 1982).

PART III

Substance

Fluency, Speech Production, Stuttering

CHAPTER 10

Fluency

When even at its most fluent, two-thirds of spoken language comes in chunks of less than six words, the attribute of flow and fluency in spontaneous speech must be judged an illusion.

> Frieda Goldman-Eisler, *Psycholinguistics* (1968)

*T*he quotation above speaks to use of the word "fluency" in its ordinary, usual sense, as a "flow of words." For centuries ordinary speaking, normal speech, was appraised in only very general terms, principally in regard to form and style: manner of delivery, choice of words, pronunciation, quality of content, and the like.[1] Throughout, "fluency" was used essentially to refer to an individual's command of a language, either his native language or one(s) acquired later. From that, the meaning of fluency as a general referent has been conceived in terms of the apparent "flow of words," of words in seemingly continuous sequence.

Although reference to fluency in this sense is of long standing, only in very recent times have the dimensions of fluency been explored. This exploration has revealed that literal fluency (words in continuous sequence) is indeed illusory, but an illusion supported by the perception of fluency as reality.

ANALYZING THE SPEECH "STREAM"

Beginning in the early 1950s, studies by Frieda Goldman-Eisler and George Mahl,[2] working independently, were addressed to what were then thought of as "extralinguistic events," as intrusions into the ordinary, typical flow of speech. It is something of an irony relative to the field of stuttering—considering its central preoccupation with fear and anxiety—that both Goldman-Eisler and Mahl originally thought such "disruptions" had a motivational origin, reflecting emotional factors that interfered with the ordinary ongoing process of verbal expression. Mahl had become interested in these seeming intrusions in speech as possible indices of anxiety in patients; he thought that perhaps different types of them might indicate different underlying psychic influences. Initially, Goldman-Eisler's ideas were similar inasmuch as her discovery of "hesitation phenomena," essentially silent pauses, had come in the course of studying interviewing techniques.[3] However, her interest soon moved on to the study of these phenomena as aspects of speech processes, and her explorations became seminal work in the emergence of the new discipline of psycholinguistics.

By the mid-1950s, research on "hesitation phenomena"—given as the generic name to these seeming intrusions in the apparent continuity of words in the speech of normal speakers—was being pursued by a number of investigators. The resulting discoveries made valuable contributions to psycholinguistics, linguistics, and cognitive theory. Within two decades, the results of a considerable amount of research had provided a reliable and stable substance of this new field of inquiry. In their individual approaches to the analysis of this dimension of normal speech, the research of separate investigators has yielded a variety of "hesitation phenomena," found to be common to the various studies even though some have been called by different names in various reports. These phenomena are summarized in Table 10.1.

DISCOVERIES REGARDING "HESITATION PHENOMENA"

In addition to identifying the variety of these occurrences to be found in normal speech, this research yielded three related findings, each of which is appropriately called a discovery. The first discovery was the frequency with which these features occur in ordinary spontaneous speech. In retrospect, earlier commentary and, more importantly, prior evidence had pointed to this reality. Some literary authors observant of verbal exchange had remarked on this nature of ordinary speech. For instance, T. S. Eliot referred to ordinary speaking as characterized by its "fumbling for words, its constant recourse to approximation, its disorder and unfinished sentences." Moreover, impressive pertinent evidence had surfaced 20 some years before the early work in psycholinguistics. French et al. (1930) reported that a full 20% of almost 2000 telephone calls

TABLE 10.1 Types of "Hesitation Phenomena"
Reported in Psycholinguistic Research Using
Normal Speakers

A. Audible
   1. filled pause
   2. sentence correction
   3. sentence incompletion
   4. repetition (of one or more words)
   5. stutter
   6. intruding incoherent sound
   7. tongue slip
   8. word change
   9. parenthetical remark
   10. drawl

B. Silent:
   11. omission (of word or part of word)
   12. silent pause

consisted of half-completed words and sentences, and "non-words."[4] Other evidence had also appeared in the intervening years (e.g., Voelker, 1944; Wyrick, 1949).

The second discovery was the revelation that, in spite of the surprising frequency of these occurrences in ordinary speech, they are hardly ever noticed. The fact that these two findings (frequency yet obscurity of the events) emerged as discoveries enlarges their significance, for they reveal what is actually a ubiquitous part of everyone's daily experience—namely, that irregularities in the flow of speech are occurring all the time, yet they are rarely noticed, by either listeners or speakers.

The third discovery was that many of these phenomena are not properly considered as disturbances or intrusions in the flow of speech, as originally thought. Instead, this research has shown that most forms of seeming intrusion in the "speech stream" are intrinsic to speech production processes. Within two decades there was substantial research documentation of this reality (see Wingate, 1988, chap. 2). The fact that so many of these phenomena are contained within ordinary, normal fluency explains why they are not noticed, in spite of their frequency.

It deserves emphasis that the routine inattention to "intrusions" in the flow of speech applies only to certain potentially observable features of spontaneous speech. The explanation for this phenomenon rests almost entirely in the realization couched in the third discovery—that most of these apparent "irregularities" are actually an integral part of ordinary speech, that is, they are aspects of normal *fluency*!

FLUENCY

MAJOR FEATURES OF FLUENCY

There are several important matters regarding fluency that are central to the meaning of the term and its use. First, as noted previously, the word is used primarily and predominantly to refer to speech. Many other words, such as "flowing," "fluid," and "liquid," are used to describe other events that move, or appear to move, continuously. However, fluent and fluency are reserved, almost exclusively, to describe the apparent continuity of speech. The *Oxford English Dictionary*, fully representative of other lexicons, gives the meaning of "fluency" as a "smooth and easy flow; readiness, smoothness, especially with regard to speech; readiness of utterance, flow of words" (Vol. 4, p. 357). Fluency is sometimes used to characterize certain other psychological functions— for example, "associative fluency" or "ideational fluency"—but such use is always in allegory to its source in reference to speech.

A second important feature of fluency is that it has both concrete and abstract significances. It is concrete in respect to what it denotes in its common usage, the "flow" of everyday speech. It is abstract in the sense that, in spite of its focal reference to the audible speech sequence, other aspects of the speaking circumstances are considered implicitly (factors such as the physical setting, the nature and size of the audience, and the content of the discourse). Similarly, the meaning of fluency is simultaneously objective and subjective. It is objective relative to the events of the speech sequence as they occur. At the same time, it is subjective in that it involves a judgment that is based on unspecified, and usually informal, criteria.

A third important aspect of fluency is that it has a broad range of reference. In general usage it refers to the ordinary speech of almost everyone, in spite of the fact that we may sometimes be aware, at some level, of the individual differences in fluency that exist among ordinary speakers. In this general sense, fluency describes the speech one is accustomed to hearing from most people in almost all circumstances. Such a broad-spectrum meaning is exemplified in the standard use of fluent to describe the level of capability in a second language. A person is considered to be fluent in a language if he speaks it in a manner comparable to the generalized, abstracted, "average" native speaker of that language. And here the broad limits are applied in two directions simultaneously—to the actual speaker in question and, at the same time, to the abstracted, "average" native speaker.

A fourth important feature of fluency is that, although having a broad reference, it also has identifiable limits that are described straightforwardly in several ways. There are several specific terms that pertain to the upper range of fluency. The adjective *articulate* indicates several favorable qualities of oral expression that encompass a commendable level of fluency.[5] Interestingly, there are other speech-specific terms that refer to a high level of fluency, but with a less favorable connotation. Thus, *voluble* refers to speech that is "characterized by a great flow of words or fluency." It carries a connotation of excess, plus the suggestion that what it describes is potentially annoying. Also, speech produced "in a manner too smooth and easy to be convincing" is described as *glib*, a word that typically carries the sense of insincerity or deception.

There are also means of describing speech that falls in the lower range of ordinary fluency. Sometimes a descriptive phrase, such as "spoke haltingly" is used, but there are formal speech-specific terms to refer to speech at the lower limit of fluency. To *hem and haw* means "to pause and hesitate in speaking." It is relevant to point out that, while these two words refer to oral expression at the lower limits of fluency, they carry no negative connotation other than that in certain contexts they might imply that the speaker is attempting "to avoid saying something definite." Most often they are simply descriptive of a lack of expected continuity in someone's speech, in which instances they are recognized as reflecting a temporary phenomenon induced by circumstances or context, such as that the speaker is nonplussed, embarrassed, or "at a loss for words."

It is of particular interest that the words *hem* and *haw* are onomatopoeic. *Hem* is "a conventionalized expression of the sound made in clearing the throat to attract attention or show doubt." The word *haw*, meaning specifically "to grope for words, to falter," is a conventionalized representation of the most common filled pause, the so-called neutral vowel /ə/, usually written as "uh" or "um."[6] This "sound" was discussed briefly in Chapter 3 and will receive considerable attention in later discussion.

The reader should recall that the word "stuttering" is also onomatopoeic. Importantly, then, the language has three different well-established and commonly used words that identify three separate kinds of occurrences observable regularly in ordinary spontaneous speech. Significantly, all three words derive from the same fundamental source of word origin, *onomatopoeia*, in which the character of the referent is reflected concretely in the sound structure of the word itself—words like "boom," "squeak," and "whirr." Such words directly represent something that is perceivable. The words "hem," "haw," and "stutter" refer to occurrences in speech that are, and have been, observed over sufficient time to have acquired special names. Two of them, "hem" and "haw," refer to occurrences that fall in the seemingly ill-defined area at the lower limits of the wide range of normal fluency—"normal" in the observational or natural sense of normal. The third word, "stutter," refers to observations falling outside the range of normal.

The existence of three different words that specify departures from actual verbal continuity constitutes compelling evidence that certain kinds of occurrences observable in the course of ongoing speech are not only identifiable but are also differentially discriminable. Such findings are all the more remarkable in view of the substantial evidence from the research on normal speech, which reveals that what is admissible as ordinary fluency contains a considerable number of "intrusions" of various kinds, most of which are rarely noticed.

A COMPOSITE STRUCTURE

The commonly held view of continuity in speech sees it as a "flow of words," as in the dictionary entry mentioned earlier and as elaborated in the quotation from Goldman-Eisler (1968) below. However, research has revealed that literal reality does not match the commonly held view. The contrast between perception and reality is recorded impressively in Goldman-Eisler's description of fluency as ordinarily perceived:

> Somehow the phenomenon of speech has become associated with images that suggest continuity of speech production. We speak of the even flow, of fluency of speech, of a flood of language, and many words relating to speech derive from descriptions of water in motion—such as gush, spout, stream, torrent of speech, and floodgates of speech. The facts, however, show these images to be illusory; if we measure vocal continuity by the number of words uttered between two pauses and call "phrase" the sequence uttered without a break, we obtain a picture of fragmentation rather than of continuity. (p. 15)

This description was based on her research addressed to nongrammatical pause, alone. It represents evidence from the instrumented analysis of her samples that 50% of the utterances consisted of three words or less, and that 75% were of five words or less.[7] Impressive as these figures are, nongrammatical (silent) pause is not the only element contributing to the literal fragmentation of "the speech stream."

There is a critical issue here: the continuity regularly perceived in speech—and which is called "fluency"—is not a continuity of words. Contrary to the commonly accepted view, fluency is not equivalent to "words in uninterrupted sequence." Something spoken does not have the same structure as if the same message were in writing.[8] Speech contains many elements other than the words of the message. Some of these other elements are an integral part of the message, such as grammatical and rhetorical pause. Others might properly be considered intrusions in some sense, in that they are superfluous, such as irrelevant word and phrase repetitions.[9] Nonetheless, whether integral to the message or superfluous, these other elements are rarely noticed—because they do not disturb the *impression* of continuity! The words, and the other elements, all together, are a composite that is perceived as continuous—all are aspects of what is recognized perceptually as *fluency*.

The point has been made several times (and it bears repeating) that elements in the speech sequence other than the words critical to the message most often go unnoticed. This phenomenon is readily explained by recognizing that the interest and involvement of both the listener and the speaker center on the message being conveyed, and therefore, under ordinary circumstances, their attention and concentration are absorbed with whatever elements are relevant to that message; other aspects, if not actually obtrusive, are "filtered out."[10] Evidence for this process was reported by Martin and Strange (1968), who found that requiring subjects to listen for nongrammatical pauses in speech samples interfered with their comprehension of the message. The reader can discover this personally while listening to any television or radio program in which individuals speak spontaneously (interviews are especially good sources). Listening for hesitation phenomena, whether focusing on various kinds or only one kind, is quite a demanding task, and one will soon realize it to be an unusual experience. In contrast, listening for the message alone is a process of which one is hardly aware—clear evidence of our customary activity. Further, if an attempt is made to register hesitation phenomena and also to comprehend the message, one will not be very successful with either objective, but will be relatively more successful at perceiving the message.

It seems clear that identifying intrusions in fluency is based on occurrences that disturb reception of the message. Under certain circumstances elements that are accepted routinely as part of a fluent utterance—such as ordinary occurrences of "uh" (a particularly relevant example)[11] or even something like "y'know"—rise out of their obscurity simply by occurring too frequently. The typical obscurity of hesitation phenomena has been noted in many sources.[12] At the same time, as Mahl (1959) noted, they are more likely to be noticed if they are "bunched." If such prominence persists, the speech begins to elicit description as "hesitant," although still accepted as within normal purview.

INCORRECT TERMS

As noted earlier, the term "hesitation phenomena," originally a reference to pauses, was accepted by sources in the psycholinguistic literature as the generic term for the full range of events revealed in that research. As should be evident regarding the items in Table 10.1, "hesitation" does not accurately describe each of the features discovered. However, evidently for want of a better term, "hesitation phenomena" has continued in use, with the implicit recognition that it is simply an umbrella rubric for the events identified.

A different circumstance surrounds the terms "nonfluency" and "disfluency." The term "normal nonfluency" emerged some time ago in the literature of stuttering as a means of designating those apparent intrusions into the speech sequence that are not stutters. "Normal nonfluencies," reflecting its underlying orientation, carries the assumption that "fluency" means a sequential flow of words, the lay view noted earlier, in which certain events disrupt that flow. However, careful observation of spontaneous speech reveals that it contains, in addition to the essential words, certain nonessential words, and non-words, that (most often) do not disrupt the ongoing character of ordinary fluent speech. From the orientation that views fluent speech as a flow-of-words, such occurrences are not a part of fluency; events other than words-in-sequence are "nonfluencies." In this schema stutters are one kind of nonfluency; the other events are "normal nonfluencies."

The use of "nonfluencies" (or similar term) reflects the persistence of the original (and the common) view that sees fluency in terms of words in sequence. However, the study of normal speech has revealed that fluency is not correctly identified as words-in-sequence; that fluency incorporates many other features of speaking—notably pauses, of both kinds, but certain other events as well. These other features are not correctly identified as *non*fluencies because they are intrinsic to the flow of speech, of *fluency*, not only as perceived but also as produced. Moreover, some of these events have demonstrable, even special, linguistic value. "Nonfluency," in this overly inclusive use, is a misnomer, and essentially self-contradictory. The terms "nonfluency," and especially "disfluency," should be abandoned, the latter because of its contaminated references. "Disfluency" is used as: (a) equivalent to "nonfluency," (b) even more comprehensively, to include stutter, and, most damaging, (c) as a substitute term for stuttering. Moreover, it is severely limited for reasonable use by being the homophone of *dys*fluency.[13]

Appropriate terms have not yet been devised to specify those hesitation phenomena that might be considered to be intrusions—notable as such because they are unessential *and* noticed to be so. It seems that proper characterization should conceive fluency to consist of: (1) *message elements*, and (2) what might be called *fluency fillers*. The message elements are significant to the meaning being expressed. Although consisting predominantly of words, the message regularly includes pauses of varying length and utility, and often certain other events such as whole-word and phrase repetitions. Fluency fillers, in comparison, are happenstances of the process of generating and expressing the message. Many of the fluency fillers often are not readily distinguished from certain message elements (because of similar form) by either listeners or the speaker. Actually, fillers are more likely to be recognized by listeners than by speakers, especially on occasions when these events rise into awareness through excessive occurrence.

It seems that, for the time being at least, it is preferable to undertake fluency analysis and description based simply on the objectively identified events, rather than to employ technically inappropriate classifications like "nonfluency" and especially "disfluency."[14] With these qualifications in mind, it is possible to derive a comprehensive list of events pertinent to a uniform descriptive analysis of fluency that is applicable to any particular sample of speech.

TYPES OF FLUENCY FILLERS

HESITATION PHENOMENA

A summary list of the types of phenomena found regularly in the psycholinguistic research is presented in Table 10.1. The list is derived from five substantial studies: Mahl (1956), Goldman-Eisler (1968), two other works on adults (Maclay & Osgood, 1959; Blankenship & Kay, 1964), and one report based on a number of literature sources concerned with speech samples from children (Levin & Silverman, 1965). The terms identifying each type of nonfluency are taken directly from these reports. In most cases, each source used the same terms; in the few instances of some difference in terms used by one source or another, the descriptor equivalences were obvious.[15]

Most of the items in the list are quite straightforward and should need no clarification. One item, "intruding incoherent sound," might seem unclear, but it is very literal, meaning simply any sound made by the speaker that is not comprehensible, such as a cough or grunt. "Parenthetical remarks," often called "asides," refers to typically brief remarks that are tangential to the main message. Regarding omission of parts of words, Mahl noted that most of such omissions involved final syllables.

The remaining item deserving notation is "stutter." This term was used by two of the reference sources as the equivalent of *sound and syllable repetition*, the descriptor used in the other three reports. Both sources listing the word "stutter" used it simply in a descriptive sense—that is, to refer to a discriminable type of fluency irregularity for which this word is a well-known and appropriate descriptor. In this purely descriptive usage the referent was understood to be benign. At the same time, this usage has relevance to the issue of stutter identification, discussed earlier, especially in Chapter 3.

THE JOHNSON LIST

This list, of "disfluencies," reproduced as Table 10.2, is brought into discussion here for several reasons. A principal objective of this chapter is to arrive at a comprehensive and adequately detailed list of filler types that will be useful for analysis of speech samples from any source. The Johnson list registers specific irregularities, from stutterers, that do not appear in the normal speech research, and therefore should be included in a comprehensive list.

As reviewed in Chapter 8, the list of "disfluencies" compiled by Johnson (1961) resulted from an attempt to meld stuttering with "normal nonfluency."[16] That list has been used widely since it was first compiled, and has dominated sources concerned with description of stuttering. It has been used even in some studies of normal speech only, by persons whose interests lay with stuttering. Evidently users of the list have found it to suit their special purposes, in view of the steadfast indifference to other lists that, importantly, have resulted from

TABLE 10.2   The Johnson (1961) List of "Disfluencies" Reported for Combined Stuttered and Normal Speech Samples

1. Interjections of sounds, syllables, words, or phrases. (Includes "extraneous sounds and words, such as "uh" and "well.")
2. Part-word repetitions. (Repetitions of sounds and syllables.)
3. Word repetitions. (Repetition of whole words, including words of one syllable.)
4. Phrase repetitions.
5. Revisions. (Change in content or grammatical structure of a phrase; change in pronunciation of a word.)
6. Incomplete phrases. (Thought or content not completed.)
7. Broken words. (Words not completely pronounced; words in which smooth flow is interrupted; words not associated with any other category.)
8. Prolonged sounds. ("Sounds judged to be unduly prolonged.")

research based on the ultimate reference source of matters pertinent to fluency—normal speakers.

As stated earlier, Johnson's list is inadequate for general use, primarily because it is incomplete, inaccurate, and based on improper procedure (see Chapter 8). The extent to which the Johnson list is unsuitable should become clear in the content of this chapter. At the moment it is germane to emphasize that to develop a list that presumably will serve as a reference, correct methodology requires that the list be based on speech samples representative of an unselected normal population. This chapter is concerned in substantial measure with the significance of lists properly developed, and the contributions they make to a meaningful description of "nonfluency." The term is entered here in quotation marks because of reservations regarding its propriety, to be considered later in this chapter.

The Johnson list also contains filler types obtained from normal speakers, an aspect of that research that raises certain notable ironies. Although the intent of the Johnson research was to link stuttering with normal "nonfluency," the most significant dimensions actually point in the other direction. We have already pointed out that the only "overlap" between the two samples (normal vs. stutterer) that could be claimed involved one normal feature—revisions. Moreover, the findings relative to the normal speaker samples simply corroborated the results obtained in the psycholinguistic research in respect to types, and the extent, of hesitation phenomena present in normal speech.[17] Beyond that, the Johnson study also revealed the considerable amounts of such phenomena in the speech of stutterers, which confirmed the point that such events occur among all speakers. Although not acknowledged in the Johnson report, it seems logical to assume that the hesitation phenomena in the stutterer samples were generally as undetected there, as they are in samples from normal speakers. More important, finding "normal nonfluencies" as well as stutters reveals that one can distinguish between the two kinds of events. Additionally, finding the substantial amounts of "normal nonfluency" in the stutterer samples presents real problems for the claim that stuttering is the effort to avoid nonfluency. That is, if that claim were true, why then all that (normal) nonfluency; why not stutters instead?

This is also an appropriate time to point out another irony, one created by the effort to normalize stuttering by pressing use of the term "disfluency." As reviewed in Chapter 7, the actual meaning of "disfluency" is "speech that does not have fluency." Now, as discussed earlier in this chapter, many of the so-called nonfluencies discoverable in samples of normal speech are not truly *non*-fluencies, simply because they are so routinely a part of normal fluency. In contrast, occurrences identified as stutters clearly create "speech that does not have fluency." Therefore, in a very literal sense, "disfluency" *is* equivalent to stuttering—although this is certainly not the sense intended by sources attempting to substitute disfluency for stuttering, or to make related claims.

Several times in this chapter, and especially in the preceding section, discussion has emphasized that hesitation phenomena, including those that are not integral to the message, are ordinarily so much a part of the speech flow that they are obscured within it. Sometimes, certain circumstances may elevate a filler into temporary prominence, after which it disappears once more into the flow of expression. In contrast, stutters are not obscure; in fact, they come into prominence quickly, and not through force of other circumstances. Most important, they do not subsequently revert to being, or thereafter become, an undetectable part of fluency, as do hesitation phenomena. Occasionally, a certain instance of stutter might not be readily distinguishable from some instance of a filler, but even on such infrequent occasions the filler too is for some reason obtrusive; that is, the event is not at that time participating as part of a vocal sequence perceived as fluent but is, on that occasion, prominent—as is the stutter to which it is being compared, even though the two remain different.

COMPARISON AND INTEGRATION

Table 10.3 presents a list of the types of filler found in the study of normal speech in comparison to the kinds of event in the Johnson list. Basically, the types reported from these two different lines of research reflect differences not only in the subject matter but also in the orientation to it. The two lists contain some evidently comparable items, but there are also real differences. Certain differences in entries are obvious (where dashes appear). Other items that are essentially comparable differ in specificity, as follows. The normal speech list contains three separate types (filled pause, intruding incoherent sound, and parenthetical remark) that the Johnson list combines as one type (interjections). Similarly, two types in the normal speech list (sentence correction and word change) are combined in the Johnson list as one type (revisions). The normal speech list combines into one type the two kinds of repetition (word and phrase) specified in the Johnson list. The different specifications in the two lists reflect the differential importance of certain items to the orientation they represent.

Hesitation phenomena items for which there are no counterparts in the Johnson list are: tongue slip, drawls, omissions, and silent pauses. Tongue slip is a reference to speech errors, which will be considered at length in the next chapter. Omission of whole words needs no comment. Regarding part-word omissions, we should recall Mahl's notation that they were of word-final sylla-

TABLE 10.3   Comparison of Items Listed in Tables 10.1 and 10.2

A. Audible

1.	filled pause	interjection	
2.	sentence correction	revision	
3.	sentence incompletion	incomplete phrase	
4.	repetition (of one or more words	phrase repetition word repetition	
5.	stutter	part-word repetition	
6.	intruding incoherent sound	interjection	
7.	tongue slip	——	
8.	word change	revision	
9.	parenthetical remark	interjection	
10.	drawl	——	
	——	broken word	[tension]
	——	prolonged sounds	[dysrhythmic phonation]

B. Silent

11.	omission (of word or part of word)	——	
12.	silent pause	——	

bles. Drawl is a common word meaning essentially a "drawing out," a lengthening of a word in ordinary speech. It too is a syllable-final phenomenon, occurring as a post-peak extension of the syllable nucleus (see discussion in Chapters 11 and 12 regarding syllable structure).

Pause is a special topic, important not only in terms of its extent but because of its roles in the speech process (see discussion in Chapter 11). Pause has been a major focus of interest in the normal speech research since the inception of that area of study. Goldman-Eisler's work was addressed only to nongrammatical pause (one form of Silent Pause). Mahl's work focused on Filled Pause,[18] which he wrote as "ah" and addressed as a separate category in contrast to all other hesitation phenomena, which he lumped together as "non-ah." The continuing interest in pause for understanding speech processes led O'Connell and Kowal (1980) to speak of a science of pausology. The important topic of pause will be considered at some length in the next chapter.

In contrast to the extensive investigations of both types of pause in the normal speech research, the bulk of stuttering research, oriented principally to the analysis reported by Johnson, has not considered silent pause, and has dealt with filled pause as simply one kind of interjection. Silent pause was omitted by Johnson because of "the practical difficulty of deciding whether or not given pauses were part of meaningful or expressive speech."[19] The reader should recognize that this description refers to difficulty in distinguishing between grammatical (juncture) and "hesitation" pause. Although the distinction may seem formidable to persons unfamiliar with the study of normal speech, the task is not so difficult as Johnson's statement indicates. For instance, Boomer and Dittman (1962) demonstrated that listeners could differentiate between juncture and hesitation pauses even when the two types were of comparable length. The matter can be resolved quite readily by attending to a number of cues. Juncture and hesitation pauses are most often not of comparable length; juncture pauses are regularly brief, rarely longer than 500 milliseconds; hesitation pauses are most often longer than a second. Beyond the variable of length, juncture pauses are of several kinds that are signaled by intonation contours—for which the various punctuation codes are attempted (but very inadequate) orthographic representations.[20]

The omission of pause in the Johnson analysis was a serious error, one whose significance has been magnified through the extent to which the Johnson list of "disfluencies" has been the reference in so much subsequent research. That research has remained insulated from other findings that reveal certain pause variables unique to stuttered speech. Probably the most compelling of these findings is the evidence, reported in several sources,[21] that the (seemingly) fluent speech of stutterers contains more (silent) pauses than normal speech, especially a high frequency of very short pauses. Such pauses, not readily discernible directly, are nonetheless significant for understanding speech production in stuttering. In addition, there are other, readily discerned, dimensions of pause, both silent and filled, that are unique to stuttering and that were also ignored by omitting consideration of pause. Discussion of these dimensions is presented most simply in reference to the most frequently occurring filled pause—"uh." In the Johnson list, "uh" is simply one of a variety of phenomena included in the general category of "Interjections" (see Table 10.2), wherein its uniqueness is obscured.

The classic Filled Pause is the ubiquitous "uh." Although certain other phenomena (see later) are appropriately included in the overall category of Filled Pause, "uh," because of its ubiquity, deserves to be considered separately. Understandably, "uh" is largely equivalent to Filled Pause in the psycholinguistic research. At the same time, there are several variants of filled pause that are demonstrably significant to fluency analysis (Wingate, 1984c) but which have received only minimal attention in the relevant literature. One important variation is locus of occurrence. The most common loci are: (1) as addition to a word, such as in the very common "anduh;" and (2) a single "uh" in isolation, between instances of silent pause. A third locus immediately precedes a word, to which the "uh" is connected.[22] This variant is rare; it is most likely to occur as a "starter" in stutter occurrences (see Chapter 3). Another important dimension of filled pause is the number per instance and their temporal sequence. Most often, in ordinary speech, several "uhs" in sequence are separated by silent pauses of a second or longer; less often the intervening silent pauses are shorter, but still perceptible as silences. In a third, infrequent, type the multiple "uhs" are immediately sequential; they are iterative.

This brings us to consider two remaining categories, in the Johnson list: the categories of "broken words" and "prolonged sounds," or the categories later substituted for them, "tension" and "dysrhythmic phonation." Either the original or the later pair of descriptors can be incorporated into a single category of prolongations.[23] Neither of these pairs, nor their inclusive category term, prolongations, has a comparison category in the Normal Nonfluency list—which indicates that they are characteristic of stuttering. This difference has been revealed consistently in the results of substantial comparative stuttering research, including Johnson's own data.[24]

The comparisons made of similarities and differences between the two lists of Table 10.3 contradict a claim asserted in the stuttering-based research, as noted earlier, namely, that all kinds of fluency irregularities are common to all speakers. Instead, the categories discovered in the study of normal speech provide a basic reference for pointing up the kinds of events that characterize stuttering. Prolongation does not show up in studies of normal speech. Another category, sound and syllable (part word) repetition, also does not appear routinely in assessments of normal speech; when it does appear there, it attracts use of the word "stutter," although in such instances the reference is benign. As noted earlier, the word stutter itself simply depicts a unique observation—of iterative speech phenomena. Again, the word is used descriptively and metaphorically in regard to various phenomena other than a curious disorder of speech, and in its descriptive reference nothing more is intended. At the same time, the essential reference of the word is to the distinctive speech disorder in which iterations of speech elements are the most obvious of the two classic markers of the disorder, as discussed in Chapter 3.

A COMPREHENSIVE LIST

The items presented in Table 10.4 are a consolidation of the items listed in Table 10.3, with certain refinements as brought into focus in the preceding

TABLE 10.4 Comprehensive List, Speech Flow Events

Code		Description	
Class I			
SP		Silent Pause 1 sec +. One may wish to record pause lengths	
FP	–a	Filled Pause	–a: as extension of a word (e.g., "anduh"
	–s		–s: single (e.g., "uh," "um," etc. bounded by SP)
	–m		–m: multiple (but not iterative; i.e., SPs are interspersed: e.g., "uh....uh....")
Reps I	–m	Repetitions Class I	–m: monosyllable word
	–p		–p: polysyllable word
	–f		–f: phrase
	[#/instance]		[number per instance, where more than one occur]
Rev	–w	Revision	–w: word
	–f+		–f+: phrase or longer
Inc	–w	Incomplete	–w: word
	–f		–f: phrase
	–s		–s: sentence
XW		Extraneous Word(s) – intrusive words not pertinent to the intended message (primarily such insertions as: "y'know; well"; etc., and also idiosyncratic or circumstantial ones)	
XS		Extraneous Sound – any oral/nasal/phrayngeal sound other than a FP (may be an isolated phone, a click, a cough, etc., or some unidentifiable noise)	
Class II			
FP –i		Filled Pause	–i: iterative (e.g., "uh-uh-uh")
Reps II	–snd	Repetitions Class II	– sound
	–syl		– syllable (incomplete; e.g., /kə- kə- kə- kæn/)
			Sound and syllable repetitions in initial positions as fragments of an intended word.*
	[#/instance]		[record number per instance]
Prl		Prolongation – involves the *early* part of a syllable, whether or not the syllable is C-initial.	
BW		Broken Word – an unnatural break in a word, in which the break may be occupied by an SP, or an FP or XS.	

*[/kə- kə- kə kæn/ as distinct from /kæn- kæn- kæn/. Special notation should be made of a syllable repetition that occurs as a bounded, or complete, syllable in a word of two or more syllables, such as /kəm- kəm- kəm- plit/. These are sufficiently rare that a category for them is not indicated.

section. The list is organized into two classes: Class I includes the types of occurrences reported in the psycholinguistics literature; Class II includes the irregularities unique to the literature on stuttering.[25] As reviewed earlier in this chapter, types in Class I also are found in the speech of stutterers; in fact, in substantial amounts. In contrast, although instances of Class II types may sometimes be observed in the speech of normally speaking individuals, such occurrences will be rare. A description of each type is entered in the right-hand column; the codes at the left are abbreviations of these identifications, primarily for use in recording.

The list omits drawls, tongue slips, and parenthetical remarks. Technically, drawls are not hesitation phenomena, even though they may be noticeable. "Drawl" is a common word, meaning essentially a "drawing out," the lengthening of a word already initiated in normal form. Importantly, it is a syllable-ending phenomenon, extending the syllable nucleus beyond its peak. Tongue slips also are a different kind of event. "Slips of the tongue," a description made famous by Sigmund Freud's account of these phenomena, has been supplanted by the designation "speech errors," which are discussed in Chapter 11. Speech errors may not be noticed by the speaker, in which case speaking proceeds apace; if noticed, they typically result in some kind of hesitation phenomenon, most likely a revision. Typically, parenthetical remarks are of more than one word, and usually have some pertinence to the message. Sometimes there is an accompanying filler, which is what merits being noted. If such remarks are not pertinent to the context, they may be catalogued as an "extraneous word." This category is also the appropriate heading for insertions such as "y'know," and the like. Although such insertions evidently serve the same purpose as "uh," they complicate the Filled Pause category; they are justifiably catalogued as a separate type.

The descriptions of the various types are quite straightforward. Silent Pauses vary in length; however, we will record only those longer than 1 second. Juncture pauses may sometimes be fairly lengthy, as in instances of rhetorical pause, but for the most part a temporal distinction corresponds to the character of the pause. The length of 1 second has become accepted in the hesitation phenomena literature as defining the lower limit of "hesitation" pauses. The limit happens to have a practical utility as well, since research has shown that human and machine recorders agree well in identifying silences longer than a second.[26]

The category of Filled Pause has been subdivided into the several variants discussed in the previous section. The first three described are normal in character and therefore appear in Class I; the fourth variant (iterative) is placed in Class II, essentially because of its iterative quality, which often is accompanied by other cues as to its nature.

Analyzing a Speech Sample

A speech sample should be obtained from an audio (or video) recording, with the objective of extracting a sample size of at least 600 words, preferably close to 1000 words.[27] The initial written transcription of the sample should concentrate on recording all verbal content. This must be done carefully, and one can anticipate having to compare the transcription and recording several times to obtain an accurate record. To this end it is advisable to transcribe in triple space, to allow adequate room for corrections and the subsequent notations of fillers. The next step is to review the transcription and recording again—as often as needed—to identify the type and locus of the hesitation phenomena, noting them by their pertinent code at their loci of occurrence.

Figure 10.1 presents a Fluency Analysis Chart for use in tabulating the frequencies with which the various fillers occur, as registered on the transcription. The headings of the chart correspond to the categories presented in Table 10.4. A simple technique for registering the frequency of each type is to first make tally marks in the appropriate boxes, then substitute number entries when finished. The chart includes spaces for totals and ratios. Total instances of Class I types and Class II types are recorded separately; the ratios express the proportion of items in each class relative to the number of words in the

Source	Class I														Class II					Totals			Ratios	
	SP	FP			Reps I			Revis		Incompl.			XW	XS	FP	Reps II		Prl	BW				# in class/ # of words	
		a	s	m	m	p	f	w	f+	w	f	s			(i)	snd	syll			Class I	Class II	# Words	I	II
1 M F																								
2 M F																								
3 M F																								
4 M F																								
5 M F																								

Source Identification

1)__________
2)__________
3)__________
4)__________
5)__________

Notes

FIGURE 10.1 Fluency analysis chart.

sample. The chart will accommodate entries for five separate subjects, if desired, but one practical use of the five separate lines is to use one line for each page of a single transcription. The source identification provides for entry of subject names, or page numbers (or other identity) and, when appropriate, whether male or female.

Figure 10.2 presents the Fluency Profile, on which the fluency analysis can be displayed graphically. Positioned immediately below the graph are the code entries corresponding to those in Table 10.4 and the Fluency Analysis Chart (Figure 10.1). For reference, abbreviated descriptions of the codes are annotated immediately below them. The three spaces directly above "SP" do not have specifications below them, as do most of the other types; the spaces were included to permit identifying levels of pause length if desired (for example, 1 second, 2 seconds, 3+ seconds). For most purposes, as discussed earlier, it is adequate to simply record SPs of longer than 1 second. The data entries called for on the first two lines at the lower part of the form are obvious. Spaces on the third line are for recording, first, the number of filler types of each class; then the Class I and Class II ratios, which represent the total number of each class divided by the number of words; and lastly the Nonfluency Index, which expresses the relative proportion of Class II to Class I types.

ILLUSTRATIONS

The remainder of this chapter presents Fluency Profiles of speech samples from 14 different individuals. All are adults, and all but one are male. Twelve speak normally, and two are stutterers.

Our principal interest is in the profiles of normal speech samples. They are presented here primarily to illustrate, as discussed earlier in the chapter, that hesitation phenomena occur in everyone's speech[28]—and concurrently, that fillers suggestive of an abnormal type occur rarely.

Figures 10.3 through 10.6 are profiles of eight individuals selected because they could represent a variety of speakers for whom normal speech, if not in fact *good* speech, is routinely expected (and routinely found). Also, they are individuals likely to be well known to most readers, and other samples of their speaking can be observed in appropriate live television programs. The next four profiles (Figures 10.7 and 10.8) are of samples from individuals who could be expected to represent ordinary speaking ability. The last two profiles (Figure 10.9) are of samples from stutterers. The latter profiles are included to provide contrasts to the normal samples and, as well, in special reference to content in

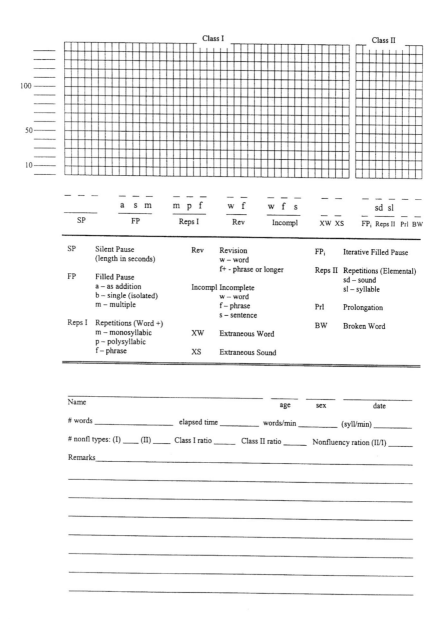

FIGURE 10.2   Fluency profile form.

Chapter 3, which was addressed to specification of the kinds of fluency features that characterize normal speech, and to which stutters stand in discriminable contrast.

THE SAMPLES OF NORMAL SPEECH

The first two samples are a serendipitous reference pair. The next six samples are from normal speakers known to be verbally capable, at least from their many television appearances; they were selected primarily because they are likely to be known to most readers. The subsequent four samples are from ordinary normal speakers whose appearance on a television program was unusual. The last two samples are from stutterers well known in the profession, speaking individually to a large audience, a routine with which each had much experience.

The profiles are presented in pairs, partly for economy of display but also, especially in regard to certain samples, for purposes of comparison. The raw data for each sample are limited to a registry of the number of words spoken, speech rate (in words per minute and syllables per minute), and the number of each type of filler. The derived ratios express the proportional frequencies of the two classes and their relative occurrence. Data for each of the various types were made proportional to a base of 1000 words in order to have their display in all 14 profiles be directly comparable to each other by visual inspection. Silent pauses of longer than 1 second were tabulated only when they occurred within a completed utterance, as reflected in a terminal juncture.

The first two samples were obtained long before my development of this approach to fluency analysis. Each of the two samples was recorded from a lecture aired on national educational television. Originally, my interest was to use the recordings for class illustrations of speech rate. That objective was prompted by having happened upon a Public Broadcasting System lecture from which the first sample below was taken. The speaker is an outstanding linguist whose "rapid delivery" has been remarked by many persons acquainted with him. The second sample, also a Public Broadcasting System program, was obtained a short time later. I saw these samples as providing a clear contrast in speech rate between two individuals who could be expected to have comparable verbal capability, considering their level of education, length of time in their chosen profession, and stature in their respective fields.

These samples have turned out to be pivotal examples for a major aspect of our concern with fluency. In respect to my initial interest, they do provide a good comparative illustration of differences in speech rate; significantly, they are equally remarkable for the contrast they provide in respect to level of perceived fluency, which is occasioned principally by a marked difference between the two samples in the amount of pause, both filled and silent. Much pause time in ordinary speech consists of brief pauses, of less than 1 second, which are not of concern in the illustrations presented here although they contributed to the computations of speech rate (see Pause discussion in Chapter 11). The relationship between pause and speech rate is quite direct and substantial. Speech rate, as measured and as perceived, is heavily influenced by the total amount of pause which, although of considerable extent in ordinary speech, is rarely noticed.

The Initial Pair (see Figure 10.3)

The first sample displayed in this figure, identified as NY, is from a lecture delivered by the linguist mentioned above, at a university in upstate New York. The second sample, identified as WA, is from a lecture given by an outstanding professor of Classics at a university in the state of Washington. Each was lecturing on a topic well known to him.

In listening to a recorded sample of NY's speech, as when listening to him "live," one is immediately impressed with his speech rate, particularly because his speech seems to be so continuous. This perception is well represented in his Fluency Profile, which shows notably few phenomena, essentially limited to a few instances of Silent Pause. Moreover, these pauses were predominantly rhetorical pauses, employed for emphasis. He has few other Class I types, and his instances of Class II types are limited to three repetitions, in which each type had only one occurrence per instance. His overall nonfluency pattern is reflected in a Class I ratio of 0.025 and Class II ratio of 0.003.

NY's sustained rate of speech, at 311 syllables per minute, is markedly above the average rate, which is generally accepted as being around 210 syllables per minute for young adults.[29] His "rapid delivery" is also characterized by brisk articulation, which contributes to the perception, as well as the actuality, of a fast rate of speech. However, as noted earlier, the extent of pause is the major determinant of speech rate (see section on Pause in Chapter 11).

The sample obtained from WA is notable for its contrast to the first sample. He evidences an extensive amount of the two most common varieties of Filled Pause (FPa and FPs), along with a substantial amount of Silent Pause. He also evidences more Class I pause types than NY, although there are few of any type. Like NY, his Class II types are rare; they consist of one instance each of the two repetition types, again one occurrence per instance. His speech pattern is reflected in a Class I ratio of 0.25, which is 10 times as large as NY's. However, his Class II nonfluencies yield a ratio of 0.003, identical to NY's.

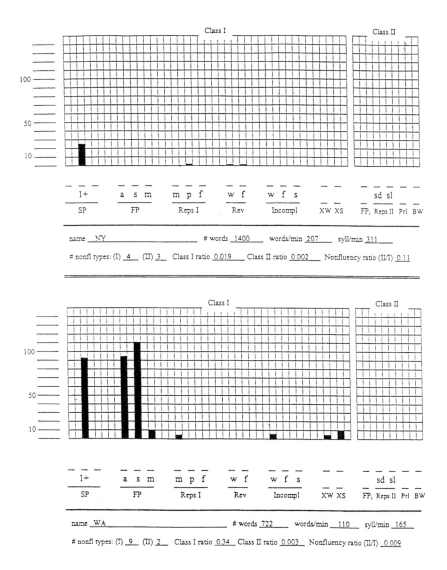

FIGURE 10.3   Fluency profile: professional speakers—1 (professors).

WA's speech rate of 165 syllables per minute is well below the reference average rate of 210. In contrast, NY's rate is twice as far above the average. Another dimension of contrast is that WA's articulation had a quality of ease and casualness. However, the clearly major determinant of his slow rate of speech is the extensive amount of pause.

A fluency pattern like WA's is not common among professors, but neither is it particularly rare. For instance, Moore (1935) found that "pausing too long in talking" was one of the most frequently mentioned "annoying habits of college professors." Silent pauses are not so likely to be remarked, but filled pauses, especially if frequent or "bunched" (to use Mahl's description), soon become noticed and then may become conspicuous. A professor of one of my undergraduate courses spoke in a manner similar to WA, enough so that occasionally several of us in the class would conspire to compare tallies of an hour's frequency of "uhs." However, and highly pertinent to discussion earlier in this chapter, most often one or more of us would become absorbed in the lecture and forget to tally throughout the appointed hour. Many readers may recall a similar experience.

WA's fluency pattern, which by computation is demonstrably below the average value for rate, and undoubtedly well above average in terms of number of pauses, would most likely fall at the lower limit of a pertinent statistical distribution. A lay judgment of such a pattern would almost certainly describe it as "below the norm" in regard to some vague lay standard (as discussed earlier in this chapter). However, one would not likely find the speaker's fluency identified seriously as *ab*normal on grounds of either the number of pauses or the rate perceived.[30]

Television Journalists

The next pair of profiles (Figure 10.4) are of samples from David Gergen and Mark Shields, nationally prominent reporters and political analysts. For a number of years they appeared together weekly as political commentators on the Public Broadcasting System's *MacNeil–Lehrer News Hour*, from which these samples were taken.

I first came to consider them for fluency illustration because they are both verbally very capable. Moreover, from casual attention to their speech there seemed initially to be some difference in the fluency of the two men, with Gergen appearing to evidence somewhat more hesitation phenomena than Shields. After attending more carefully, concurrent with extracting and transcribing these samples, this initial judgment was seen to most likely have resulted from three influences: as revealed in the analysis, Gergen does have a faster rate; typically he speaks rather energetically and with a seemingly more

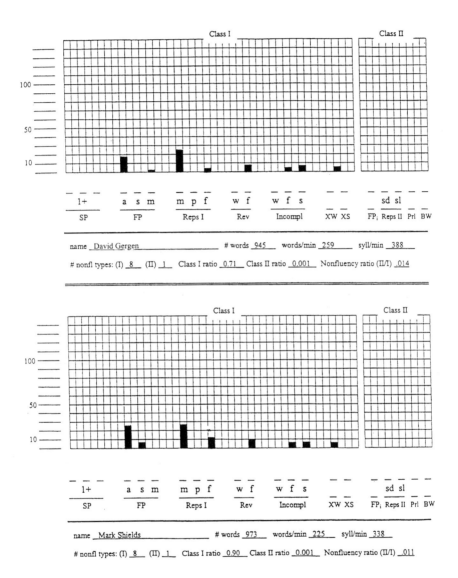

FIGURE 10.4 Fluency profile: professional speakers—2 (political analysts).

intense manner; but also, and probably most influential of the three, his fillers were more often "bunched." As discussed earlier, such occurrence tends to bring fillers to notice.

It is, then, particularly instructive to find the considerable similarity in fluency pattern of these two speakers, which is clearly Class I. They evidence similar numbers of several types, and comparable frequencies within each type. Although each evidenced one Class II repetition, in both cases it is limited to a single occurrence for that instance. Their summary ratios are very similar. Of special interest, contrary to the original casual impression described above, Shields actually has the higher Class I ratio.

National Figures

The fluency profiles next in sequence (Figure 10.5) are for speech samples from Billy Graham and William F. Buckley. Graham, the well-known evangelist, should need no introduction. Buckley is a writer, editor of the magazine *The National Review*, and host of a regular television program, *Firing Line*, addressed to current affairs.

The sample of Graham's speech was obtained from an interview with David Frost in which the content centered around Graham's beliefs and relevant biographical matters. Graham characteristically speaks in an easy manner; somewhat sonorously, with pronunciation often having a quality of drawl. It should be noted that he was speaking about things well known to him, much of which he probably had expressed in at least similar form and manner many times before. His speech rate of 171 syllables per minute is considerably below the reference average. The range of his nonfluency types is small, the narrowest of the samples presented here; the range is almost limited to the most common form of filled pause, and even these are few. Consequently, his Class I ratio is the lowest of the samples presented here. Also, he evidenced no Class II irregularities. This speech pattern would seem to reflect, beyond idiosyncrasy, the effect of his particular, and lengthy, professional experience. Briefly put, although this sample is of truly spontaneous speech, it is unique inasmuch as having come from a practiced, polished speaker talking about long-familiar material.

Buckley is widely recognized as an assertively articulate spokesman for political conservatism. This sample was taken from a *Firing Line* program in which he and two knowledgeable guests discussed the problem of illiteracy in the United States. As always, the discussion was impromptu.

Buckley expresses his views clearly and precisely, speaking in an assured, decisive manner that varies in tempo, at times seeming a bit hurried. He evidences an excellent vocabulary and careful word choice. Occasionally he

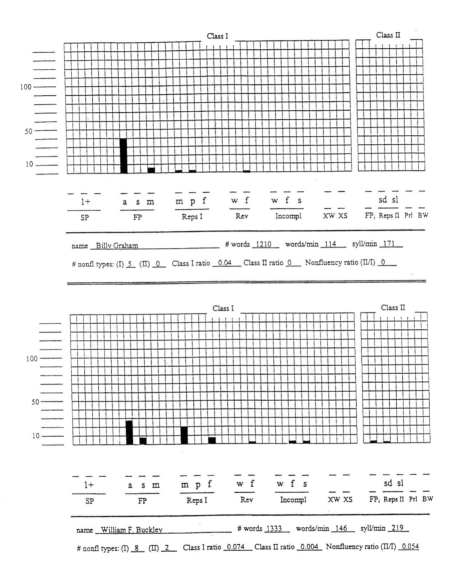

FIGURE 10.5   Fluency profile: professional speakers—3 (national figures).

seems to be at a momentary loss for the exact word or phrase to express a point with the desired precision. It is at such points, and in the context of increased tempo, that an iterative filled pause may occur. The three instances registered here were each of three "uhs" per instance. His one sound repetition had only a single repeat. These occurrences give a measurable Class II ratio, which, though slight, is notably greater than in the other normal speech samples presented here, and leads also to a higher nonfluency ratio—which is, however, still negligible. His Class I types, and frequencies within certain types, are similar to other normal speakers sampled, and his Class I ratio is well within the range of most of the other normal speakers. His speech rate is just above the reference average.

Of particular pertinence to issues in the identification of stuttering, presented in Chapter 3, it is important to note that Buckley evidences, while speaking, what would generally be described as "little mannerisms." These vary in kind and frequency. Among the more prominent are: raising the eyebrows, which is sometimes one aspect of retraction of the full scalp; protrusion and lateral movement of the tongue; and retraction of the corners of the mouth, which sometimes eventuates in a genuine smile. These movements occur most often during brief silent pauses, and at times they seem possibly relevant to expressed content. However, there is no indication that they are aspects of, or involved with, speech production itself.

Sportscasters

The next pair of profiles (Figure 10.6) are samples from notable persons intimately associated with American football: John Madden and "Pat" Summerall. Madden was for many years head coach of the Oakland Raiders; Summerall played with several professional teams over a period of 10 years. Both men became live-broadcast announcers and commentators for televised professional football games, and often work together. The samples on which these profiles are based were obtained during one of these events. Both men know their subject thoroughly and are well able to speak expertly about it.

Speech samples from these men were selected for illustration especially because of the contrast in their speaking patterns. Madden is characteristically vigorous and animated in expression, thorough and explicit in his descriptions and analyses. One is vaguely aware that he speaks rather rapidly, but his speech is always readily intelligible. Summerall is much more casual in manner, speaks more calmly, reflectively and seemingly much slower.

One's casual impression regarding the comparative rates of these two speakers is clearly confirmed by the rate figure of 204 syllables per minute for Summerall, compared to Madden's rate of 365 syllables per minute. The latter

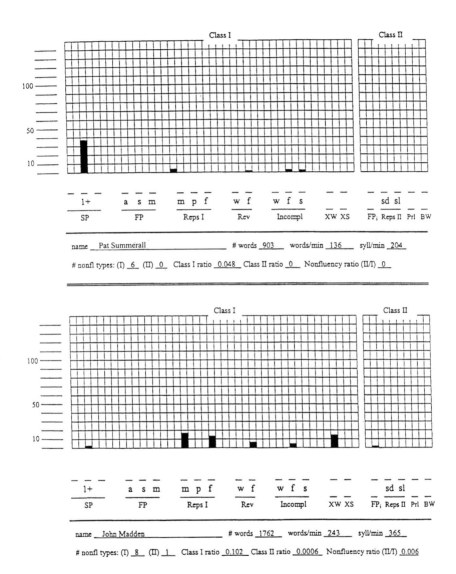

FIGURE 10.6   Fluency profile: professional speakers—4 (sports announcers).

rate, highest of the samples presented here, is considerably higher than one might expect[31] from listening to live broadcasts of his commentary. The difference in pattern between these two speakers also is reflected in the data regarding types and amounts of fillers. Although both speakers evidence a similar range of types, Madden's are predominantly audible, whereas Summerall's are primarily silent pauses, which are not as noticeable. Madden's greater number of fillers yields a Class I ratio twice as great as Summerall's; however, their Class II and nonfluency ratios are essentially identical—minuscule for Madden and zero for Summerall.

Cartoonists

The next four profiles (Figures 10.7 and 10.8) will be considered as a group. The four speakers—Steve Kelley, Doug Marlette, Michael Ramirez, and Ann Telnaes—are editorial cartoonists for widely read sources.[32] They were interviewed by Elizabeth Farnsworth of *The News Hour with Jim Lehrer* regarding their retrospection of a year's events that had prompted each of them to create certain memorable cartoons.

These four samples were selected as being very likely to represent speech patterns to be found among "ordinary citizens," for whom speaking in public is not a frequent, certainly not a familiar, event and whose fluency might be adversely affected by being interviewed on a national-level television program. Other features about them that increased the value of their speech samples for purposes of illustration were the following. All four are of similar age; they have achieved comparably in the same profession, especially one that does not rely upon or make specific use of verbal capability. At the same time, fulfilling the expectations of their profession requires familiarity with current events as well as the ability to select and "comment" about certain of these events in conceptual terms, which, though often expressed graphically, they were well able to cast into verbal form.

These samples contain certain notable similarities and differences. All speech rates are above the reference average of 210 syllables per minute; in fact, three of the four are considerably higher. As with the other samples, all four evidence a range of Class I types, and for each individual the pattern varies in respect to both types and the frequencies within them. Three of the four evidence a Class I ratio considerably above that of other normal samples, except for WA. As with most of the other normal samples, there is little silent pause to register. Also like the other normal samples, Class II irregularities are rare: two samples have only one repetition each; in both instances the repeat was single.

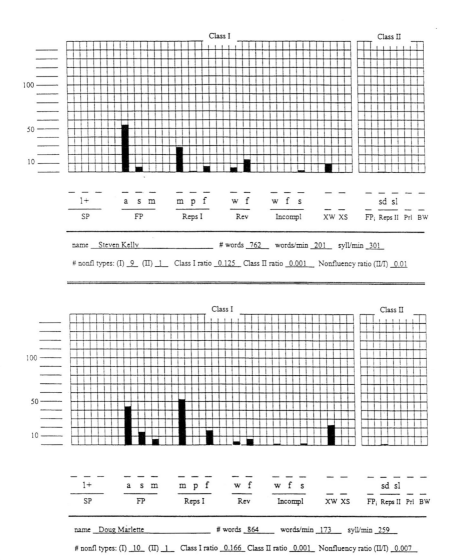

FIGURE 10.7   Fluency profile: ordinary speakers—1 (cartoonists).

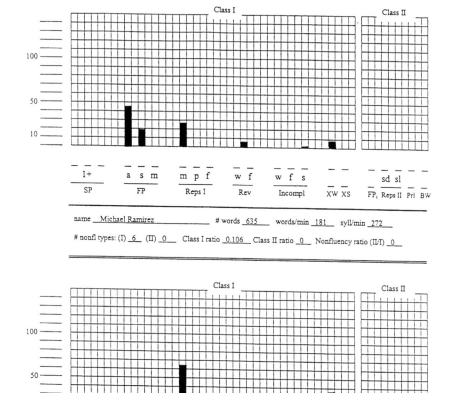

name __Michael Ramirez_____ # words _635___ words/min _181___ syll/min _272__

nonfl types: (I) _6_ (II) _0_ Class I ratio _0.106_ Class II ratio _0_ Nonfluency ratio (II/I) _0_

name __Ann Telnaes_____ # words _502___ words/min _188___ syll/min _282__

nonfl types: (I) _9_ (II) _0_ Class I ratio _0.159_ Class II ratio _0_ Nonfluency ratio (II/I) _0_

FIGURE 10.8   Fluency profile: ordinary speakers—2 (cartoonists).

NORMAL SAMPLES REVIEW

The 12 samples just presented provide clear illustration that certain "nonflu-encies" are a part of normal speech. At the same time, as one might well expect, there is considerable variation in the expression of such events.

The extent of nonfluency is revealed in the Class I ratios, which ranges from 2 to 34%, with an average of 11% for these 12 speakers. Moreover, these values do not include silent pauses of 1 second or less, which previous research has indicated constitute almost three-quarters of silent pause occurrences.

The types of hesitation phenomena observed in individual samples range from 4 to 10, with an average of over 7 types. The two most prevalent types are monosyllabic word repetitions [Reps 1 m] and filled-pause-as-word-addi-tion [FPa]. Monosyllabic word repetitions, marginally the most common event, occurred in 11 samples, with an average occurrence frequency of 24. Filled-pause-as-addition occurred in 10 samples, with an average occurrence fre-quency of 36. Phrase revisions [Rev f] also occurred in 10 samples, but with an occurrence frequency of only 5.

The next most prevalent nonfluency types are: phrase repetition [Reps 1 f], in nine samples, with an average frequency of 6.6; extraneous words [XW], in eight samples, average frequency of 13; and single filled pauses [FPs], in seven samples, with an average frequency of 27.

Class II irregularities are rare. Although observed in eight of the samples, the average occurrence frequency for all types combined is only 1.2. Moreover, they are qualitatively unremarkable.

Several aspects of speech rate in these 12 normal speech samples are notable. The range of rates is extensive, from 165 to 388 syllables per minute—a range similar to those reported in other research. The average rate (238 syllables per minute) is considerably higher than the reference average (210 spm). The two slowest are less than half the fastest, yet only three rates fall below the reference average.

Overall, these samples show hesitation phenomena to be commonplace features of spontaneous speech, although expressed through a notable amount of individuality in actual patterns of their occurrence. The patterns of types and their relative frequencies constitute a major dimension of what may be called individual "speech style."[33] To consider a speech style to be characteristic of an individual, one should anticipate analyzing more than one sample of the person's speech. However, there is reason to expect considerable stability in speech style, as revealed in the work of Goldman-Eisler (1968) and others, and attested by the following report.

One might expect that speech content and speaking circumstances are likely to influence measures of fluency. Schachter and colleagues (1991) found that the frequency of "uhs" in the lectures of college professors varied systematically with subject matter, being lowest in the natural sciences, considerably more in the social sciences, and highest of all in the humanities.[34] The investigators had predicted these results on grounds that there are differing options in the working vocabulary of these three disciplines, with sciences likely to have the fewest expressive options and humanities the most; therefore, more points of decision in the latter, leading to more "uhs."

At the same time, clear evidence of individuality was found by comparing the frequency of "uhs" in the speech of these same individuals in interview. For each individual, the "uh" frequency in interview was higher than in lecture. The frequency varied slightly among individuals, but this variation was not related systematically to the respective discipline each speaker represented.

SAMPLES OF STUTTERED SPEECH

The first eight samples of normal speech, selected to serve as a sort of reference, were obtained from individuals who, from preparation or achievement, could be assumed to be capable in word knowledge and usage and to have had experience speaking in public. The individuals from whom the stuttered speech samples were obtained, Wendell Johnson and Charles Van Riper, clearly meet such criteria. Both were professors whose credentials include an earned doctoral degree, extensive professional writing, and years of presentations at public gatherings in addition to delivery of class lectures. They are well known in the profession.

These samples (displayed in Figure 10.9) are the full recordings of presentations made to a large audience at a national convention of the American Speech and Hearing Association. Johnson and Van Riper were participating, with several other individuals, in a program featuring "recovered" stutterers, each of whom spoke about his own stuttering and what he had done to improve his speech. The word "recovered" is placed in quotation marks (as it was in the convention program) because, although the speech of the participants evidently had improved considerably, it was not the speech of a normal speaker.

Johnson's speech has a measured quality. Although fairly resonant, there is a cautious, rather constrained quality to the delivery and at certain points a clearly tentative manner of proceeding, often with noticeable pause that, from time to time, is associated with an evident Class II irregularity. In contrast, Van Riper's speech has a fuller sound and gives the impression of moving more slowly. Both of these features reflect Van Riper's employ of a form of controlled prolonging, which he acknowledges openly. This form of control enables him to slide through many potential "blocks," although in many instances the

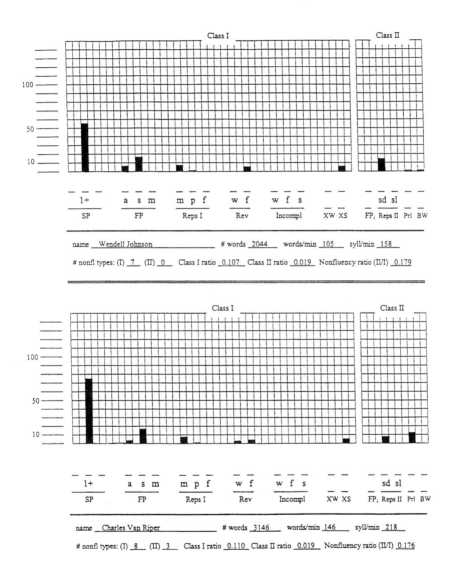

FIGURE 10.9   Fluency profile: professional speakers—5 (stutterer professors).

blocks are not completely obscured. Also, as his profile shows, a number of prolongations discernible as stutter are evident.

The fluency profiles of these two men have several notable similarities, two of which are particularly compelling in contrast to the other samples presented here. One of these features is the impressive frequency of silent pauses lasting 1 second or longer. In comparison to the normal speech samples illustrated here, in which silent pauses of longer than 1 second were seldom observed, the pattern in these two samples shows the reverse; most of their Class nonfluencies are silent pauses. This finding is consistent with the evidence from certain previous research, mentioned earlier in this chapter, regarding the extent of pause in the speech of stutterers. The other notable feature, which could have been expected, is the amount of Class II irregularities.

Both samples have the same number of Class II irregularities, but they differ in type—a difference that is discernible in the manner of speaking observed for the two men, as described above. The very substantial amounts of silent pause have a significance related to the matter of Class II events. It seems evident that the pauses recorded here are reflections of the control being exercised by each speaker. To a certain extent, these silent pauses are substitutes for some type of Class II irregularity. This pattern exemplifies a point made in Chapter 3, namely, that some stutterers mask a potential stutter by being able to substitute what could be considered a normal speech irregularity[35] (of which silent pause is the simplest).

These two profiles also show similar numbers of other Class I types, and very similar frequencies in certain of those types: filled pauses and repetition forms. The two samples also yield very similar summary values as represented in the Class I, Class II, and nonfluency ratios.

However, there is a notable difference in speech rate between the two speakers, Johnson's measured rate being considerably the slower. This difference, relative to his lower number of recorded silent pauses, suggests that those pauses were generally of longer duration than Van Riper's. This inference is consistent with the direct impression of Johnson's speech, as described early in this section. The difference in rate may also reflect differences in amount of (unmeasured) brief silent pauses, which always contribute to measures of speech rate. (This matter is discussed in Chapter 11.)

SUMMARY

To be fluent in a language means that one is able to express oneself in a manner comparable to the ordinary speaker of the language. There are many variables that contribute to the identification of a nonnative speaker of a language, such as pronunciation, accent, and the like. The typical native speaker is usually at least subliminally sensitive to most of these variables in the speech of another person, even though he may not consciously take note of them. However, even when such deviations are evident, if they are not so obtrusive that the speaker can convey his message well, he will be accepted as being fluent in the language. The judgment of fluency in a language overlooks immaterial departures in the kind of variables just noted (minor aberrations in pronunciation, regional dialect, etc.). The essential focus of a judgment of fluency centers on the perception of the words spoken, the major carrier of the message.

Universally, both listeners and speakers are intent upon the speaker's message, which is borne substantially through words, typically uttered in an appropriate sequence. With attention focused on the message that is emerging through the words that carry it, the sequence of words is regularly perceived as continuous. This perception is well supported by the fact that, on the whole, there is a certain real continuity within sequences of a speaker's words. However, the extent of this continuity is illusory. Contrary to common belief, fluent speech is not literally a flow of words. In fact, ordinary spontaneous speech is largely discontinuous in the literal sense of words in extended sequence.

A speaker's word sequences, of varying lengths, are interspersed with both silent and audible events, some of which are integral to the message, but many of which are not. The latter, which most often are not actually part of the message, are nonetheless part of "the speech stream"—incorporated in the perception of fluent speech. They occur with notable frequency in everyone's speech, yet both speakers and listeners are hardly aware of most of them. Because such events are routinely accepted as part of ordinary fluent expression, the extent of their occurrence went unrecognized in the long history of interest in speech.[36] Actually, their extent and significance is still not properly acknowledged, even though the variety and frequency of these events has been well reported since their discovery in the middle years of the twentieth century.

Among the variety of these phenomena, seven major types, with certain subtypes, are identified here as Class I. These types are characteristic of normal speech, found in anyone's speech. The commonality of their occurrence is well illustrated through recording speech samples of verbally capable, experienced normal speakers, as well as in samples of individuals presumably more representative of ordinary speakers. Individual differences among speakers are clearly revealed by displaying occurrence frequencies of the several types in a profile format.

Certain other speech phenomena, identified here as Class II, represent the classic markers of stutter events, as discussed in Chapter 3. As expected, they are prominent in samples of stuttered speech. Samples of stuttered speech also contain many instances of Class I events—consistent with the observation that instances of Class I occur in everyone's speech. In contrast, instances of only certain Class II types (elementary repetitions) occur but rarely in samples of normal speech, in which occurrences they also are most often perceptibly different in character from what might seem to be comparable instances in stuttered speech.

The utility of the classification, and the analytic procedure presented here, have been demonstrated in successful use by undergraduate students at two different universities. While careful use of the procedure does require time, it has been found easy to use.

NOTES

1. See Wingate (1997, p. 32 ff).

2. See references under these names.

3. Silences in psychotherapeutic interview have long been recognized as likely to signal unexpressed content having special significance.

4. Primarily Filled Pauses; see later in this chapter and in Chapter 11.

5. Other favorable qualities of oral expression are: "to utter distinctly; pronounce carefully; enunciate; expressing oneself clearly; well formulated; clearly presented." These descriptions, and those for the other italicized words in this paragraph and the two that follow, are taken from Webster's New World Dictionary, Second Concise Edition (1982). Similar entries will be found in any standard dictionary.

6. Although written as "ah" in Mahl's extensive reports (see review in Wingate, 1988). Standard dictionaries (as the preceding) also include "er" as a conventionalized writing of this "vocalized pause."

7. See also Figure 11.4 and pertinent discussion.

8. The reader is reminded of discussion in Chapter 9 regarding the influence of literacy.

9. Certain word and phrase repetitions, intended for emphasis, are not superfluous.

10. See discussion of meaning in Chapter 11.

11. See later discussion regarding various expressions of "uh."

12. See review in Wingate (1988, pp. 47–54).

13. Critical review of these terms is presented by Wingate (1984a, 1987).

14. Or such faulty expansions as "within-word disfluencies" and "between-word disfluencies" (reviewed in Chapter 7).

15. Readers interested in details of the list collation are referred to chapter 2 of The Structure of Stuttering (Wingate, 1988).

16. See later in this chapter regarding reservations about this term.

17. The extent to which this was actual discovery was not acknowledged in the Johnson report.

18. Which consists almost entirely of some variant of /ə/, the so-called "neutral vowel," variously spelled as "uh," "um," "m," and "er," (Mahl's "ah" is not found often).

19. Johnson & Associates (1959, p. 201).

20. The standard juncture marks are also inadequate.

21. See Love & Jeffress (1971), Watson & Love (1965), and Zerbin (1973).

22. As in items 5 and 7 in Table 3.1.

23. Wingate (1964, 1976, pp. 44–46). As developed in Chapter 3, "protractions" is a preferable term.

24. See Wingate (1962a, 1976, pp. 52–60); also, Johnson's own data in Johnson (1961, table 6); Johnson & Associates (1959, pp. 134–135; 206–207).

25. These classes correspond, respectively, to the designations Type N and Type S used in *The Structure of Stuttering*. Class I and Class II are used here to avoid the possible interpretation that Type N are found only in normal speech, and conversely, that Type S would never be observed in normal speech.

26. See, for instance, Hargreaves & Starkweather (1959), Siegman (1978), and Weintraub (1981). Of course, depending upon one's interests or objectives, different lengths of silences can be recorded, but instrumentation is needed for the shorter durations.

27. Ordinarily, 8 minutes should be adequate to obtain a sample of this size.

28. The companion feature of this fact—that such "nonfluencies" routinely are not detected—cannot be shown directly for these samples, but one can appreciate from the accompanying descriptions of the speakers' manner that in most of these samples too it is likely that at least many "nonfluencies" went unnoticed.

29. See Brigance (1936), Cotton (1936), Howes & Geschwind (1969), Lieberman (1973), Ptacek & Sander (1966), and Yorkston & Beukelman (1980).

30. Even though one might be prompted to think of comedian Tim Conway's "The ...... Slow .... Talkers .... of .... America .... Association."

31. To casual, and retrospective, assessment I would have judged his rate as much like that of "NY" (first sample). Actually, it is 17% faster.

32. Respectively, the *San Diego Union Tribune*, *Newsday*, the *Memphis Commercial Appeal*, and *USA Today*, and the *North American Syndicate*.

33. Such as in the comprehensive analyses done by Sanford (1942).

34. Represented in some measure in the contrasting speech samples of NY and WA, the first two illustrations presented here.

35. And that is, moreover, a form of control.

36. See O'Neill (1980) and Wingate (1997).

CHAPTER 11

Normal Speech Processes

Talk implements conscious life but it wells up
into consciousness out of unconscious depths.

W. J. Ong, *Orality and Literacy*

Specifically, we are more than ever baffled by how
language performs its primary function, to convey
meaning. All our understanding of the mechanics
of language, built up from real or fancied elementary building blocks, stops dead before the
question of meaning.

A. C. Oettinger, *The Semantic Wall*

A central theme of this book is that stuttering is a disorder of speech. This
theme follows initially from the obvious fact that "stutter" is, and has
always been, recognized as a unique anomaly in speaking, wherein
"speech" is understood in its comprehensive traditional reference, not simply
as the activity of making oral movements (see pertinent discussion in Chapter
9). There is now a substantial body of evidence that dimensions of the process
of generating and producing speech are significantly involved in the disorder
of stuttering. It is, then, necessary that serious students of stuttering become
conversant with what is known about (normal) speech processes. Much of such

content does not appear in sources especially relevant to the study of stuttering, which is a major reason for giving the subject special coverage here.

The content of this chapter is addressed to findings, derived from study of normal speakers, regarding various aspects of speech and speech processes with which persons interested in stuttering should be familiar. This knowledge will serve as a foundation reference against which to view pertinent findings in the speech of stutterers, to be considered in Chapter 12. Our coverage of this very important content cannot be comprehensive since the literature pertinent to each of several areas in the field is itself extensive. However, synoptic review and discussion of major lines of inquiry in the field should provide the student a foundation adequate to appreciate the complexity of its several dimensions. The objective in discussion of these topics is to acquaint the reader with the many functions that careful analysis and deduction suggest must be operative in the production of ordinary spontaneous speech. Little attention will be given to attempts to explain the operation of this marvelous capacity, since it is not really understood, contrary to the presumption in certain sources.

FIRST OF ALL

One matter of fundamental importance, deserving emphasis at the outset, is that speech is *not* automatic! As discussed in Chapter 9, the commonplace lifelong experience with speech underlies the practically universal casual attitude with which speech is regarded. Certainly this attitude is standard among the laity, whether or not well-educated. Unfortunately, it also is evident in orientations within some areas of speech or language study, especially notable in some discussions of stuttering, as revealed in the stated objective of aiding stutterers to regain "the automaticity of speech." The assumption that speech is somehow automatic appears, as well, even in recent reports of stutter research that make reference to normal speech (e.g., Andrews et al., 1983; Christenfeld, 1996; de Nil et al., 2000).

As should become evident through material presented later in this chapter, it is doubtful that any aspect of speech production occurs automatically. The description "automatic" dismisses many very important functions, including: intent, planning, analysis, judgment, adjustment, and other operations as well. Conditions conducive to thinking of speech in terms of it being "automatic" are set up by our life experiences with speaking in which our own speech, and that of others as well, seems to occur so readily and effortlessly, through actions of which we are largely unaware. However, "automatic" is also misused in describing many other human activities that are much less preconditioned than is speaking, in which "automatic" dismisses the role of processes of which the average person should be aware. One simple example should suffice as relevant illustration.

Many times I have heard someone say, in describing an averted mishap while driving, something like "I automatically hit the brake and swerved to the right." The reactions being reported were by no means automatic; they were not even at a reflexive level. Certain reflex actions undoubtedly participated, but the whole event involved a number of complex determining processes such as, at least: perception, memory, recall, analysis, judgment, decision, and appropriate motor adjustments. The fact that everything ran off so well and so rapidly does not in any way make the process "automatic," although the ease of performance makes it seem so. No doubt the reader can think of many comparable events, and in other areas, that would yield the same illustration.

The example of a musician's performance is especially appropriate to elucidate how "automatic" cannot possibly describe ordinary speech. For instance, a skilled pianist will rehearse any particular composition many, many times before giving a formal performance, on which occasion(s) it will almost certainly proceed without error. Although the activity is highly practiced, well rehearsed, performed many times, even "routinized," it is by no means automatic. Each time performed, even according to the score, it is a little different, and in many tiny ways undetected by the audience or even the performer. Beyond that, the artist may intentionally alter the "interpretation" of the selection.

For our purposes, the crux of the matter, to be considered in more detail later, is that processes analogous to those reflected in musical performance occur continuously within the complex activity of speaking. Playing a musical composition, and speaking, are both serial phenomena, but that is the sum of their identity. Speaking is an infinitely more complex activity, and typically is not only unrehearsed, but created anew for the occasion. The complex processes of speech, many times more intricate than the sequences of activity represented in examples of any other human skills, most certainly do not run off automatically.

Persons in speech pathology, in particular, should be knowledgeable about the ultimate reference for the only permissible use of "automatic" in regard to speech, found in the area of aphasia. In the late nineteenth century, the outstanding British neurologist, Hughlings Jackson, from his study of the speech of aphasics, developed the classifications of *propositional speech* and *automatic speech*.[1]

PROPOSITIONAL SPEECH

Propositional speech will be discussed first because it sets the framework against which "automatic," as applied to speech, is properly understood. The classification "propositional speech" taps the essence of normal, ordinary speaking. In Jackson's words, it "states a proposition," meaning that what is uttered is newly created by the speaker and conveys an intended, meaningful message, pertinent in context and understandable as such by listeners. It reflects intellectual processes participating in a specially created verbal communication, as conveyed in Jackson's reference to the "clear preconception" inherent in it. Most propositional speech consists of words in sequence, which, *in toto*, may be fairly lengthy sequences. However, propositionality is not necessarily qualified by length of utterance; single-word utterances, even "yes" and "no," may be propositional if they are pertinent to context and reflect an intended message. The essential requirements are those stated above, which pertain most often to connected speech, that is, word sequences of some length.

Nonetheless, varying levels of propositionality can be identified, the various levels representing differing degrees of "cognitive complexity." Increases in cognitive complexity pose greater demands on the speech production system relative to word selection, word sequencing, and overall verbal organization. For instance, describing a simple machine is a much less demanding task than explaining how the machine operates. Importantly, especially for our interests, fluency is clearly related to cognitive complexity. This interaction was well illustrated in some of the early psycholinguistic study (see Goldman-Eisler, 1968), wherein several differences in verbal expression, especially "hesitation phenomena," were revealed through the tasks of interpreting, as compared to describing, uncaptioned cartoons. More recent work, such as that of Dillon (1983), has identified an extended range of cognitive complexity levels[2] and concurrent decreases in fluency.

Propositionality is also interlaced with prosody, wherein stress is the agency for signaling the relative importance of words in sequences. Stress is applied not just to words to be emphasized but also to other "non-redundant" words (Liberman & Prince, 1977)—that is, words that are used infrequently, which almost certainly identifies them as words of the "content" category (see later in this chapter). This pattern of interrelationship between propositionality, linguistic stress, word frequency, and word type will reemerge in later contexts.

"AUTOMATIC" SPEECH

"Automatic" speech, in contrast to propositional speech, is best described as being devoid of the characteristics just noted. The classic example is cursing, or other similar emotional exclamations. Some sources have included within descriptions of automatic speech what has been called "old" speech, that is, verbal utterances that are well-practiced, routinized, expressed without evident contextual formulation. The examples usually given are the routine, simple expressions that are an aspect of what has been called "social lubrication," the widely used, informal, spontaneous greetings and replies, and the salutations at departure. These expressions are for the most part simple, brief, oft-repeated, well practiced, sometimes even routinized. However, despite such aspects of their occurrence, they do not regularly exemplify automatic speech. They embody certain characteristics that, in most circumstances, lift them out of this category. First, they are most often appropriate and pertinent to context. They also may vary in form of expression, thereby reflecting processes of judgment, decision, selection, etc. At the same time, they clearly do not fit the requirements of truly propositional speech. Such expressions occupy a position between automatic and propositional; they are best described as *phatic*.

PHATIC EXPRESSION

The word phatic is an abbreviation of the description "phatic communion" originated by the anthropologist Malinowski (1923) specifically to identify speech of the type just described. "Phatic communion" refers to speech that is used to establish social relationships rather than to impart information. For this reason the word "phatic" has become extended in meaning to denote speech having formal or trivial verbal content. In a practical sense, "phatic" describes speech of a low level of propositionality, as reviewed above.

PROPOSITIONAL LEVELS

Examples of "naturally occurring" variation in levels of propositionality can be found in some aphasic efforts referred to as "word salads," and certain more intelligible utterances of recovering aphasics. Diminished propositionality characterizes some psychotic communications as well. Also, it is possible to construct or modify (written) verbal sequences, for experimental purposes, that yield varying levels of approximation to a fully propositional expression, as in Taylor and Moray (1960). Simpler means of eliciting low levels of propositionality include having written material spoken in reverse order, or creating material in which word order is jumbled, or constructing lists of words varying in "connectedness." Actually, even reading aloud ordinary prose is at least one step below full propositionality, inasmuch as the oral reading of prepared material lacks the features of newly generated, spontaneous utterance—and, most often, immediate pertinence as well.

Ordinary spontaneous speech is typically unrehearsed—it is created anew for the particular immediate occasion. Many of the same words are used repeatedly, but with varying frequency and with considerable variation in their context and in how they are said. Moreover, some phoneticians contend that, as an expression of allophonic and free variation of phonemes, a person never says something in the exactly same way twice—to the extent that even individual phonemes are not reproduced exactly.[3] The inclination to view "speech sounds" as being always the same reflects lack of phonetic sophistication that, as emphasized in Chapter 9, is deepened by the insidious influence of our extensive experience with print.

The claim that even phonemes are not reproduced exactly may seem extravagant, but its plausibility can be readily appreciated with a simple demonstration from the analogous function of writing. If one's name is written 10 times in succession, one below the other, the signature is clearly "the same" in all 10 samples, as would be attested by any viewer. Yet variation in the whole and in its parts will also be evident to even casual inspection. In comparison, the phones of spoken words are subject to many more influences than in writing the sequential letters of the same words.[4] A comparative illustration would be to note the differences between a sequence of 10 typewritten word groups and the same words handwritten 10 times.

Ordinary spontaneous speech is the antithesis of "automatic." The hallmark of spontaneous speech is *planning*. Long-term study of the process has led to the realization that speech production must, in fact, involve several areas of planning.

There is no need, or space, to review in detail what is now known about these processes. However, a reasonably comprehensive survey should provide the reader an adequate basis for appreciating the extent and complexity of the processes that must occur when someone speaks.

AN OVERVIEW

We need not address here certain matters that are considered in linguistics and psychology, such as questions regarding the nature of thought and how speech may participate in thought, including the concept of "inner speech." However, it is worthwhile to direct brief attention to the age-long belief that speech embodies, or "clothes," thought. This belief, still current in lay awareness, has been dismissed for some time among those who are sophisticated in the subject.

Some years ago Vygotsky (1934) emphasized that what is called a thought is not truly a mental entity, as assumed but, through several processes of formation, *becomes completed* through speech.

The nature of thought is still not understood, despite years of inquiry addressed to it. What lies behind (actually, *before*) a propositional utterance is not at all clear, except for one feature not often mentioned—motive. Vygotsky (1934) and later Luria (1961, 1981) emphasized the central importance of motivation, pointing out that without a motive to say something, speech does not occur. This profoundly important aspect of the generation of speech, often disregarded, finds extreme illustration in cases of mutism.

Speaking originates in an intention to convey meaning, and from this "state" there is generated a set of plans that, rapidly and marvelously, become an acoustic signal that carries the intended meaning.[5] Although the full process remains a mystery, certain of its dimensions have become plausibly understandable through extensive study and analysis, inference, and deduction. The credible conceptions regarding speech processes are based in substantial measure on reliable data regarding the structure and use of words, to be reviewed shortly.

More than anything else, attention to the initiating condition for utterances gives an appropriate sense of the marvel and mystery of spontaneous speech. The evanescent, yet perceptible, quality of this condition was well described over a hundred years ago by the psychologist William James (1890):

> And has the reader never asked himself what kind of a mental fact is his *intention of saying a thing* before he has said it? It is an entirely definite intention, distinct from all other intentions, an absolutely distinct state of consciousness, therefore; and yet how much of it consists of definite sensorial images, either of words or of things? Hardly anything! Linger, and the words and things come into the mind; the anticipatory intention, the divination is there no more. But as the words that replace it arrive, it welcomes them successively and calls them right if they agree with it, it rejects them and calls them wrong if they do not. It has therefore a nature of its own of the most positive sort, and yet what can we say about it without using words that belong to the later mental facts that replace it? The intention *to say so and so* is the only name it can receive. One may admit that a good third of our psychic life consists in these rapid premonitory perspective views of schemes of thought not yet articulate. (p. 253)[6]

James' description conveys in essence the states involved in generation of an utterance plan which, beyond the motivation to express a meaning, includes processes of selection, judgment, decision and revision.

SPEECH PRODUCTION MODELS

Late-nineteenth-century interest in speech production was associated largely with work in aphasia,[7] wherein attention focused largely on various speech deficits and probable loci of responsible cerebral lesion. It was the neurologist Arnold Pick who, in his book on aphasia (Pick, 1973), presented the first detailed model of speech production, a model that reflected the concepts and deductions of Hughlings Jackson.[8] Other models have been proposed during the twentieth century, the more recent ones emanating from psycholinguistics. The reader is encouraged to gain some acquaintance with these efforts by reviewing proposals presented by Fromkin (1971), Butterworth (1982), and Levelt (1989). All three models contain some fairly general ideas about what may occur in the speech production process, and offer graphic representations of the complexity of speech production that these hypothetical models try to encapsulate. The three differ considerably; each has properties not presented in the other two. All the properties specified are, or course, conceptual and tentative; some of them are questionable.

   Although conceptions such as the foregoing direct attention to probable intricacies of speech production, reference to the process in terms of hierarchy and the levels projected is rather misdirecting. The terms used indicate that the proposed dimensions of utterance planning are stages that are layered in a top-to-bottom structure and, especially when depicted in flowchart diagramming, that the proposed hierarchy unfolds in the temporal sequence depicted. Such models evince a predilection to view things in a parts-to-whole schema; they reflect the heavy influence of a background awareness of mechanical or electronic systems made up of parts, each of which does some special task performed in a certain order. Models of this sort present a linguistics counterpart of "the diagram makers" criticized by Head (1926) in his treatise on aphasia. In the models noted here, for example, one finds entities such as "articulator" and "comparator," that bespeak special processing by isolatable units.[9] However, there is no evidence that such units exist in the system they are conjectured to represent—speech. Just because speech can be analyzed to contain what may seem to be "parts" that even have been given names (words, phones, morphemes, etc.), does not mean that speech is created or organized in the same fashion as some familiar system that has palpable parts. Speech production may well be of a much more holistic nature than is portrayed, or even suggested, by such models. It is quite likely that the several conceivable marvelous functions of speech process occur simultaneously, or in some imbrication(s), which are not reflected in such models.

A Common Failing

A serious limitation common to all three conceptions is their inadequate treatment of what must be the core component of utterances and utterance planning—words (words/syllables).[10] Especially in view of what is known about the course of speech development in the individual, words are not well conceived as amorphous entities having some independent, precursor existence to which phones are then fitted.[11] Words as phonetic patterns are readily discerned as such introspectively, in that amorphous "inner speech" of which we can be partially aware. Moreover, there is good evidence that words exist similarly as plans, and as parts of larger plans. The identity of words rests in their phonetic pattern, their phoneme sequences, although the identity of individual phonemes is obscured in, and by, the sequences into which they become organized in connected speech. Importantly, the sequences embody a prosodic pattern, which is a salient dimension of their form.

For some time, research addressed to word access (see later in this chapter) has indicated that words are stored as assemblies. Although the nature of such storage is not known, it would seem that the stored entities must have a phonological configuration, because that is the form in which they were acquired and entered into memory. There is ample research basis to believe that words are stored morphemically in a speaker's "lexicon" (vocabulary memory/storage), whatever that may be. The bulk of these forms are "free" morphemes, the root-word form of open-class (content) words.[12] In addition, there are the, proportionally few, "bound" morphemes that are used as modifiers; prefixes, such as un-, mis-, dis-, and suffixes such as -ly, -ness, and -ity, and the plural and possessive markers. Nonetheless, it would seem that many words must be stored "whole," that is, consisting of both free and bound morphemes; again, the structure of words as stored must depend upon how they were learned. For instance, "man" is learned early, as an independent form, and underlies the later acquired modified meanings of "manly" and of "unmanly." In contrast, a word like "ungainly," acquired later than the word "gain," has a meaning in present day use that is quite apart from its free morpheme "gain." Moreover, it is likely that most speakers of modern-day English are not even aware of such words as "ungain" or "gainly." Of course, many words remain completely independent of bound-morpheme modifiers; prominent among these are the function words.

Even though (content) words can be taken apart intentionally and their constituents manipulated, and although, under certain circumstances they may come apart inadvertently, there is good evidence that words are stored as assemblies whose plans are ready to be implemented. Moreover, and of special importance, when words do come apart inadvertently, or are taken apart intentionally, the separation does not occur just anywhere—they come apart at predictable loci. These matters are of particular import for understanding stuttering. Their occurrences in ordinary speech are addressed in detail in the final sections of this chapter, which deal with word games and speech errors. Their significance for stuttering is presented in Chapter 12.

When considering schemas proposed to describe the speech production process, such as the modern ones noted above, one should keep in mind that all such efforts omit the matter of meaning, and overlook the central role of words in the transmission of *meaning*. The issue is well cast in the sobering statement by A. C. Oettinger, speaking to the tentative nature of linguistic theory. The statement, presented as the second epigram for this chapter, bears repetition here.[13]

> Specifically, we are more than ever baffled by how language performs its primary function, to convey meaning. All our understanding of the mechanics of language, built up from real or fancied elementary building blocks, stops dead before the question of meaning.

At the present level of knowledge about speech production, certainly at least for our purposes, the schema of Figure 11.1 is a more comprehensible representation of the speech production process than the detailed schemas presented

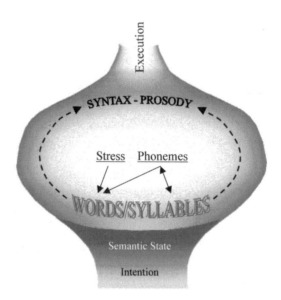

FIGURE 11.1   Major sequences of the speech process.

in the sources mentioned above. Simply described, that figure depicts the process as beginning with a subjective sense of a "meaning" that is to be expressed, coincident with the intention to generate a (propositional) utterance to convey that meaning. The shading in Figure 11.1 is designed to represent that the processes involved are intimately interleaved.[14] The large swelling at the center is intended to reflect that a lot is happening during that progression of the process, whose operations we can only infer or conjecture.

An ideal graphic representation would show that the intent to express meaning continues throughout the production process. To actualize the intention to convey a meaning, words appropriate to the sense of that meaning, extant as assemblies of phonetic structure and stress pattern, evidently are selected from storage in one's lexicon, whatever that might be (see later in this chapter). Clearly, word accessibility is critical to planning a propositional utterance. The selected words are arranged into sequences that are planned according to rules of grammatical relationship pertinent to the words selected.[15] The resulting sequence constitutes the syntax/prosody of the utterance, which completes the propositional construction. The final operation involves transducing the plans into acoustic signals.

For other than very brief messages, the overall production is organized and executed in relatively brief sequences (tone groups) that, remarkably, may proceed while succeeding plans are being generated. (See later discussion involving Figure 11.3.)

ILLUSTRATION BY CONTRAST

An appreciation of the normal speech production process should be gained by recognizing that it is impossible to spontaneously speak complete nonsense, the level of nonsense epitomized in Chomsky's classic formulation: "colorless green ideas sleep furiously." The word "nonsense" (literally, "no meaning") is applied to many things spoken or written, ranging in extremes from statements with which a person does not agree (wherein the word is used inappropriately) to the irrational fabrications of a psychotic individual (in which there is a lack of full coherence). Yet all of such statements will be found to have at least some amount of meaningfulness. In complete nonsense there is no coherence whatsoever in terms of meaning, even though the sequence may be grammatically proper (the point intended in Chomsky's example).

The reader will find it instructive to attempt a brief sentence that is complete nonsense. Even if using the Chomsky example as a model, one will find that generating a sequence of five words in which no word is meaningfully appropriate to any other, requires considerable time and application—with many necessary revisions. Nothing like such effort is involved in generating an ordinary spontaneous five-word utterance, which typically will take less than two-and-a-half seconds. In spontaneous speech, word selections are made within a context that proceeds from a meaning to be expressed; appropriate words are selected and arranged in proper sequence(s) to express that meaning.

DIMENSIONS OF THE PLANS

Earlier it was noted that, since words are acquired as phonological forms, it is reasonable to deduce that they must be "stored" (and therefore accessible) in that form. The likely composition of word plans and assemblages is thus suggested by description of the constituents of ordinary speech, and what is known of normal speech development in the individual.

The foundation of (audible) speech lies in phonation, the sound generated at the larynx. To emphasize the centrality of this dimension of speech as expressed, one might offer the comment that "audible speech begins at the larynx" as an aphorism that pertains not only to the development of speech in the individual but, more comprehensively, to what occurs in any utterance. However, speech does not simply begin with laryngeal actions; what happens at the larynx provides the continuous substance of speech.

In particular relevance to the subject of this book, the aphorism above has unique value to the analysis of stuttering, and special pertinence to management of the disorder.

The Structure of Speech

There are several closely related processes identifiable in the structure of intelligible speech. In ordinary speech these processes are so merged as to seem inseparable. Although it is difficult to provide clear illustrations to exemplify each of them, they can be adequately identified descriptively. The first three processes merit special attention, because the terms that refer to them often are used interchangeably.[16]

Phonation

Phonation is the fundamental dimension of audible speech; in fact, it is identified as such—"the fundamental"—in acoustic descriptions of speech. Phonation is produced when air from the lungs, pressed upward through the trachea through action of the diaphragm and muscles of the rib cage, sets into vibration the approximated ("brought close together") vocal folds, stretched within the larynx.

With one's mouth held closed, phonation is perceivable as a sort of "rumble" in the throat. If, while phonating, one allows the jaw to lower, thus opening the mouth, the resulting resonance yields a continuous "uh" sound—/ə/, the so-called "neutral vowel."

The basic sound of phonation is modulated, elaborated, and refined, eventually becoming intelligible speech through the action of various muscle systems that: (a) vary the air pressure into the trachea, (b) alter the vertical position of the larynx, (c) control the tautness of the vocal folds, and (d) modify the shape and volume of the cavities above the larynx.

Vocalization

Vocalization is used here to designate a "first level" in the elaboration and modifications that eventuate as audible speech. The term is understood here to refer to modulations of phonation occasioned by the first three actions noted above: (a) variations in air pressure, (b) vertical positioning of the larynx, and (c) adjustments of the vocal folds. These modulations are perceived as changes in intensity, duration, and pitch of the sound generated at the larynx.

The simplest vocalization is a brief sound, usually called a "grunt," produced by a brief pulse of air pressure that activates the lightly approximated vocal folds. Muscle systems other than those involved in the increase of air pressure and adjustment of the vocal folds are passive. The minimal resonance is generated in the immobile supralaryngeal (above the larynx) cavities as the "excited" pulse of air passes through them and exits through the nose. The critical role of air movement (pressure) in this process can be illustrated by obstructing the nares (nose openings), which immediately stops the sound.

This brief audible pulse can convey differing meanings through variations in intensity, duration, and pitch that range from expression of alarm to one of pleasure. More specific meaning is carried simply by producing two pulses in sequence, which can mean some variant of "yes" or "no," depending upon whether the first or second pulse is the more prominent (stressed). The meaning of these gestures also can be elaborated substantially by variations in vocalization control, listed as (a), (b), and (c) above. Opening the mouth alters the resonance of the basic sound, yielding "the neutral vowel" and now the double-pulse versions of "yes" and "no" will also contain a minimal consonantal segment; the expressions are transcribable as /əhʌ/ and /hʌʔə/, respectively.

Ordinary speech contains myriad elaborations of the two forms just noted—namely, the resonances of cavities and the introduction of consonantal segments, which yield syllables/words. These elaborations are considered in the following two headings. However, all of this elaboration is founded on actions at the larynx and below, which generate the basic laryngeal sound and control the variations in its expression. These actions yield the "undulating tone," known as the prosody of speech. Vocalization is the essence, the carrier, of speech in its audible realization.

Voicing

Partly from lack of a more adequate word, "voicing" is used here to refer to a third degree of elaboration: the refinements that result from shapings of the oral, nasal, and pharyngeal cavities, which yield the vowel forms. (The term "voicing" is intended to emphasize that vowel forms characterize this process.) Identifiable as varying modulations of the tone they shape, vowel forms occur in speech as sequential pulses that form the nuclei of the basic units of speech—syllables. Syllable nuclei are, in essence, individual expressions of the undulating tone.

Articulation

The complete product, intelligible speech, involves the inclusion of consonants, which establish syllable boundaries. By briefly obstructing or impeding the air stream bearing the vowel-embellished vocalization, syllables of the standard (CVC) form result.[17] To suggest articulation as the ultimate process in the elaboration of audible speech follows readily from extensive records of the progression in speech acquisition evidenced by young children. "Articulation defect," which refers essentially to limitations in consonant production, is the most common type of speech disorder, well recorded in the history of speech correction in the United States alone. Although typically of limited scope, in some youngsters the defect is remarkable in extent, resulting in what is called, simply, "vowel speech," in which the quality of many consonants is poor. However, although the syllable boundaries may be degraded, the syllable pulses are discernible—they are the substance by which the undulating tone is expressed.

The foregoing descriptions of several "processes" might suggest a progressive sequence in their occurrence, which is not intended. While the early era of speech acquisition lends itself to such description, the several processes properly characterize the structure of ordinary speech, analyzable as such in any particular speech sample.

FROM THE BEGINNING

In the development of the individual, the laryngeal sound appears initially as cries. However, it relatively soon modulates into gentler and more continuous, even mellifluous, sounds that are traditionally called "babbling." Vocalization continues to be the predominant dimension of this sound-making, and gradually elaborations discernible as at least rudimentary vowel forms appear.

Speech of a primitive nature appears in the form of this phonologically indefinite sound-making that, through prosodic modulation, conveys differing meanings even before the occurrence of "first words."[18] A child's first words clearly are laid in a prosodic substrate, and this core of primitive speech extends through the holophrastic period and on into the era of connected speech, whose onset is signaled in the achievement of expressing word combinations. As words emerge in this progression, certain phonetic constituents of the words, particularly the consonants, may be inaccurate, yet the substance of word plans is evident. A recent pertinent study with young children (Goodell & Studdert-Kennedy, 1995) indicates that children first build a repertoire of words as integral sequences of oral-vocal gestures, which become differentiated some time later. The plans for words are basic to, and become integral with, plans for what follows in the speech production process—namely, the prosodic/syntactic[19] sequence.

THE SALIENCE OF WORDS

Words are the central reference in discussions of each of these areas of the speech production process. Words, with their sound-pattern coding, are the ultimate carriers of meaning.[20] The meanings inherent in words may be qualified or elaborated by their position in a sequence of words, that is, by syntax; yet words remain the essential vehicles of the meaning conveyed in the sequence.

Publication of Chomsky's *Syntactic Structures* in 1957, followed by his *Aspects of the Theory of Syntax* in 1965, received extensive consideration in linguistic circles for some time. In the years that followed, this conception, with its focus on grammatical structures and transformations, spread to other disciplines having some level of interest in linguistics. In some of the latter fields it has continued to have a certain influence. However, in time, as noted by Hudson (1984), linguistics began to return to the view that words are the central component in language and that syntax is secondary. Marin (1982) remarked that he had always been more impressed with "the capacity of the human brain to discriminate, characterize and store in memory the thirty-plus thousand words"[21] than he was with the complexity claimed for "a few dozen syntactic algorithmic rules." Certainly the nature of words and their use—their sheer number, their differences in type, their variation in structure, their formal yet flexible roles—merit more awe than they typically receive. Without words there is no syntax; and, in contrast, many meaningful communications can be, and are, achieved without syntax. Moreover, the words of a message can convey the same meaning even though syntax is altered.

Words also are obvious entities that, amenable to important manipulations and analyses, are central to a wide range of language study and description. In many respects, words constitute the central focus in the study of speech. Familiarity with the attributes and uses of words is requisite to any effort to appreciate the processes of speech production—and to the effort to understand stuttering, addressed in Chapter 12.

Words have several attributes by which they are separable into several interrelated classifications that are significant for the generation, planning, and execution of utterances. It is important to not only identify these attributes but to keep in mind their close interrelatedness, a matter that should emerge as the following discussions progress, since it is difficult to discuss any of these attributes without referring to another.

WORD TYPES

The principal feature of words is their type, traditionally identified as the "parts of speech." The conventional eight major categories are: noun, verb, adjective, adverb, article, preposition, conjunction, and pronoun. Most of these types have subordinate categories, which are not of particular concern here. However, a broader classification of these categories is of special interest and value, in this chapter and the next.

The parts of speech are separable into the broader classifications of Content words and Function words. Nouns, verbs, adjectives, and adverbs make up the class of Content words, so-called because these words have a referential content; they have a meaning, or content, in and of themselves. Articles, prepositions, conjunctions, auxiliary verbs, and infinitives are called Function words because they function to relate content words to each other. Some sources refer to words of the two classifications as, respectively, "open" and "closed." These terms reflect another important aspect of the difference between the two categories, one that bears pointedly on the matter of frequency of use. Content words are referred to as *open class* words, indicating that this large category is open to new items—well reflected in the fact that new nouns, verbs, etc., continue to be added to the vocabulary of the language (also that, less frequently, some drop out). In contrast, the small number of function words remains unchanged—it is a *closed class* of words.[22]

The Content–Function distinction does not signify absolute categories that are mutually exclusive. Many individual words, in isolation, cannot be fit invariably into one or the other of the two categories. This is true even of words most often identified as function words. Some of the words standardly considered to be function words are invariant, even within classes of this category; such as the prepositions "of" and "at." Certain others may take different roles within the function word category; for instance, "for" and "unless" may be used as prepositions or conjunctions. Still others will cross categories; for instance, "in" and "under," used predominantly as prepositions, occasionally occur as adverbs, and in certain circumstances as adjectives.

The final determinant for classification of words is, of course, their role in connected speech. In spite of the vagaries of classification just noted, words listed in either category in isolation ordinarily are found in that role in connected speech. The identification of Content and Function word categories, although not perfect in a literal sense, has utility in several important ways. Ultimately, for our purposes at least, the categories have special value for identifying other important speech production variables, as will become evident in discussions to follow.

It is of particular interest that, in some sources, function words are called "structural" words, inasmuch as they provide the structure within which the content words assume their relevance in the message.[23] The roles of Content and Function words in connected speech are well illustrated in the following "nonsense" passage, the first stanza of Lewis Carroll's "The Jabberwocky":

> 'Twas *brillig*, and the *slithy toves*
> Did *gyre* and *gimble* in the *wabe*.
> All *mimsy* were the *borogoves*,
> And the *momeraths outgrabe*.

The italicized words are nonsense words fabricated by Carroll. While not real English words, note that they are phonetically possible English words. They have no meaning in themselves, yet they occupy "slots" ordinarily filled by content words of various types that are appropriate to certain slots. Moreover, importantly, content words of certain types are unique to certain slots. Thereby we subliminally accept the nonsense words of this stanza as content types and, in fact, are able to identify the category to which each one must belong if they were real words—what "part of speech" they must be. We are able to make these decisions, intuitively, because of the structure provided by the function words, and also from our knowledge of the "rules" of word sequencing.

The following skeleton version of the stanza illustrates the foregoing description. In it, the function words are left intact and the content words are represented by abbreviations: Noun, Verb, adJective, etc.[24]

```
(It)  V    J  , and the  J    N
Did   V  and   V   in the   N
All  J   V   the   N  ,
And the    N     V  .
```

One could use the Jabberwocky structure as a template and, by substituting appropriate real content words in their respective spaces, create many different passages, each of which could be thoroughly meaningful.[25] The procedure would involve changing the content words only; the function words would be used indefinitely.

The next section of this chapter will emphasize that function words, actually few in number, are used very often, and that many of the vast remainder of words in one's vocabulary, which are content words, may occur only infrequently. The "Jabberwocky" illustration reveals this disparity very clearly: it is the function words that are few in number but occur very often. In contrast, content words, drawn from a very large word pool, appear in varying frequency, some of them rarely.

Note that in the Jabberwocky selection there are 12 content words, each of which occurs only once. There is an almost equal number of function words—11, one of which occurs four times, another three times. This proportion of function words to content words is not unique to poetry, nor to written prose; it has been found in studies of ordinary speech as well. This fact of word use is revealed in Table 11.1, which reports the relative proportions of content and function words occurring in several substantial samples of ordinary spontaneous speech. Clearly, function words, although few in number, are used (repeatedly) much more often than any of the (differing) words from the vast number of content words in the lexicon.

The proportions of content and function words in spontaneous speech reflect the level of sentence structures. The simple sentences of early childhood consist almost entirely of content words, which continue to predominate in the utterances of the preschool years. In those years, content words make up

TABLE 11.1 Proportions of Content and Function Words in Various Samples

Source	Nature of corpus	Number of words	Percentage Content	Function
Howes & Geschwind	Interviews	5,000[a]	54	46
H. Fairbanks	Interviews	30,000	55	45
Blankenship & Kay	"Speeches"	(extensive)[b]	54.5	45.5
French *et al.*	Telephone	79,390 conversations	43	57
Miller, Newman, & Friedman	Various prose	36,300	41	59

[a]The authors refer to average samples or this size obtained from normal speakers.
[b]The corpus consisted of "5 hours and 54 minutes or American-English speech."

about 70% of the child's speech, a proportion that will gradually decrease to about 50%. The articles soon come into use, but prepositions, and especially conjunctions, are few and infrequently used. As noted in Chapter 10, syntax is implicit in early, basic word combinations. As the more mature sentence forms gradually predominate, syntactic relationships become explicit through use of function words, and the content–function ratio moves toward the proportions of approximate equivalence recorded in Table 11.1.

It is important that the reader appreciate the remarkable contrast between the numbers of words in the two categories relative to their actual use in utterances. Referring to Figure 11.2, the very center represents the most common words in an individual's "use vocabulary"; heavily represented by the function words and pronouns—words that are used again and again, as reflected in Table 11.1. This fact of differential (content vs. function) word use in ordinary spontaneous speech is of central significance in the analysis of stuttering as a disorder of speech, addressed in Chapter 12.

WORD LENGTH

Words vary in length, measurable in terms of phones, or, more meaningfully and therefore most often, in terms of syllables.

The length of words is clearly related to their type. Content words are on the whole longer than function words. Although some English content words

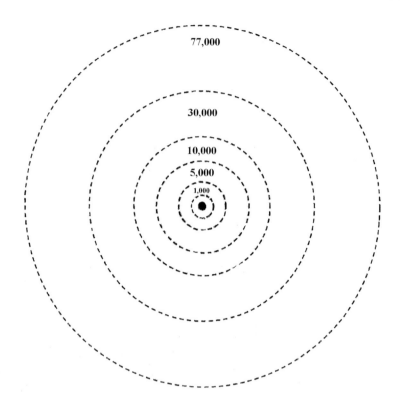

FIGURE 11.2   Representation of use-frequencies of words in individual vocabularies. The most common words are at the center (see text).

may have as many as seven syllables (see Roberts, 1965), words as long as five or six syllables occur only rarely in actual use. In fact, words of four, or even three, syllables do not occur very often; most multisyllabic words in connected speech are of two syllables or less (see Wingate, 1988, chap. 5).

The several categories of content words differ substantially in length. Verbs are generally shorter than the other three content types, with approximately 82% of verbs being monosyllabic. In comparison, one third of nouns, adjectives, and adverbs are two syllables or longer. Function words, in contrast, are predominantly short. Pertinent data are presented in Table 11.2.

Many content words of a "use vocabulary" may be stored primarily in root word form. In a typical utterance, actual word usage may require certain adjustments to a root form, which include: (a) the appropriate use of bound morphemes such as "un-," "-ly," "-ness," and the like; (b) correct adjustment

TABLE 11.2 Syllabic Structure of Conversational Vocabulary

| Parts of speech | Percentage of words having number of syllables shown | | | | | | Average number of syllables |
	1	2	3	4	5	6	
Nouns	53.3	33.8	9.7	2.7	0.47	0.03	1.63
Verbs	81.9	15.0	2.8	0.3	–	–	1.21
Adjectives & adverbs	57.8	30.7	8.0	2.8	0.66	0.02	1.58
Minor	94.8	4.7	0.6	0.1	–	–	1.06
All words	82.0	13.8	3.2	0.86	0.15	0.01	1.23

Data from French *et al.* (1930, tab. VI).

regarding verb conjugation; c) expression of contractions; and (d) inclusion of singular or plural markers, and possessive markers. These modifications are incorporated with the root word plan. Function words, few in number but frequently occurring, evidently are stored for the most part "as is." The few requirements for modification would be limited to certain changes in grammatical form of pronouns, and the tense of auxiliary verbs.

Stress pattern is probably the most significant aspect related to word length. Of course, word stress is a variable only in words of more than one syllable; also, it varies somewhat as a function of word length. Two-syllable English words tend to be stressed on the first syllable; with increasing word length, stress tends to move to a later syllable. The description "tendency" is very *a propos*, as revealed in Table 11.3. Although movement of stress to later syllables is evident, most often early syllables are still more likely to receive stress. In connected speech the stress pattern of the utterance must accommodate, and incorporate, the stress patterns of the words within it; in fact, the prosody of

TABLE 11.3 Locus of Stress in Polysyllabic Words in Percentage Occurrence*

| Word length | Syllable bearing stress | | | |
	1st	2nd	3rd	4th
2 syllables	74	26	0	0
3 syllables	55	39	6	–
4 syllables	33	36	29	2

*Data from DeLattre (1963).

the utterance is based upon the stress assignments of the words within it, in terms of the relative significance of the several words to the intended message. For example, the full meaning of the short sentence, "he's got your pen" depends upon which word is stressed.[26]

NUMBERS AND FREQUENCIES OF WORDS

Estimates of the approximate overall size of the individual lexicon[27] are derived from individual measures of vocabulary, many of which are available from studies of all age levels. It should be noted that, in keeping with standard usage, "vocabulary" means essentially content words.

Vocabulary assessments have revealed that, in normal individuals, the lexicon is of impressive extent. Data presented in a number of reports on vocabulary acquisition[28] indicate that, on average, vocabulary increases from about 10 words at 18 months to over 100 by age 4, that vocabulary is at least 1000 before the time of school entrance, and continues to expand to 15,000 or more at the 12th-grade level. For most persons, vocabulary growth continues. Several authoritative sources have reported data indicating that the average adult vocabulary ranges between 30,000 to 77,000 words,[29] the larger sizes generally reflecting higher levels of education. These values represent "recognition" or "knowledge" vocabulary, meaning words that a person understands, a substantial portion of which a speaker may not (ever) use. An individual's knowledge vocabulary is always considerably larger[30] than one's "use vocabulary," contained within it, which consists of words to which a speaker has ready access and will employ, with broadly varying frequency, at some time when speaking.

A person's "use vocabulary" itself is usually of considerable size even though much smaller than the vast number of words potentially available in his vocabulary—that is, those words the individual understands and could, with some attention and effort, use in at least certain circumstances. A Study by Denes and Pinson (1993) led to an estimate that 95% of the time we select words from a pool of between 5,000 and 10,000 words. This pool varies among individuals, and undoubtedly varies somewhat from time to time in the same individual, reflecting circumstantial influences. Although it is considerably smaller than an individual's potentially accessible range of known words, it is nonetheless of remarkable size (see Figure 11.2), especially in view of the conditions of word usage. The words in this large pool are not used with comparable frequency: most of the words are used only in the special contexts to which they are especially relevant; several hundred words (the "common" content words) are used fairly often; a very small number (the function words) are used repeatedly and with remarkable frequency.

Figure 11.2 illustrates the proportional relations of the vocabulary amounts just reviewed; the circular areas encompassed are proportional to the values cited. The outer two circles represent a basic full range of individual vocabulary estimates, as noted earlier in this section. The area encompassed within the border at 10,000 represents the range of the word pool reported by Denes and Pinson, noted above, which gives an approximate representation of an individual's "use vocabulary"—those words accessed for most discourse. Word counts reported by several different sources are quite comparable below the first 500 words, but begin to differ notably by the first 1000, indicated in the figure by the second circle. At the center are the "common" words, those used frequently by everyone. The most frequently used, of course, are the function words, represented in this figure by the center spot.

Measures of vocabulary and data on word-use frequency provide only a minimally adequate picture relative to the "task" of word selection and use in the generation of an utterance. One must also take into account that most content words have more than one meaning—and a word's meaning is the determinant of its use in any utterance. The values in Table 11.4 give some idea of the extent to which word meanings enlarge the actual word-count figures. As the data in Table 11.4 indicate, even the most common words have a number of different meanings. In addition to the tabled values, the authors of this analysis, Fries and Traver (1950), found that only 3 of these 850 words have only a single meaning. Also, in elaboration of the evidence that verbs have the highest number of different meanings, they noted that 18 of the verbs have an average of 50 different meanings each.[31]

TABLE 11.4   Separate Senses for 850 Basic English Words*

Division of basic English	Average number of senses per word
100 "Operations" (verb forms)	26.0
600 Things	
400 General	12.0
200 Picturable	14.8
150 Qualities	
100 General	12.7
50 Opposites	14.0
Total	14.6

*Data from Fries & Traver (1950, p. 81). See text.

Compilations of the words produced in extensive samples of spontaneous speech reveal that only 3 to 10% of the words within any sample are different words. Moreover, close to half of these different words are used only once. Even more astonishing is the finding that between 30 and 70 words account for half of word occurrences in any particular sample. Clearly, relative frequency of word occurrence is a remarkable feature of word use in ordinary spontaneous speech: a few are used very often, some occur with moderate but varying frequency, others are rarely used. The few that are used with greatest frequency are the function words. Again, this differential is of special significance for the analysis of stuttering in terms of speech processes.

In the generation of an utterance, words from all frequency levels must be selected, and arranged appropriately, within a very brief time. Most often the speaker is not aware of selecting words. However, the fact of selection is revealed in instances when the "right," or appropriate, word is not immediately forthcoming and the speaker must undertake a consciously initiated search. Significantly, this search is always for some content word; function words are readily accessed.

ACCESS TO THE LEXICON

James' description of the "arrival" of words, quoted earlier in this chapter, expresses an experience familiar to anyone who has paused to reflect on it. A companion reflection carries the assumption that, certainly, words must be stored somewhere in "the mind"—that is, in the brain. The matter of word storage remains an enigma; we can deal with the topic only abstractly, through the concept of a "mental lexicon," a kind of multiple-entry dictionary. This hypothetical entity is conceived as an organizational system, some of whose properties have been estimated, and certain others credibly inferred, from the results of pertinent research.

The means by which words are ecphorized to fit appropriately into an utterance is by no means very well understood. Concurrences within extensive data from varied sources regarding use-frequency of words have led to the deduction that some sort of semantic relational base serves as a vehicle for what might be called search-and-selection. As noted above, these processes pertain essentially to content words. Still, function words also must be sought and selected, for they must be fitted well into an utterance, and often are critical to its meaning. However, ordinarily function word access must be relatively easy in view of their limited number and frequency of use, as discussed earlier.

Several lines of research have shed some light on the nature of the processes involved in word search and retrieval, and together lead to the concept of a multidimensional cross-referencing system of organization of the lexicon. These inquiries have been implemented through: Word-Association procedures, "Tip-of-the Tongue (TOT) research, and Word-Fluency achievement. As might be expected, these inquiries have dealt only with content words.

WORD SEARCH AND RETRIEVAL

WORD ASSOCIATION

In word-association procedures the subject says the first word that comes to mind in reply to each of a number of words (called "stimulus" words) said by the examiner. Word-association tests, whether of some standard type or created for some special procedure, regularly consist only of *content* words—understandably, because individual content words have specific references (meanings), to which related references can be expected, a matter of considerable value in psychodiagnostics. Function words, in contrast, do not have such specific properties; associations to function words are predominantly syntagmatic (see below), which clearly reflects their status as structural dimensions of verbal expression.

Several formalized word-association tests have obtained associations from large numbers of subjects, the findings being then accepted as essentially a normative reference. The associations used as illustration here, in Tables 11.5 and 11.6, were reported by Postman and Keppel (1970), a frequently cited reference. Their findings were obtained from administration of a widely used word-association test, the Kent-Rosanoff, to slightly over 1000 subjects.[32]

Some stimulus words elicit the same association from many people, and although these are referred to as "common" associations, the commonality varies considerably. This point is evident from an overall review of Tables 11.5 and 11.6. The data in the two tables were selected for illustration because they are, respectively, the high- and low-frequency extremes in the data reported by Postman and Keppel. The most frequent associations listed in Table 11.5 were given by 67 to 84% of the normative subjects. Much less frequent "common" associations are listed in Table 11.6; these proportions range only from 9 to 16% of the normative associations

Among the words elicited in a word-association procedure, one finds many that are classifiable as "paradigmatic" and some as "syntagmatic." These two designated classes are not, however, mutually exclusive. Paradigmatic associations,

TABLE 11.5 Words Given in Association to the Ten "Stimulus" Words Eliciting the Most "Common" Associations (see text)

Word	Associations		Word	Associations	
black	white	751	king	queen	751
	dark	54		England	20
	cat	26		crown	18
	light	22		pin	13
	night	20		George	11
	sheep	11		ruler	10
boy	girl	768	long	short	758
	man	41		fellow	11
	scout	37		narrow	10
	dog	10			
dark	light	829	man	woman	767
	night	55		boy	65
	room	33		girl	31
	black	31		dog	18
				lady	17
				mouse	10
girl	boy	704	slow	fast	752
	woman	49		car(s)	23
	friend	18		stop	22
	young	17		down	17
	dress	14		snail	12
	pretty	13		sign	10
high	low	675	table	chair	840
	school	49		food	41
	mountain	32		desk	21
	up	18		top	15
	chair	17		leg(s)	11
	tall	17			

the most usual of the two types given by adults, are primarily a word of the same grammatical class as the word spoken by the examiner (the "stimulus" word). Examples in Table 11.5 are "black–dark," "boy–man," and "girl–woman"; in Table 11.6, "baby–child," "butterfly–moth," citizen–man." Especially among common paradigmatic associations, there is a strong antonym/synonym dimension. This phenomenon is well illustrated in the most common associations given to the 10 stimulus words of Table 11.5. Paradigmatic associations, by their nature, reflect a hierarchical system of concepts.

TABLE 11.6 Words Given in Association to the Ten
"Stimulus" Words Eliciting the Fewest "Common"
Associations (see text)

Word	Association	
baby	boy	**162**
	child	142
	mother	113
butterfly	moth	**144**
	insect	117
	wings	104
citizen	U.S.	**114**
	man	112
	person	105
	America	92
	country	87
	alien	79
child	baby	**159**
	mother	117
comfort	chair	**117**
	bed	99
	ease	76
	home	71
	soft	69
earth	round	**130**
	dirt	118
	ground	108
head	hair	**129**
	foot	126
memory	mind	**119**
	remember	99
	forget	80
	think	58
trouble	bad	**89**
	shooter	49
	worry	45
	danger	41
working	hard	**132**
	loafing	99
	sleeping	79
	playing	65
	man	48

"Syntagmatic" refers to associative words that reflect elementary syntactic relationships. Examples are found in the lists of both tables. For instance, In Table 11.5, "black–cat," "dark–night," "high–school"; in Table 11.6, "baby–boy," "butterfly–wings." Note that the latter two are also paradigmatic. Other items also show both associative types: "girl–friend," "king–pin," "trouble–shooter"; and also, "boy–(and his)–dog," "head–(of)–hair," "head–(to)–foot." A syntactic relationship is also reflected in such inverted sequences as: "girl–young," and "trouble–bad." Syntagmatic associations have been shown to often be like the transitional frequencies between words in connected speech. It is, then, more than simply interesting that such associations are related to age level, reflecting the cognitive and speech developments as the child matures. Syntagmatic associations, given more frequently by children of kindergarten age, are gradually replaced by the paradigmatic type during the grade-school years.[33]

Other associations, not easily identifiable as either paradigmatic or syntagmatic, nonetheless have a clear, often contextual connection that centers in meaning, the principal feature of word associations. Clearly, the connections between words vary in nature and strength, variables that are affected by certain features of words beyond their, often multiple, meanings. For instance, the marked difference in frequency of associations in the two tables reflects a difference in the frequency with which the respective "stimulus" words occur in ordinary usage. The 10 stimulus words in Table 11.5 occur much more often than the 10 words in Table 11.6. Nonetheless, the early view of "associative bonds," accepted literally for many years, has been modified by evidence that associations are evidently "generated by rule," influenced by certain other verbal relations as well.

Further, the different word types (grammatical classes) differ in the form of associations elicited. Associations to nouns are largely paradigmatic; in contrast, adverbs elicit many syntagmatic associations. Verbs and adjectives elicit both types. In general, the average probability of a word occurring as an association is found to be the same as its probability of use in ordinary discourse, a finding especially pertinent to the matter of use-frequency of words. Overall, several separate dimensions of word association analyses, corroborated by studies of word recall, show significant "clustering," which indicates that there is a basic category structure of vocabulary that underlies word accessibility and use.

Ordinarily, word associations are rarely a function of phonetic structure as the sole, or central, dimension. For example, associations such as "black–tack," "dark–lark," or "high–my" are rare. In psychodiagnostic assessment, items like these are referred to as "clang" associations. They occur occasionally among very young children, but are rare beyond age 6. If given by adults, they are considered, psychodiagnostically, suggestive of aberration in mental function. Associations given to the phonetic structure of a word are anomalous because they clearly depart from the essential character, and use, of words—their meaning.

An unusual procedure in association testing yielded findings especially pertinent to evidence that word-initial sound is focal in lexical access. Under instructions to give the first word coming to mind in association to each of various letters of the alphabet, most of the words given in association began with the "stimulus" letter presented (Anderson, 1965). These results add to other findings regarding the significance of word-initial position.

TOT RESEARCH

The reader undoubtedly can remember personal experiences of being unable to recall some particular word, for the moment, although at the same time having a sense that the word is about to "appear"—an experience in which the word is said to be "on the tip of the tongue." Findings from inquiry into this phenomenon (Brown & McNeill, 1966; Yarmey, 1973; Rubin 1975; Brown, 1991) indicate that success in ecphorizing the latent word is frequently achieved through one, or both, of two avenues: identifying the initial sound of the sought word, or the number of syllables in it. As might be expected, in view of the discussion in Chapter 9 regarding the literate person's extensive experience with words in print, the initial-sound clue is strengthened when phone and letter agree but is confounded in instances of disagreement, such as words spelled with "c" but pronounced as either /s/ or /k/ (e.g., city and cat). On the other hand, the clue regarding the syllabic length of a word is aided considerably by concurrent recollection of the stress pattern intrinsic to the word.

In view of the large proportions of single-syllable words occurring in ordinary connected speech (see Table 11.2), there is good reason to assume that word-initial phone is the more extensively used single cue in word retrieval. It is also pertinent to recall here that consonants occur more than twice as frequently as vowels in word-initial position, a disproportion that is even greater in the shorter words. Certain particular features of word structure, especially phonetic composition, are introduced in Chapter 12, where they are especially pertinent to issues considered there.[34]

WORD FLUENCY

Measurement of "word fluency" originated as one of the subtests in *Tests of Primary Mental Abilities* developed by psychologist L. L. Thurstone. Word

Fluency turned out to be among the most clearly defined of the six "primary abilities" assessed in Thurstone's test battery, separate dimensions identified through factor analysis of a large variety of mental tests. The Word Fluency test is described as a measure of the speed and ease with which words can be used, a clearly important function demonstrated to be independent of other verbal dimensions such as knowledge of word meanings (that is, vocabulary). Facility in word access is understandably vital to propositional generation, and to continuity of speech production.

Word Fluency is measured by having a person list, within a brief time period, all words that come to mind that meet certain criteria. The original, and most frequently used, requirement is to list words beginning with "s," a criterion selected because "s" is the most frequently occurring initial consonant of content words. The test is thus a measure of word-access function that employs the well-known avenue of word recall—word-initial phoneme. Relative to our particular interest, one must be impressed that this function has been identified as a separate special dimension of an individual's verbal capability, one that concerns the speed and ease with which words can be used rather than the understanding of verbal concepts. It is described as reflecting "the ability to write and talk easily."

OTHER ASPECTS OF RETRIEVAL

Word selection in spontaneous speech involves processes in addition to those suggested in the preceding sections. Word Association and TOT involve almost exclusively content words, predominantly nouns. Word Fluency elicits words of more grammatical classes, yet also predominantly content words. As revealed in data presented earlier, roughly half the words of spontaneous speech are function words. Moreover, speaking is not simply the production of words in sequence, but words in interrelationships that elaborate their meanings through qualification, expansion, and specification. Also, one should recall here that most words have multiple meanings; and, as well, that many words can serve in more than one role of word-type (noun, verb, etc). Selections of words, including functions words, are made to fit the meaning of an intended utterance. Words suitable to the meaning of an utterance are not equally accessible, even if they are among those more frequently occurring words of one's "use vocabulary." Still, the entire process is accomplished with remarkable speed, which must be facilitated by organization that binds individual words into a meaningful structure.

In support of the foregoing deduction, consider the following illustration from Oldfield (1966). Speaking the name of a familiar (real or pictured) object requires only 0.6 seconds. If this rate of access could be sustained, one should be able to name 100 familiar objects within 1 minute, a rate well below the average speaking rate of around 140 words per minute. However, to produce unrelated words at a rate that is only about two-thirds the average rate of speaking is a quite impossible task. Oldfield reported that attempting it results in "speech blockage, naming errors, and even attempted circumlocution."

Along somewhat similar lines, a speaker who is asked to say as quickly as possible whatever words come to mind typically will produce words in groups that vary in length, with the sequences manifesting both paradigmatic and syntagmatic associations. During the task, subjects intermittently adopt a silent reflective manner or look about to find things to name, actions that are then followed by another group of words. Notably, unless instructed or cautioned not to do so, subjects are prone to expand words into meaningful phrases.

CONNECTED SPEECH

Speaking is aptly described as words produced in connected sequence. Although the child's first words are eagerly anticipated, and a regular source of parental satisfaction, "putting words together" is the milestone that signals emergence of a child's verbal capability. With the appearance of two-word combinations, and beyond, the child is acknowledged to then be "really talking." Thenceforth, expression in word sequences will be the reference for his speaking ability, and concurrently, considerable attention will be addressed to the number and variety of words used. However, as discussed in Chapter 10, there is more to speech than saying words in sequence.

WORDS IN SEQUENCE

Words, the essential carriers of meaning, are accessed as needed to implement an intended message, their structures organizing into sequences of tone groups embodying a prosodic line. The needed words must "arrive" at the right time to incorporate into the utterance plan of which it is an integral part. The arrangement of words in sequence is determined largely by their grammatical class relative to the intended meaning of the utterance being generated. In a basic, simplified description, content words are the major substance of these sequences, with nouns and verbs being the salient foci, modified as necessary by adjectives and adverbs, all framed in an appropriate structure of relationships provided by the function words. These verbal arrangements are portrayed in the "Jabberwocky" stanza presented earlier.

The essential aspects of this production sequence are highlighted by noting the progression in children's verbal expressions. In general, nouns (naming) appear earliest and continue to predominate, occasionally with an accompanying modifier. Such productions are followed by addition of verbs—the noun–verb sequence generally accepted as the beginning of "connected speech." Gradually, more modifiers are added, lending to description of speech in terms of noun-phrase and verb-phrase, in which syntax of an elementary level is implicit. Later, the more complex relationships between words are signaled *explicitly* by function words, which, on the whole, are the last word types to be incorporated in the child's verbal achievements.

It is relevant to note that, in keeping with a child's developing cognitive capacity, vocabulary growth in children is moderate at first, then rapid between ages 4 and 8, after which it becomes proportionately slower. As noted earlier, it is in this era that children's word associations shift from the syntagmatic to the paradigmatic type.

The structure of connected speech is well illustrated in the sequences portrayed in Figure 11.3. The complete statement, a normal fluent utterance, is expressed in relatively short groups of words. This particular figure was selected because of its clear visual display of typical connected speech, and because the narrative it depicts spells out succinctly many of the points being made in the present discussion. Also, various features of the figure are relevant to content previously addressed (especially in Chapter 10) and that pertain as well to content yet to be considered. These features are described in a subsequent section addressed to the topic of pause.

In contrast to the ever-present preoccupation with words as being the stuff of connected discourse, students of the speech process must recognize, and keep in mind, the first sentence of the narrative of Figure 11.3, that,

> "We speak in phrases, not in words; in thought units, not in parts of speech."

The rest of the statement is also particularly germane to the matter being developed in this chapter, and deserves special attention here:

> A more or less obvious phrase is spoken quickly, and with reduced emphasis, so that the important phrases stand out clearly, strongly, and with real contrast. The length of phrases varies, because speakers vary in their habits of speech, and in the meaning which they wish to give to phrases. In other words, phrasing depends upon the meaning of what you say, and also upon your whims as a speaker. And although there is an element of logic in the process, there are no definite rules.

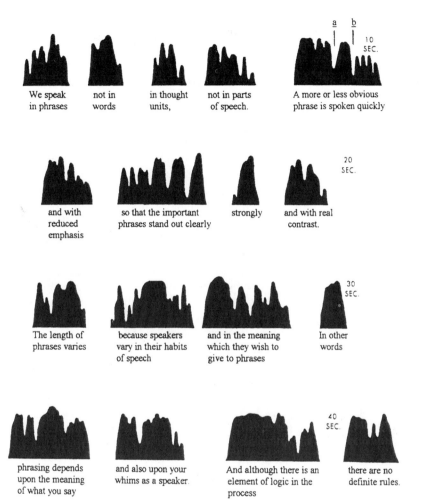

FIGURE 11.3   Phrasing as shown by intensity variation. Data from Fairbanks (1960, fig. 13.1).

One change in the quotation is in order. Rather than "phrases" or "thought units," it is more fitting to use one of several equivalent terms from the linguistics literature, such as "phonemic clause," "syntagma," or "tone group," in reference to these brief sequences of words.[35] These three terms are equivalent descriptions of the typical form of connected speech, which is produced in relatively short sequences of words that are separated by silent intervals of varying duration. The term "tone group" is preferred here because it makes clear reference to the essential prosodic substance in the organization of each sequence.

The silent intervals are identified linguistically as "open junctures." As discussed in Chapter 10, these junctures are the Silent Pauses regularly present in ongoing fluent speech; most of these pauses go unrecognized, because they are part of the ordinary flow of speech. It is at these loci that Filled Pauses also may occur; most of these pauses also go unnoticed, for similar reasons. As explained in Chapter 10, pauses of both kinds come into awareness only when they become, for various reasons, obtrusive. Ordinary pauses, of either kind, have an integral role in the flow of connected speech, roles revealed through analysis of the processes involved in the production of a verbal message.

The three descriptive terms introduced above, designating groups of words within an utterance, all speak to the evidence that the overall plan of an intended message is generated in sections, small coherent aggregates of words that are assembled prior to final expression, and uttered in connected sequences. Some silences, typically brief and clearly identifiable as grammatical pauses, may be part of an assembly—for example, those indicated at "a" and "b" of Figure 11.3. Other longer pauses occur as intervals between syllable groups during which the next section of the message is being assembled and readied for expression. When the next assembly is for some reason not quite in final form, a silent pause may be fairly long. In fact, it is in such circumstances that a filled pause is likely to occur, as a form of adjustment for the delay in preparation of the next section.

One of the points made in Chapter 10 was that something spoken does not have the same structure as if the same message were in writing. One must expand that point to emphasize that words spoken in isolation differ, in their expressed form, from the same words spoken as part of a connected utterance. The contrast is most evident in many brief expressions, such as when "How are you?" (/hau ar ju/) becomes /hə'warjə/, but similar changes occur in much less casual speech. The last two phrases displayed in Figure 11.3 provide good illustration.

Line number 1 below is a transcription of the words in those two phrases spoken as connected utterance. Line number 2 contains transcriptions of those words as spoken in isolation.

1. /ændal'ðo:ˌðə'rɪzn'ɛləmnt + əv'ladʒɪk + ɪnðəpraˈsɛs | 'ðɛrəno + dɛfnət + rulz #/

2. ænd aldo ðɛr ɪz æn 'ɛləmənt əv 'ladʒɪk ɪn ðə 'prasɛs ðɛr ar no dɛfənət rulz

The graphic contours of the phrases in the figure reflect the stress pattern and junctures of the connected utterance. The differences in pronunciation of the words in the two lines of the above illustration reflect the elision and compression typical of connected speech, which in this example results in several instances of phoneme reduction, in some cases to actual omission. The most marked examples occur with the word "definite," in which there is loss of the median vowel—a fairly common occurrence called "syncope"—and, as well, reduction of the last syllable of that word. Note also the shift in stress for the word "process" from the first to the second syllable. These two pronunciations of "process" (stress on either first or second syllable) are not common alternatives; in this instance, the (actually infrequent) pronunciation may reflect personal style, but a major influence would seem to be the anticipation of expressing an emphasis (note the extent of juncture after the first phrase, followed by the falling contour pattern of the last phrase, which, however, ends with clear stress on "rules.") The reader should be able to notice certain other alterations in pronunciation occasioned by the words being expressed in connected utterance as compared to words spoken individually. However, other important changes occur that are beyond analysis here, such as changes in coarticulation and the transitions that occur in connected speech; this matter was touched upon briefly in discussion of palindromes in Chapter 9.

Of the three descriptors, given above, that refer to the sequential word groupings in typical connected speech, "tone group" is the most comprehensive because it includes reference to the underlying continuity within the group of words, the "prosodic line" that is expressed in the stress pattern of the syllable sequence.

SYLLABLES

Just as a focus on individual words diverts attention from lengthier assemblies of words, it also precludes appropriate consideration of the more fundamental dimension of spoken utterance—the *syllable*, which must be recognized as the basic unit of speech. Although we intuitively sense that we generate speech as a series of words, and also perceive it as such, speech is organized and expressed in sequences of syllables, which vary in lengths and "textures."

The essence of the syllable is a resonant vocal pulse, the nucleus of the syllable, perceivable as a vowel-form.[36] In most cases this nucleus is bounded by consonants, which in ordinary connected speech constitute transitions between the nuclear pulses. The salience of the syllable pulse (its prominence in the speech signal) is well illustrated in the sonagram of six familiar monosyllabic words, displayed in Figure 11.4. The thick dark horizontal bands,

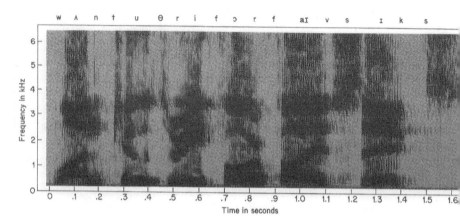

FIGURE 11.4   Sound spectrogram (voice print) of the spoken words "one," "two," "three," "four," "five," "six." Vertical scale shows *frequency* in kilohertz (kHz), or thousands of cycles per second. *Time* can be read from the horizontal scale (total time of sample about 1.6 seconds). The darker the voice print mark, the greater the acoustic energy at that point in time and frequency. Reprinted with permission from Carrell & Tiffany (1977, fig. 4.7).

called "formants" that appear below their respective vowel symbols represent the resonances of the vocal tract that characterize each vowel. The irregular tracings that appear mostly in the upper portion of the record represent the consonants pertinent to those words. One must be impressed with the extent and intensity of the vowel representations, appropriately noted as massive relative to consonant registration. Tracings like these reveal clearly that the principal substance of speech is borne in these vocal pulses.

Ordinary spontaneous speech consists of a series of these pulses that vary in frequencies, duration, and intensity, the essence of the series being audible as an *undulating tone*. As noted earlier in this chapter, this undulating tone is the central substance of speech; it is represented graphically in the contours of Figure 11.3. It is a distinctive sound pattern, readily perceived as human speech in contrast to all other sound patterns, and recognized as human speech regardless of whether produced by a man, a woman or a child. It is recognizable even when degraded by conditions that reduce or eliminate many finer acoustic features of the speech signal (essentially, the higher frequencies, representing most consonants). In fact, this fundamental dimension of speech—which ordinarily receives so little direct attention—becomes elevated into awareness under circumstances of acoustic degradation of the speech signal. It comes into prominence when the refinements of the signal are less perceptible. This undulating tone is what one hears as the so-called "hum" of conversations at gatherings; or the unintelligible talking of persons in an adjoining closed room, or the like.[37]

PROSODY AND STRESS

The undulating tone described in the preceding section is the prosodic dimension of speech, sometimes called speech melody. Prosody is expressed through variations in syllable stress—perceptible changes in some combination of intensity, duration, and pitch of the vowel forms that comprise the syllable nuclei.

It has long been known among phoneticians that stress contours in English constitute a most complex aspect of the sound pattern of the language (Chomsky & Halle, 1968). The contours are recognized to vary considerably in extent, so that many degrees of stress should be recorded if one is to give a fully adequate phonetic transcription. Occasionally an effort is made to record graphically the actual stress variation heard. However, most often the practical resolution in transcription, sufficient for many purposes, is to make notation of several perceived "levels" of stress. A four-level system, of "primary, secondary, tertiary, and unstressed" seems to be the most suitably manageable, although some authors use only three levels.

As noted, stress variation is describable as some combination of changes in intensity, frequency, and duration. A major dimension of the complexity of stress lies in what is called the "trading relationships" among these three variables—that is, some varying interplay in their expression. There is, as well, an interaction with vowel quality; for instance, vowels of stressed syllables are produced closer to their citation (idealized) form. Although stress is an acoustic reality that has an evident perceptible unity, pertinent research indicates that stress is best described in physiological terms, since there is no single acoustic event that occurs in all stressed syllables. At the same time, it is difficult to identify stress physiologically, because muscular involvement apparently differs in different expressions of stress. Nonetheless, significantly, one central feature is that every stress is accompanied by some extra increase in subglottal pressure.[38]

As just reviewed, although prosody is the basic dimension of speech, it is typically given minimal consideration in discussions of speech and language. This typical focus on words and their relations reflects the principal concern with meaning, in which the prosodic dimension typically is viewed as a rather subordinate and tangential aspect of the speech sequence, conveying primarily affective qualities of speech. Prosody does serve that function well, but prosodic variation conveys nonemotional meanings as well, principally in its ubiquitous function of signaling points of emphasis in an utterance. This regular prosodic contribution to meaning is exemplified in the first two peaks in Figure 11.3, corresponding to the words "phrases" and "words."

Moreover, a speaker may alter the meaning of a message, as contained in its words, by intentionally manipulating the prosody of the utterance. The meaning of a complete utterance may be changed markedly, even inverted, by prosodic variation identifiable as sarcasm, or simply as qualifying innuendo. Actually, as noted earlier, a brief utterance may be spoken with as many meanings as it has words, depending upon which word is given the major stress, for instance, giving major stress to either word of "My coat is gone."

Earlier it was pointed out that, in connected speech, the stress pattern of the utterance is built upon and incorporates the stress patterns of the words within it. A central qualification in this accommodation involves the distinction between content words and function words. Except for very special circumstances, only content words are "eligible" for assignment of the higher stress levels; function words are typically unstressed. The rules of stress assignment in English[39] are clearly stated by H. L. Smith (1959):

> It is necessary to bear in mind that the various classes of words in the language can appear only with certain stresses and not with others. For instance, excepting "compounds," nouns, adjectives, adverbs, and main verbs never occur with less than secondary stress; auxiliary verbs, prepositions and conjunctions never appear with more than tertiary. Articles almost always occur with weak stress—never more than tertiary—and personal pronouns regularly with no more than tertiary though they quite frequently are "nominalized" by virtue of being said with secondary. Of course, any word can be said with primary stress when a higher degree of pitch is shifted to it for reasons of emphasis, in which case the word that would normally carry the primary stress in the sequence is reduced to secondary. These are *facts* of the structure of the language, internalized by all native speakers outside of awareness. (p. 3).

Typically, verbal expression is viewed as a succession of words which, in certain respects, it is. Both speaker and listener are oriented to an utterance as a string of words. However, speech is described more realistically, and correctly, as a sequence of syllable groups and silences, as illustrated in Figure 11.3. Within any syllable group (tone group), the consonant boundaries of the syllables constitute transitions to and from sequential syllable nuclei of the group, through which variations in the stress pattern are expressed. The phone sequences and appropriate stress patterns, of words *and* of word sequences, become an amalgam that is produced and perceived as a meaningful series of words, organized into tone groups. A speaker conceives of his own verbal expression as a series of words he has intended to use. He is not likely to realize that, in differing utterances, he alters his production of those same words due to the assimilations[40] resulting from coarticulation. A listener, through his knowledge and intimate experience with the language, is able to discern *words* in the flow of sounds and silences uttered by the speaker, even though most often the words are not pronounced as they would be if said as separate entities—in citation form.[41] Further, he perceives those words as being the same when they occur in different utterances, in spite of modifications due to their context, as noted above.

The sequential tone groups constitute the prosody of an utterance—the undulating tone discussed earlier, discernible as recurring stress patterns, and often referred to as the rhythm of speech. The rhythm of speech is aptly described as a "*basically* regular" recurrence of stress patterns, implying a certain contrast to the literal (strict) recurrence of cadences ("time," or beats) found in music; for instance, the 2/4 time of marches, the 3/4 waltz time, and the 4/4 time of jazz. However, it is this "basically regular" character of ordinary speech that renders it expressible in the more literal regularity of certain poetry forms, which have a clear cadence or "time." Familiar examples are: trochaic (abababab), iambic (babababa), dactylic (abbabbabbabb), and anapestic (bbab-babbabba), sequences.[42] These patterns of poetic meter are built from the patterns of ordinary speech; the common dimension of the two modes (speech and poetic meter) is that, in both, stressed syllables are focal.

PAUSE

Pause is a ubiquitous and substantial part of ordinary connected speech, and an appreciation of its role is crucial to understanding speech production process.

The importance of pause has been recognized in at least some sources over a very long time. In his review of Sanskrit literature regarding speech, Savithri (1988) found the following quotation: "care should be taken with regard to pauses, since they clarify the meaning—in fact, meaning depends on pauses." In mid-twentieth century Stetson (1951) wrote, "Indeed, in ordinary speech, silences are quite as important in any phonetic pattern as are the neighboring sounds." Nonetheless, until the turn of the century, the matter of pause received little direct attention in sources interested in speech. Then, due to psycholinguistic research concerned with "hesitation phenomena," beginning in the 1950s, pause has come to attract more extended interest in regard to its linguistic significance.

"Pause" is understood generically as "silent interval." This is the sense in which it appears in the Sanskrit and Stetson sources; also in general references of a similar kind. However, the psycholinguistic interest in pause led to specification of three forms of pause, which may be classified in several ways. Acoustic reference gives a basic classification of Silent Pauses and Filled Pauses. Silent Pauses, the more common, include two major subcategories: grammatical and non-grammatical. Filled Pauses consist essentially of "uh" (/ə/) or some occasional variation, such as "um" or "er."

SILENT PAUSE

Silent pauses are the more frequently occurring of the two major pause types. Ordinary spontaneous speech contains an abundance of silent pauses, the vast majority of which are not noticed, essentially because of the pervasiveness of grammatical pauses.

Grammatical Pauses

The preponderance of silent pauses are grammatical pauses. These silent intervals are called "grammatical" pauses because they are part of the grammar embodied in the message being conveyed. These silent intervals are typically brief, but vary somewhat in length depending upon their role. They occur as junctures (joinings) between words or phrases and are referred to as "open junctures" because they occur between phonemes that might otherwise be immediately sequential. The shortest of these silent intervals, called a "plus juncture," refers to standard, very brief, barely discernible breaks between words or word combinations. Two slightly longer silent intervals (identified as "single bar" and "double bar" juncture), are regularly accompanied by a change in intonation contour (prosodic modification) that conveys a unique meaning relevant to the message. The longer of these two latter intervals often assumes the role of a "rhetorical" pause. The longest grammatical pause, identified as "terminal" juncture, is accompanied by a typical intonation contour that signals (at least momentary) "finish." Except for the shortest interval ("plus juncture"), the other grammatical pauses correspond roughly to standard orthographic notations of commas, semicolons, and periods.[43]

As might be expected, the latter three forms of grammatical pause often come to notice, but not so much because of their length as from their associated prosodic contours, which carry information. The very brief plus junctures pass by undetected; however, as noted in Chapter 10, they are an important dimension of speech rate.

The statement represented by Figure 11.3 exemplifies many of the structural features of speech production discussed earlier, including good illustration of grammatical pauses. The statement contains 101 words, produced as 138 syllables, completed in 42 seconds. These figures yield a speech rate of 197 syllables per minute, slightly below the average rate noted in Chapter 10. In the statement represented by Figure 11.3, 30% of the elapsed time is taken up with grammatical pause alone. If this pause time were excluded from the calculation of speech rate, the value would be 256 syllables per minute. As noted in Chapter 10, speech rate, as measured and as perceived, is heavily influenced by the amount of pause, which is considerable in ordinary speech.

The proportions of word types are consistent with typical distributions reported for spontaneous speech (see Table 11.1); 52 content words and 49 function words. A substantial majority of the words (69) are monosyllabic; 26 words are bisyllabic, of which 21 are stressed on the first syllable; six words are three syllables in length, five of them stressed on the first syllable (cf. Table 11.3).

The seventeen syllable sequences (phrases/tone groups) vary in length from 2 to 13 syllables, with an average length of 8 syllables. In most of these sequences, the syllables are in "closed" juncture—that is, the syllables are "run together," which is so typical of connected speech. Within this common pattern there are occasional instances of the very brief "plus" junctures, clear examples of which are indicated at points "a" and "b" in Figure 11.3.

The 16 silent intervals between the phrases, all open junctures, range in length from 0.25 to 1.5 seconds. Only three of these intervals are 1.0 second or longer; these are the three terminal junctures (the ends of sentences) at the fourth, ninth, and fifteenth intervals.[44] A fourth terminal juncture, at the 12th interval, is relatively brief; at 0.77 seconds it is similar in length to the second and fifth (non-terminal) pauses. The average length of the 13 non-terminal open junctures is 0.61 seconds.[45]

We might insert at this point a suggestion that should help the reader appreciate the relevance and value of grammatical pause as emphasized in the Sanskrit statement and in the point made by Stetson, mentioned earlier. Try speaking the narrative of Figure 11.3 continuously, omitting all of the pauses recorded. Two phenomena should quickly become obvious: (1) almost immediately one is induced to speak very much in monotone, and (2) one cannot continue very long without taking a breath. The attempt should also yield, vicariously, a potential listener's perception that, spoken in this manner, it is not as easy to make sense of what is heard, as when the selection is read normally.

Non-Grammatical (Silent) Pauses

As this designation indicates, some of the silent intervals that occur during speaking are not integral to the message being expressed. Pauses of this kind are identified, from psycholinguistic inquiry, as one type of "hesitation phenomena." Typically, these intervals are considerably longer in duration than grammatical pauses. However, length alone is not the defining dimension; the two types have been shown to be discriminable even when they are of the same length (as noted in Chapter 10). Moreover, rhetorical pauses, those employed intentionally to enhance meaning, and which therefore have grammatical value, are regularly of notable length.

The speech sample of Figure 11.3 does not contain any examples of a non-grammatical silent pause, those identified as "hesitation phenomena." As noted earlier, such pauses are typically longer than grammatical ones, but, more important, they cannot be accounted as part of the message structure. Nonetheless, under ordinary circumstances listeners are routinely indifferent to such silences too, unreflectively accepting them for what so many of them appear to be—common lulls in speech during which forthcoming assemblies are being generated. Conversely, some non-grammatical silent pauses occur for other reasons—for example, a momentary external distraction, an intruding thought, etc., as discussed in Chapter 7.

Earlier discussion called attention to the fact that pause is the major determinant of speech rate. One could then expect that speech rate and extent of pause would co-vary, and together reflect capability for generation and production of speech. This deduction is substantiated in Figure 11.5, which shows significant changes in the variables of rate and pause[46] in spontaneous speech, from kindergarten through adulthood. The progressive increase in speech rate, and decrease in hesitation phenomena, reflect the rapid development of linguistic skills and cognitive abilities of young children, and their continuation through adolescence. The indication of some decrease in rate and pause at adulthood are interpreted as representing increase in reflective and rhetorical dimensions of adult speech.

FILLED PAUSE

Filled Pauses, of which the most common is /ə/, or a variant, occur with surprising frequency in ordinary speech; "surprising" because, as discussed in Chapter 10, so many of them go unnoticed, by both listeners and speakers, unless they are somehow brought to attention. Filled pauses can also be described as non-grammatical, since they are not grammatically relevant. Along

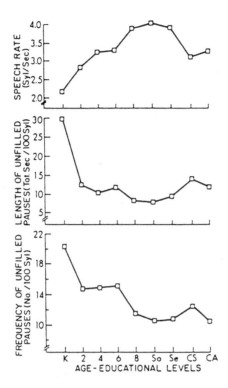

FIGURE 11.5   Speech rate (syllables/second), length of unfilled pauses (total sec-
onds/100 syllables), and frequency of unfilled pauses (number/100 syllables) based on
spontaneous narratives at nine educational levels: kindergarten (K); grades 2, 4, 6, 8;
high school sophomores (So); high school seniors (Se); college seniors (CS); and college
alumni (CA) of 25 years. Reprinted with permission from Sabin *et al.* (1979).

with non-grammatical silent pauses, they have been identified as "hesitation
phenomena." Also, like non-grammatical silent pauses, filled pauses occur for
various reasons. Many reflect internal activities of planning the forthcoming
verbal sequence(s). Filled pauses often appear when the duration of a silent
pause is insufficient for generating the plans of a forthcoming sequence, in
which case both of these "hesitation-phenomena" pause types are likely to
occur in the same locus.

Several variants of Filled Pause, identified in pertinent research (Wingate,
1984b), were discussed in Chapter 10. The variant, "Filled Pause-as-Addition,"
coded FPa in the composite list (Table 10.4), was identified as the most

common type of Filled Pause. A frequently observed expression of this variant occurs in the extension of a linking word between two phrases, for instance, "anduh..." or "butuh..." and the like. Another common occurrence is the insertion of /ə/ as extension of the first word in a syllable group, for example: "Theyuh ... descended..." or "Theseuh ... properties." Such occurrences provide one line of evidence that planning is under way while speech is ongoing.

Of course, filled pauses also occur in isolation, and in combination with silent pauses. In many instances their function is indeterminate, and must be deduced from context or other cues.

WORD/SYLLABLE UNITS

Some discussion of syllables, presented earlier in this chapter, focused on syllable nuclei, emphasizing their central role in speech. The present section is addressed to syllables as units, with particular attention to their components and the stability of their organization.

The word/syllable prototype, or "template," is CVC—a vowel nucleus with initiating and terminating consonants (a fully "bounded" syllable). A very few words, in isolation, consist only of a vowel, and a few more have only either an initiating or a terminating consonant of the vowel nucleus. However, most words, by far, are some variation of the CVC prototype—that is, one or more consonants in both initial and final positions. The majority of words duplicate the prototype, but a substantial number are "unbalanced" in this respect, some having more final than initial consonants, or *vice versa.*

Additionally, words have a more common unevenness in respect to initial and final consonants. Apparently, the prominence of the nucleus effects a differing relationship between itself and its bounding consonants. Transitions from consonants *to* the nucleus (vowel form) are of a different order than transitions *from* the nucleus (vowel form) to trailing consonants. Regardless of the number of consonants in either position, final consonants evidently are more attached to the syllable nucleus than are initiating consonants; evidently the pulse of the nucleus carries over and subsides into the following conso-nants. Syllable-initial consonants, in contrast, are notably more "independent," and isolatable, than are syllable-final consonants, a matter broached earlier in this chapter in discussion regarding syllable asymmetry. It is well exemplified in sections to follow, addressed to Word Play and to Speech Errors.

The uniqueness of syllable-initial position is revealed in relevant findings from a variety of sources, reviewed in the following sections. These findings are of particular significance for the study of stuttering, in view of the recurring evidence that *stutters are in some way a phenomenon of word/syllable-initial position—but not of word/syllable-final position.*

THE SYLLABLE STRUCTURE HYPOTHESIS

This hypothesis, proposed by Hockett (1967), describes syllables as consisting of two parts: (1) initial consonantism, and (2) all that follows. "Initial consonantism" includes instances of consonant clusters and, as well, the few instances in which there is no initial consonant. As proposed by Hockett, the "all that follows" includes the syllable nucleus (the vowel form) and whatever consonants follow. Subsequently, these two syllable parts have come to be called, respectively, "onset" and "rime." Some sources have divided the "all that follows" into "peak" (the vowel form) and "coda" (the syllable-final consonants). In most discussions, little attention is paid the matter of "coda," since it is typically of marginal significance—a matter of considerable pertinence to the fact that stuttering does not occur in word/syllable-final position. Most often, then, syllable structure is viewed simply in terms of onset and rime. It is especially noteworthy that the syllable nucleus is identified as the "peak."

Syllable Structure is more than a hypothesis, or even a linguistic construct. There is a considerable range of evidence to support its reality. Two familiar verbal constructions clearly exemplify syllable structure as described. One is alliteration ("sly, slouching, slob…"), which emphasizes word-initial position (onset); the second is its counterpart, rhyming (score, floor, drawer), which features the last part of words (the "all that follows"), in which the nucleus (and its coda) become the dominant element.[47]

Many other lines of evidence support this analysis of syllabic structure. The most impressive corroboration is found in the prominent role of initial consonants in word retrieval—and its commonplace counterpart in the standard organization of the ordinary dictionary. Other sources also reveal the linguistic uniqueness of the initial part of the syllable, as expressed in the analysis of "syllable asymmetry." A compelling indication of such syllable asymmetry is the evidence that in most languages the syllable-initial phone is more distinct than the phone in syllable-final position (Osgood & Seboek, 1959). The same asymmetry is revealed in evidence that any initial consonant can occur with any vowel nucleus, but, in contrast, there are marked restrictions regarding occurrence of final consonants and certain vowel nuclei (Halle & Vergnaud, 1980). Syllable asymmetry also finds expression in an influence on phones. Considerable evidence from this line of inquiry shows consistently that phones in syllable-initial position are stronger than in syllable-final position. Initial consonants ordinarily coarticulate with "all the rest" of the syllable, particularly with the syllable-nucleus vowel form, with which it is routinely inseparable in normal connected speech.[48] As usually produced, the initial consonant and the vowel nucleus are merged in one continuous blend in which the adjustments for production of the vowel are under way during production of the initial consonant(s), which are released ballistically into the syllable nucleus (the vowel form). In contrast, production of the syllable-final consonant does not require such preparation or adjustment.

These facts of syllable production are particularly significant to the analysis of stutters. As emphasized throughout earlier chapters, various sources have consistently pointed to the concurrence of stutters and word/syllable *initial* position; in other words, onsets. In contrast, word/syllable-final position has been acknowledged as of no consequence in stutters.

The several sections that follow speak pointedly to the uniqueness of initial consonants—their critical contribution to the identity of the word/syllable as a unit, and yet their remarkable independence of "all that follows." In each of the topics to be reviewed, it is clear that "initial consonantism" can be readily separated from "all that follows," even though these two word/syllable constituents are ordinarily melded.

WORD PLAY

Certain intentional alterations of words reveal significant features of word structure and speech production. Although, as discussed above, it seems most likely that words are stored as entities and ordinarily produced as such, the word games to be considered here show that words can be taken apart and reassembled in novel ways, quite spontaneously and by individuals having no special sophistication about the language they speak.

The first two illustrations have a property in addition to word play, namely, use as a form of code. Pig Latin is a word game found most often among preteen children for whom it also is employed as a form of communication code. Significantly, some youngsters can speak in Pig Latin at a rate that is at least close to their normal speech rate.

The technique of Pig Latin is rather simple: transfer the initial consonant of each word to final position and then add the sound "ay" (/e/, often /eɪ/) at the end of the word, as follows:

/ɪgpe ætnle ɪze oknspe ute ɑkte aɪbe odke/

Importantly, the alteration is fully phonologic; that is, it operates on the sounds of words, not on how the words are spelled. This point becomes clear if one attempts to record Pig Latin orthographically. In the following spelled version of the example above, the words with an asterisk do not give the proper pronunciation

igpay atinlay isay* okenspay otay* alktay ybay* odecay*

It is particularly significant that the alteration operates on word-initial—actually syllable-initial—position; a clear instance of syllable-structure description. Note, in particular, the /sp/ cluster of /spokn/ and the zero-consonant treatment of "is." It is also important to note that the transposed initial consonants cannot, readily or usually, simply be inserted at word-final position of the Pig Latin version, but require instead the addition of a vowel form, which creates another syllable.

There are other similar forms of word play contrived by children. A most elaborate one that recently came to my attention is called "Elephant Language." In this code, the phonetic alteration requires inserting the phone sequence /ɛləf/ (the early portions of "elephant") immediately after *syllable*-initial consonants, a maneuver that is considerably more demanding than the changes required in Pig Latin. Reportedly, this code too was spoken at normal rate by many of the youngsters who used it. My informant, now an adult, can still speak lengthy sentences in Elephant Language at a rate indistinguishable from her ordinary speech rate.[49] Because words of more than two syllables often presented a formidable challenge (as might be expected), speakers of the language were allowed to alter just the first two syllables of a long word, but in any instance must alter at least the first syllable.

The first transcription below is part of an illustration spoken by my informant. The second transcription is the same statement as ordinarily spoken:

1. /ðɛləfis ɛləfiz ɛləfe sɛləfæmpɛləfl ɛləfəv ɛləfə lɛləfæŋgwɛləfidʒ wɛləfi jɛləfuzd tɛləfʊ spɛləfik hwɛləfɛn ɛləfaɪ wɛləfʌz ɛləfə tʃɛləfaɪld/

2. /ðɪs ɪz e sæmpl əv ə læŋgwidʒ wi juzd tʊ spik hwɛn aɪ wʌz ə tʃaɪld/

This word-play/code shows, even more elaborately than Pig Latin, the spontaneous, ongoing, and facile alteration of the structure of meaningful words that can still be produced as connected speech. Significantly, the alterations of Elephant Language also focus on separation of the word at syllable-initial consonantism. Again, note the /sp/ of /spik/ and the zero-consonant treatment of several words ("is," "a," "of," etc.). In this code, however, the initial consonants, when present, remain in place but are now brought into coarticulation with a different syllable nucleus.

Another word game that reappears intermittently among persons of any age involves transposing the initial consonants of nearby words. This activity duplicates a naturally occurring phenomenon in which the initial sounds of words are accidently exchanged (see next section). These occurrences are widely known as "Spoonerisms," in the name of the Reverend William A. Spooner, a distinguished clergyman and warden of New College, Oxford, in the latter part of the nineteenth and early twentieth centuries. Reportedly, such transpositions were an idiosyncrasy of Dr. Spooner's speech, but there is reason to question whether such errors were so distinctive an aspect of his expression (Potter, 1980). However, "Spoonerisms," which came into colloquial use in Oxford from about 1885, has persisted as the casual reference for these errors.[50]

Intentional transpositions of this sort often are pursued briefly as a passing fancy, frequently prompted by a spontaneously occurring exchange. At other times, the play may be extended among a group of friends as a transient form of humor (see Squire, 1961). In recent times, one member of the cast in a nationally broadcast comedy program, called "The Capitol Steps," frequently gave a soliloquy on some current topic in which transpositions of initial consonants were the vehicle of humor. In one soliloquy the topic was "the *sti*fe *ly*les of the *fi*ch and *ra*mous," which ended with "the *sto*ral of my *mo*ry" being that even the "*fi*ch and *ra*mous" might go "*el*ly *bu*p."

Clearly, this game of transposing phonemes also involves separating initial consonantism from "all that follows." Note especially that the alterations in all of the above examples were (and typically are) performed only on content words.

SPEECH ERRORS

Speech errors make a special contribution to knowledge about speech processes. The fact of their occurrence is *prima facie* evidence that speech is not automatic, for they reveal the number of ways in which the process may go astray. At base, speech errors give evidence that planning takes place in several aspects of the speech production process.[51]

Speech errors are sometimes called "slips of the tongue," the reference to tongue reflecting the widely accepted association of the tongue with speech. The point has been made that speech errors are more properly identified as slips of the mind, which better represents their nature. "Slips of the tongue" is a description that became popular following the attention given to certain speech errors by Sigmund Freud (Freud, 1914). Subsequently, speech errors in general were often, improperly, called "Freudian slips," a description that should be reserved for only a certain type of speech error, those that appear to embody a property emphasized by Freud, namely, that they reflect some motivation within "the unconscious." At the same time, Freud recognized that many speech errors are not of this nature, but simply represent more mundane speech anomalies.

At the present time, thousands of speech errors have been recorded and studied by linguists, psycholinguists and psychologists. The errors have been analyzed, their features classified, and hypotheses advanced regarding what they reveal about speech processes.[52] We will cover here, in synopsis only, the major outlines of this field of inquiry and give a few representative examples.

Speech errors occur in various parts of the speech process, and vary in extent. The most frequent errors involve syllabic structure, predominantly with initial consonants (see above). Importantly, throughout this range it is clear that the errors follow grammatical and word-structure principles; the various errors are consistent with one or another feature of different areas of speech production. These consistencies have been described formally as a set of speech-error regularities; these "rules" are discussed below.

The various kinds of error are not all equally detectable. Many errors are corrected by the speaker,[53] but many are not and go unnoticed by both speaker and listeners. One form of error that seems more likely to be noticed by the listener involves the substitution of an improper or inaccurate word—for example, if someone, having told of traveling from New York to Chicago, were to say, "After we arrived in New York." A not uncommon occurrence of this type involves the unintended use of an antonym: saying "up" for "down," "good" for "bad," "late" for "early," etc. Such errors reflect a dimension of verbal organization tapped by the word-association procedure. The listener's detection of antonym errors is often dependent upon the clarity of the context in which they occur, which will influence how obvious the error is. As noted often in the relevant literature, many errors are not noted because listeners "fill in" or make the necessary correction implicitly. As is the case with hesitation phenomena (Chapter 10), listeners are intent on the message and are most likely to notice errors only when they are in some respect obtrusive. It is important to note that often the listener is more likely to notice an antonym error than is the speaker who produced it. The intention to make sense of what one hears also accounts for the observation that even clearly noted speech errors fade easily from one's awareness; they slip quickly from recollection if not recorded when they occur.

The following numbered examples were selected to illustrate errors in various areas of speech production. Items 2 and 3 are selected from recordings of radio "bloopers" collected by Kermit Schafer.[54] The remainder are from my personal collection.

1. A covey of quail, established in cover near the stock tank in our west pasture, had become increasingly bold in their excursions, eventually venturing near the place where the driveway joins the lane, an area frequented by our part-time bird dog, Tippy. One day

my wife observed the whole covey crossing the driveway no further
than five feet from the dozing dog. In relating the incident she
finished by saying,

> "They just *drove* right by Tippy."

Note that the error, appropriately representing terrestrial motion, was also a
word of the proper type (verb) and proper tense (past) inserted in the proper
grammatical/prosodic locus, but the content clearly was determined by association to *driveway*.

2. In the featured introduction at a celebration in the Virgin Islands,
   the master of ceremonies evidently intended to say,

> "Ladies and gentlemen, it gives me great pleasure to
> introduce to you the Governor of the Virgin Islands."

Instead, he introduced:

> "the *virgin* of *Governor's Island*."

Two frequent features of speech errors are evident in this example:
anticipation and transposition. In this particular instance, the exchange
involves whole words. Note that each is a content word bearing syllable-initial
stress. Further, the prosodic pattern of the intended utterance is preserved
in the error version. "Governor," although spelled as a three-syllable word,
is hardly ever pronounced that way. The second syllable is either said as a
very reduced schwa or, more often, omitted. Certain alterations of the
grammatical structure were necessary to accommodate the error: (a) addition
of the possessive marker to "Governor"; (b) omission of (the much reduced)
the before "Governor"; and (c) deletion of the plural marker of "Island." As
noted, the prosodic line of the whole tone group remained unchanged, a
feature common in speech errors.

3. The next example involves syllables, the error showing anticipation
   and transposition, in this instance of unstressed syllables; again
   with preservation of stress pattern. The radio announcer's intended
   network identification went awry in the last two words. His intended

> "This is the Dominion Network of the Canadian
> Broadcasting Corporation"

became

> "This is the Dominion Network of the Canadian
> broad*corp*ing *cast*ration."

Pronunciation of the word "corporation" commonly omits the second vowel, (syncope) yielding a three-syllable pronunciation (/kor'preʃən/).[55] Thereby, the prosodic plan of the intended word is matched by the prosodic plan of the error word, in syllable number and stress pattern. Note that the exchanged syllables have the same initial phone, /k/, and that both syllables are unstressed (which is relatively infrequent in speech errors). This example also illustrates another significant feature of speech errors—namely, that in spite of the jumbling of syllables or phones, at least one of the error distortions is most often an actual, or possible, English word—although often hardly appropriate for the context. This finding is one of the "regularities" that have been noted about errors, to be reviewed below.

4. The following example is included to illustrate an error in which the semantic/prosodic plan perseverates, but with differing lexical/syllabic insertion. This example occurred during a casual discussion about gardening in which the topic at the time was how to destroy an especially troublesome worm pest. Said one experienced gardener,

> "You have to chop them to *cut* them."

Clearly, "cut" was intended to be "kill"; the intended word and the error word are both monosyllabic words with the same initial consonant (/k/). Note also that the prosodic plan of the whole utterance remains intact, clearly based in the two primary stress peaks. Notably, this clear error was not corrected by the speaker, nor evidently noticed by other listeners (including his wife, generally not reluctant to correct).

5. This next item represents a relatively infrequent kind of error involving syllable exchange. The two source-words have very similar meaning, under which the exchange and blending are a product of their similar structure. The two words have the same number of syllables and, importantly, the same stress pattern.

> "I believe it will *perdure*." [persist/endure][56]

6. As noted above, the most numerous speech errors involve phones, which figure in various instances of anticipation, perseveration,

transposition, blending, omission, and substitution. The following
are illustrative. All of these examples involve syllable-initial consonantism (which often is also word-initial):

> a—"Another category is His*n*oric Names"
> b—"...at Mons*t*ana State"
> c—"...and he's p_aying in p*l*ain"
> d—"...plenty of sunshine at Sunny*sh*ide"
> e—"How much are you willing to *s*pay?" [spend/pay]
> f—"...in this collection of *sh*ories" [short stories][57]
> g—"He's not that *k*ype of person." [kind/type]

7. The following, final, example is a good illustration of a "Freudian
slip." A small group of faculty from several disciplines had met in
a classroom to discuss a topic of common interest. The meeting
had gone beyond the expected duration, due largely to the latest
speaker who, already having had the floor several times, was again
speaking at length and seemed not to notice the noise, coming
through the partly open door, of persons moving about in the
interval between classes, which signaled the end of the hour. A
member of the discussion group, arising and moving to the door-
way, was hailed by the speaker with the question, "Oh Dr. _____,
are you leaving?" To which came the reply:

> "No, I'm just going to shut the *bore*."

A psychodynamic interpretation of this error would explain that it represents
both an unverbalized judgment that the speaker is boring, and a latent wish
that he would shut up, a judgment and wish that slipped into expression
through the nonconscious motivation to select /bɔr/ instead of /dɔr/—two words
with the same rime but critically different onsets.

The foregoing examples are only a representative sample of the multitude
of errors that occur in everyday speech. As noted earlier, irregularities in speech
are most likely to come to attention if they are obtrusive, like the more dramatic
error examples given here. However, most speech errors are rather mundane,
such as the several items in number 6. Except for such memorable errors as
those of numbers 2, 3, and 7, many errors, as represented in the remaining
examples, may be unheeded; and, most of those will not be remembered.[58]

Study of large numbers of speech errors has found certain regularities
of their occurrence that tell much about operations involved in utterance
planning. Essentially all errors involve content words. In instances of word
transpositions, both words will be of the same grammatical class (noun–noun,

verb–verb, etc.). The syllable nucleus is pivotal. The salience of stress, noted earlier in so many aspects of speech production, emerges in respect to speech errors as well—errors most often involve stressed syllables. Where stress participates in an exchange, both syllables will be stressed, or (infrequently) unstressed; there are no exchanges between stressed and unstressed syllables. The greatest number of errors involve syllable-initial consonants—actually consonant*ism*, as occurs in the consonant combinations of items 5b, 5c, and 5e. In phoneme exchanges and substitutions, the phonemes involved will be of the same class, as in 5a and 5g. Almost always, at least one of the two words resulting from phoneme transpositions will be a real word; and even if one is not an actual word, it will be a phonetically possible word in the language. Significantly, it will match in structure the word for which it substitutes.

Speech errors not only attest to the reality of syllable structure; they confirm the syllable as the basic unit of speech production. The dominant status and role of the syllable is evident throughout the range of speech errors. In the simpler errors (the most frequent), as in the various forms of word play, the initial consonantism is detachable and transferrable. The syllable onsets are exchanged; the rimes remain.[59] In errors involving words that have several syllables, the prosodic pattern (a syllabic phenomenon) of the error is the same as of the word intended.

Speech errors occur in the planning process, not simply in execution; whether simple or compound, the errors are produced whole. This principle is quite evident in exchanges involving full words or syllables of words. However, it is clearest in the most frequent errors, those involving only the syllable-initial consonant(s), because even when errors result in "non-words" they are nonetheless properly structured and complete. In these instances too, the altered syllables obviously are produced as integral units, even though the shifts or exchanges of onsets require altered coarticulations with the rimes. One must be impressed that throughout, the prosodic dimension, borne principally through syllable nuclei, is focal in these occurrences.

SYNOPSIS

The objective of this chapter has been to acquaint the reader with matters fundamental to an appreciation of speech and its production. The central theme is that speech is an intricate and highly complex function, properly recognized as an inherent human capability, whose essential role is to convey meanings. How this marvelous process is accomplished, seemingly with minimal effort, remains a mystery. Knowledge derived from many avenues of study, reviewed briefly in this chapter, give some appreciation of all that, it seems, must be involved in the process of producing meaningful utterances. Still, we have little idea of how it is done. Most (especially modern) efforts to explain the process make use of models whose structure is clearly suggested by mechanical or electronic systems. Viewed circumspectly, such models seem not to appropriately represent the nature of the functions inferred. Findings from various sources support certain deductions regarding activities that possibly may occur in the overall process of speech production; however, the manner of their organization and execution is recondite. Nonetheless, it seems evident that the processes are organized throughout, and that the central organizing principle is *planning*, of which the speaker usually is almost completely unaware. The speaker typically recognizes an "intention to say a thing" (see the James quotation, earlier in this chapter), and is usually aware of the level of success in expressing the intended meaning, but organization of the utterance typically proceeds below awareness.

Considerable evidence has accrued which indicates that there are several conceivable areas of planning, within an organizing system that extends from the intent to generate a message, through a range of assembly processes. In this chapter, attention has been directed especially to the interrelated matters of: propositionality; its intrinsic vehicle, prosody; syllables, the basic units of speech through which the foregoing are realized; and the unique feature of syllables, namely, their asymmetry wherein the initial portion has special qualities. The latter finding, in particular, is of special interest for the study of stuttering, in view of the recurring evidence, presented in preceding chapters, that syllable-initial position is the locus of stutter occurrence.

NOTES

1. These terms, proposed by Jackson in 1878, are more focal than others suggested later (Head, 1926; Goldstein, 1948).

2. Defining, interpreting, fact stating, giving opinion, explaining, justifying—in that order.

3. See, for example, Carrell & Tiffany (1977).

4. Which, pertinent to our interest, includes speaking one's own name. This particular matter is of special interest in Chapter 12.

5. Very often more like a reasonable facsimile of the intended meaning. (The reader should reflect on the many instances in which his/her expression has not accurately represented what was "in mind.")

6. A similar, though less lyric, description will be found in Luria (1981). His summary statement (p. 152) is very much the same.

7. The more prominent figures were: H. Jackson, P. Marie, P. Broca, C. Wernicke, and A. Pick.

8. Pick's book was republished in 1973. The student should consider reading this model and its rationale.

9. One should remain fully aware that such designations are simply names for *inferred* functions. Note the evident emulation of computer concepts. One can also discern the probable influence of literacy, as discussed in Chapter 9.

10. I use this combined term to keep in focus the facts that: (1) words are composed of syllables, and (2) most words used are monosyllabic.

11. A central dimension of Levelt's schema. Giving such hypothesized phantoms a name, such as "lemma" (featured in Levelt's model), does not make them real, or more credible. The notion that the appropriate phones are fitted to a preexisting amorphous word-form might be dubbed "the typesetter conjecture," which seems to provide more evidence of "the literacy complication" discussed in Chapter 9. In casual inquiries, I have found that laypersons are at a loss to accurately reproduce the phones of even relatively simple words, although they are most often successful at spelling the words. (Interestingly, comparable results are routinely obtainable from students who have passed a phonetics course.)

12. Called *lemmas* in some sources (see Francis & Kucera, 1982). In certain other sources (Levelt, 1989), "lemma" appears to have a much broader reference.

13. "The Semantic Wall" appeared as Chapter 1 in David & Denes' *Human communication* (1972).

14. Possibly the whole process is simpler than described in current conjectures, yet still a marvel.

15. To avoid clutter, these rules and other hypothetical details of the process are not depicted.

16. The reader will find that dictionaries are not of much help in resolving the matter, a circumstance undoubtedly occasioned by the fact that the pertinent etymology is confounding: *phon*, a root word from Greek, means "voice"; *vox*, a root word from Latin, means "voice."

17. "CVC" (Consonant–Vowel–Consonant) is the basic syllabic form. See, for example, Carrell & Tiffany, 1977, table 2.2).

18. See especially Brown (1973), Crystal (1976), and Halliday (1975).

19. This combined term makes the point that, in speech, prosody is integral with syntax.

20. Because we are concerned here with speech, I exclude consideration of meanings conveyed by gesture, even formalized gesture as in "sign language."

21. See a later section of this chapter regarding estimates of individual vocabularies.

22. Pronouns constitute a special case. As their name [*pro-noun*] reveals, they are words that stand for nouns, yet their independent meaningfulness is less than that typical

of content words. On the other hand, neither do they have the characteristics of function words. However, they fit the specification of a closed class.

23. Function words are also called "interstitial" since they occur in the "spaces" between content words.

24. In this abbreviation scheme, the first letter in each word that discriminates it from the other parts of speech is used to represent that word. Thus: Noun, Verb, adJective, adverB, aRticle, Conjunction; Preposition; prOnoun; auXiliary. The ∞ symbol seemed appropriate for "infinitive."

25. Actually, some of the nonsense words in the Jabberwocky suggest a meaning, derivable from some phonetic similarity to an actual word.

26. Further, any version could be embellished by the intonation employed.

27. It is impossible to accurately measure anyone's actual vocabulary. In most of the values to be noted in this section, one must be, and can be, satisfied with approximations.

28. Gale & Gale (1902), Doran (1907), Drever (1915–16), Brandenburg (1918), Nice (1920, 1925, 1932), Horn (1926), Smith (1926, 1941), McCarthy (1930), and Adams (1932).

29. Some sources give an even higher upper limit; for instance, Oldfield (1966) reports 90,000; Seashore & Eckerson (1940) report 156,000!

30. This proportional contrast between word comprehension and word use exists from before a child begins to talk.

31. Although the many different meanings of words enlarge the speaker's task of word selection, this also provides an additional creative dimension in speech, as in *double entendre* and puns. It is also a source of unintended humor, as in certain errors of spontaneous speech, and ones found in print, such as the headlines featured in the *Columbia Journalism Review*.

32. College students, 60% male/40% female.

33. See Ervin-Tripp (1961).

34. Compilations of data regarding structural aspects of English words, as used, are presented in Wingate (1988, chap. 5).

35. These three terms were proposed, respectively, by Trager & Smith (1951), Kozhevnikov & Chistovich (1965), and Halliday (1967).

36. "Vowel-form" refers to vowels, diphthongs, and the occasional triphthong. It should embrace, as well, the relatively frequent syllabic consonant. Such consonants, always voiced, have an identifiable resonance and serve as a reduced syllable.

37. Or what one hears in an airliner immediately after having barely made out "This is your captain speaking."

38. See Fonagy (1966), Ladefoged (1963), and Liberman & Prince (1977).

39. For a four-level system of recording stress. Some sources have used a three-level system. Actually, even four levels do not accurately represent acoustic reality.

40. The several influences neighboring sounds may have on each other.

41. According to dictionary pronunciation, as might be said in isolation.

42. The letter "a" indicates stress, the letter "b" means unstress. Carrell & Tiffany (1977, p. 139) give the following as examples:

    Trochaic (ab)   Frankie Dinkle thwarted Bessy
    Iambic (ba)   Collapsed upon the pickle bush
    Dactylic (abb)   Corpulent Cadillacs padded in chrome.
    Anapestic (bba)   It's a fact that he talks to himself all the time.

43. "Correspond roughly" because the orthographic marks are quite inadequate representations of the actual pause features.

44. Intervals 5 and 9 could not be properly rendered graphically due to space confinements.

45. Recall here the omission of pauses of less than 1 second in the profiles of Chapter 10.

46. The measure of pause was based on three kinds of hesitation phenomena: Filled Pause, Revisions, and Word Repetitions. Inclusion of measurable Silent Pause would have inflated these values, especially at the younger age levels.

47. The term "rime" is an alternative, sometimes preferred, spelling of "rhyme."

48. See Wingate (1988, chap. 6).

49. Of interest is the observation that the spoken samples had a perceptible, though mild, rhythmic quality. My informant, Ms. Carol Robinson, is a native of Moscow, Idaho.

50. Kenneth S. Wherry, a United States Senator from Nebraska in the mid-twentieth century, evidenced similar errors—which were called, of course, "Wherryisms."

51. Although there is a heavy conscious element in their planning, word games also contribute to evidence that speech is not automatic.

52. Tweney et al. (1975) point out similarities between speech errors and TOT phenomena, reviewed earlier in the chapter.

53. Corrected speech errors are properly a form of "revision," a hesitation phenomena category.

54. See Kermit Schafer's *Blunderful World of Bloopers.*

55. Another instance of syncope.

56. The kind of product that, in humorous reference to his word "frumious" in *The Jabberwocky*, Lewis Carroll described (in *The Hunting of the Snark*, p. x) as reflecting "a perfectly balanced mind."

57. Note also the /ʃ/ (sh) in the word /kə'lɛkʃən/ preceding the error.

58. It is of interest that similar, sometimes identical, forms of error turn up in newspaper headlines. Examples of these errors appear often in "The Lower Case," a regular feature of the *Columbia Journalism Review.*

59. "Onset" and "rime" from the Syllable Structure Hypothesis.

CHAPTER 12

Speech and Stutter

It is the disturbed relation and the antagonism
between the vocal and the articulating mechanism
which give rise to stuttering; ... It is, therefore,
during the transition from one mechanism to
another that the impediment chiefly takes place.

James Hunt, *Stammering and Stuttering* (1860)

*T*he objective of the present chapter is to review certain findings and observations about stuttering, principally psycholinguistic in substance, that relate particularly to the content of the preceding chapter. Currently there exists a considerable amount of information pertinent to certain speech variables in stuttering, much of it from within the field itself, accumulated over the past 50 years. However, much of the content dealing with aspects of speech production presented in Chapter 11, which stands as the pertinent foundation reference, has received relatively little recognition in writings concerned with stuttering.

OVERVIEW

Interest in what are considered to be "language" dimensions of stuttering appeared in two separate eras of recent times. The initial expression of interest, emerging in the mid-1930s, was couched in the belief regarding "difficult

293

sounds," which prompted a study undertaken to discover which sounds are most difficult for stutterers. That inquiry, as envisioned, was essentially a failure because, in the extensive data collected, no particular sounds were found to be most difficult for stutterers. However, the effort led to further analyses along these lines that, in a few years, yielded clear evidence that stuttering is related to several attributes of words, attributes that came to be called "the language factors" in stuttering.

This early expression of interest, essentially from two sources, lasted less than 10 years. It then fell dormant, and for almost 20 years aroused no interest. Attention to language dimensions reappeared in the 1960s and has continued, although somewhat sporadically, since then. However, the most recent expression of interest along this line has been addressed largely to motor aspects of speaking, which seems to represent a lingering extension of the persuasion regarding "difficult" sounds.

The initial work done in the first era, originating at the University of Iowa, was a series of studies by S. F. Brown, under the direction of Wendell Johnson. This historical notation is important because of a significant, obscurant shift in conception of stuttering from the orientation extant in this first period to that which pervaded the later era, beginning in the 1960s. The series of studies reported in the initial period may be accepted as having been mounted reliably in regard to stuttering, a matter well reflected in the objective and realistic description of stuttering contained in the first report of the initial series (Johnson & Brown, 1935). That description read,

> A stuttering spasm was taken to be any interruption of the normal rhythm of reading. It might take the form of a complete block, undue prolongation of a sound, a repetition of the initial sound of a word or syllable, saying "uh-uh-uh," repetition of the *previous* word or words, or a complete cessation of all attempts to speak for a moment. It was necessary to interpret these various interruptions of rhythm carefully for each case, in the light of what was known about the type of stuttering characteristic of each stutterer. For example, saying "uh-uh-uh" before beginning a word was a definite indication of a spasm in some cases, while other stutterers never hesitated in this way before words in relation to which they had spasms. In these latter cases the "uh-uh-uh" was either a mannerism or an indication that the stutterer had momentarily lost his place, while in the former cases it was marked as a spasm in relation to the word *before* which the "uh-uh-uh" came. (p. 484, italics added)

This straightforward, realistic, unrestrictive description, which appeared early in the modern era of professional interest in stuttering, merits careful attention.[1] Note the use of "normal rhythm" in regard to speech, another form of reference to undulating tone and prosody as discussed in Chapter 11. In the description of stutter, note: (1) clear reference to the elemental features,[2] (2) specification of word/syllable-initial position, (3) distinction between variants of "uh-uh-uh", and (4) the specifications of locus. The latter feature is especially pointed in the reference made to "repetition of the previous word or words" ("words" = phrase). Note that such repetitions are specified as occurring just *prior to* the stutter; that is, they are not the stutter, but occur immediately before it. Such description regarding stutter occurrence was featured, and elaborated, in Chapter 3. Specification of the status of word repetitions is especially pertinent because of the continuing present-day effort, made by some sources, to press monosyllabic word repetitions into the "stuttering" classification, a matter discussed in Chapter 8.

Especially because the description of stutter quoted above is consistent with the identification of stutter as reviewed in earlier chapters (especially in Chapter 3), one can be assured that the work reported in that early era actually did deal with stuttering. However, during the 20-year interim between this era and the second one, the persuasion that stuttering is a psychological problem expanded dramatically. That orientation was especially characterized in the viewpoint formulated and elaborated by Wendell Johnson over a period of many years following the initial work on "language factors."[3] In this later, personally based formulation, the identification of stuttering was shifted from the straightforward, realistic description noted above to the essence of his "definition" of stuttering recorded in Chapter 2, in which objective features are completely ignored. As discussed earlier, this shift blurred the identification of stuttering, a confounding that has been expressed in the policy, widely followed since that time, of endeavoring to not distinguish stutters as unique irregularities of fluency, but instead to meld them with speech features that psycholinguistic research has identified as "hesitation phenomena" in normal speech. The extreme expression of this policy has been to call stuttering "disfluency." (See again pertinent discussions in Chapters 6, 7, and 8 regarding obstructions created by the persisting use of this confounding term, and other contentions of the orientation it epitomizes.)

Because of the orientation described in the preceding paragraph, it is important that one be circumspect regarding studies of "language factors" in stuttering that have been published in the second era. In many cases, one can be comfortable that stutter is the only focus of inquiry and discussion. However, in other cases one can discern probable, sometimes clear, admixture with other "nonfluencies." In particular, any report speaking of "disfluency" should be read with particular scrutiny since there is frequently a shifting back and forth between proper versus inaccurate use of the term. One must keep in mind that "disfluency" is certainly *not* equivalent to "stuttering," unless one has a very clear understanding of the proper meaning of "fluency" as developed in

Chapter 10. It is equally important to be clear about the reference for "stuttering" in these works. One particularly misleading practice has been to include certain hesitation phenomena, particularly monosyllabic *word* repetitions, along with elemental repetitions as instances of stutter. Unfortunately, this practice not only persists but has been elaborated in a number of current sources (e.g., Yaruss & Conture, 1996; Au-Yeung *et al.*, 1998). In some sources it is expanded into more flagrant departures. For example, Au-Yeung and Howell (1998) write that the most common disruptions in stuttering are "part-word, word or phrase repetitions, sound prolongations and blockages."[4] The findings of research in which stutter is mingled with a variety of "disfluencies" are invalidated as specifically pertinent to stuttering, and are therefore at least of questionable value for understanding the disorder. Readers are referred to the discussions of stutter identity presented in Chapters 3 and 10.

Except for certain especially pertinent work that has appeared in recent years, the relevant findings from inquiry into linguistic dimensions will be reviewed here largely in synoptic form, to cover the important material efficiently. Readers interested in more detailed reviews of work reported up to the late 1980s are referred to Chapters 3 and 4 in *The Structure of Stuttering* (Wingate, 1988).

THE "LANGUAGE FACTORS"

The original findings in this area were reported by Spencer F. Brown in a series of publications between 1935 and 1942. Through those studies he identified, in the following order, five "language factors" that were clearly associated with stutter: type of phoneme, type of word, word "accent," words in early sentence position, and word length. Significantly, there was a sixth feature, about which we will have much to say, even though it was dismissed by Brown and has routinely been ignored in later writings—word-initial position.

These findings were soon corroborated by Eugene F. Hahn (1942a,b), whose work was the other relevant source of investigation during that early period. In view of the ensuing lengthy interval of apparent disinterest in this area, Hahn's results evidently were accepted as confirmation and consolidation of the initial findings reported by Brown, rather than simply as a corroboration.

In summary of his findings, Brown (1945) concluded that just four of the factors were "adequate to account for the loci of stuttering." These four were: (1) type of phoneme, (2) grammatical class of words (word type or "parts of speech"), (3) word length, and (4) words in early sentence position. It is curious that he omitted "word accent" from this summary list, since it was more closely associated with stutter than certain other factors. While that omission is curious, ignoring the feature of word-initial position is difficult to understand. Initial position had been clearly noted in his reports—as one would certainly expect, not only in view of its frequent mention in so many contexts, but because it was criterial in identifying the presumably "difficult sounds"[5] being sought.

Brown interpreted the full range of his findings in psychological terms—specifically, that these "language factors" reflected the stutterer's reactions to the "prominence" embodied in each of the dimensions he identified (including those not recognized in his summary). Evidently this explanation was readily accepted within the field (and elsewhere). Certainly the account is consistent with the belief that stuttering is "something psychological," a belief that, essentially universal at the time, has continued to be widely accepted. The explanation given by Brown had assimilated the "language factors" into the general body of psychological explanation of stuttering.

When interest in this area reappeared in the early 1960s, inquiry took this early work as its point of departure. Importantly, it proceeded largely in reference to the four "factors" emphasized by Brown in his summary. Soon an additional dimension, word frequency, was identified in other research. Interestingly, the prevailing conception regarding these several dimensions continued to view them as being separate, essentially independent, variables in spite of occasional recognition of a relation between certain of them. In fact, the eventual expression of this view was the effort to assess the relative importance of the several "factors," to order them into a hierarchy of importance. The effort was unsuccessful. This conception reflected the persisting orientation to stuttering as a psychological problem, in which these "language factors" were viewed in terms of emotional reaction and learning. The preoccupation with psychological interpretation precluded an orientation that could view these several dimensions as linguistic features per se. This limiting constraint is well reflected in the failure to realize that all of the "language factors" are closely interrelated. The interconnections among these several dimensions—portrayed graphically in Figure 12.1—might have been recognized had investigators been interested in the relevant psycholinguistic sources addressed to these variables, reviewed in Chapter 11. The substantial interconnections shown in Figure 12.1 should be kept in mind throughout the discussions that follow, relative to the interdependence of the several "factors."

As discussed in previous chapters (especially Chapters 3 and 6), the attempt to find "difficult sounds" in stuttering, although failing in its initial objective, eventually yielded several matters of great significance for understanding the disorder, which emerge when looking more carefully at the "factors" and their interrelationships. Actually, as we shall see, all of the "factors" identified by

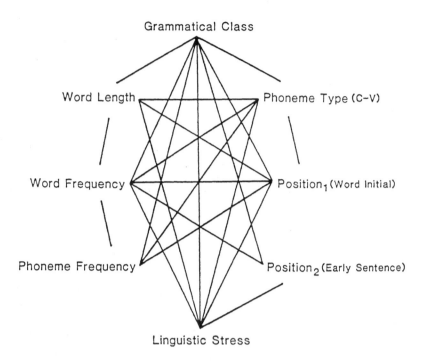

FIGURE 12.1   Interrelationships among "the language factors."

Brown (and later work) are encompassed within the first two, intimately related, "factors" listed above—type of word, and type of phoneme *in word-initial position.* The matter of word-initial, actually *syllable-initial,* position is critical; it has been mentioned earlier in this book, and will come into focus many times more.

TYPE OF PHONEME

The search for "difficult sounds" failed largely because no particular sounds were found to be difficult for all, or even most, stutterers. The only way in which "type of phoneme" emerged as an identifiable variable in this research was in terms of a comparison between consonants and vowels. These results simply confirmed what had been reported for many years,[6] namely, that stutter is more often associated with consonants than with vowels, as in K-K-K-Katy or K------aty. This differential consonant–vowel relation to stutter has remained evident in later experience as well. However, the description of stutter "on" those initial sounds is a misconstruction, based on surface appearance and testimony, rather than objective analysis. If considered carefully, it seems evident that, whether a sound is repeated or prolonged, the sound itself is being made, either in repetition or protraction—as in the example above. So, the difficulty cannot be with the sound per se; the crux of the anomaly is the evident failure (better, transient inability) to move on, into the sound that should follow. This crucial issue will be discussed later in this chapter.

The Johnson and Brown (1935) research regarding stutter "on" the various phonemes was reported as a rank order of phoneme difficulty, represented by the relative frequency with which each phoneme was stuttered in the extensive speech samples assessed. This rank order came to be of considerable value, although not in terms of individual phonemes as such. This matter will be discussed shortly in a second section about phonemes, the Phoneme–Word Connection, wherein they are considered in relation to another "language factor" with which they are most intimately connected—word types ("parts of speech," or grammatical classes).

Before proceeding further, special attention should be directed to what might well be called "the forgotten variable"[7]—word-initial position. Unaccountably, initial position has been largely foregone as a variable meriting attention. Ironically, it seems most likely to have been ignored because it serves so routinely as the criterial feature for identifying stutter occurrence. Significantly, this criterion for stutter occurrence has not been contradicted by any findings in either research or observation. Even more than the consonant-vowel contrast, the observation that stutters occur in word-initial position is massively confirmed by pertinent research. Its use as a criterion should not have precluded attention to its continual verification.

As discussed in Chapters 3, 10, and 11, "initial position," although commonly implying word-initial position, is actually *syllable*-initial. Syllable-initial position as the essential locus of stutters is further confirmed in research findings that the rather rare instances of stutter in other than word-initial position occur in the initiation of a word-internal syllable.

It is curious that the ubiquity of *where* stutters actually occur (syllable-initial position) has been so blandly ignored—obscured first by the focus on "difficult" sounds, and then by the preoccupation with the "language factors," especially the type of word.

TYPE OF WORD

The disappointment in not finding a true phonetic factor prompted analyses leading to the discovery of other attributes of words that clearly are associated with stutters. The first of the other attributes studied, and the one that turned out to be pivotal, was word type—grammatical category.

It was discovered that stutters occur much more frequently with certain "parts of speech" than with others. An extensive ranking of these numerous word types in terms of stutter frequency revealed that types classifiable as content words crowded the upper portion of the list, whereas words classed as function words were near the bottom. Although certain exceptions could be discerned, it was clear that, in general, more stutters were associated with content words than with function words.[8] This finding, corroborated extensively, has been accepted as a principle in the "language factors" research. At one time efforts were made to identify a "gradient" of stutter occurrence among content word types, but none materialized.

The discovery that stutter occurs much more often with content words was quickly assimilated to the belief that stuttering is due to emotional reaction, as follows. Proceeding from the assumption that it is content words that carry the meaning of whatever is expressed, it was claimed that stutterers are therefore more anxious to say those words well which, supposedly, results in stutter. Thus, the purported reactive psychology of the stutterer is presumed to predispose him to stutter on content words because they are held to be the more important words in what is said. This contention regarding the importance of content words, in contrast to function words, was supposedly buttressed by the "telegram" and "headlines" arguments; namely, that telegrams and headlines contain mostly content words. We will consider such matters shortly, after first noting the remaining "language factors."

OTHER "LANGUAGE FACTORS"

The first three items to be included under this heading are the remaining three "factors" identified by Brown, two of which were among those he identified as adequate to account for stutters (see above). The fourth item, word frequency, was contributed from research undertaken in the second era of interest in this topic.

As noted early in this chapter, all of the "language factors" were viewed for some time as being independently associated with stuttering. However, it was eventually pointed out (Wingate, 1988) that these presumed factors are not independent dimensions but are, in several ways, overlapping aspects of the content word-function word difference, as portrayed graphically in Figure 12.1. The nature of these interrelationships will be discussed shortly in following sections of this chapter addressed to analysis of the several "language factors."

Word Accent

This dimension is more properly identified as linguistic stress. Although identified by Brown in one study of his series as a "language factor," he did not mention it in his summary of the factors importantly related to stutter. Stress also has been largely ignored in the subsequent literature dealing with linguistic dimensions in stuttering. However, the significance of this feature merits separate discussion, to be presented shortly.

Word Length

This "factor" represented the finding that stutter is more likely to occur with long words. The discriminant length specified was five *letters*, which reflects the fact that so much of the research in stuttering has dealt with written prose. Measurement of word length by letters is inaccurate in respect to length by phoneme in the same words as spoken.[9] However, in this instance the difference evidently was not material.

Word Frequency

The word frequency factor was derived during the second era of "language factors" inquiry through reference to large compilations of the frequency with which various words occur. The reference compilations were, defensibly (see Chapter 11), accepted as a generalized representation of individual vocabularies. Thereby, the relative frequency with which various words were listed in the large compilations was taken to represent their relative frequency in an individual speaker's use. In application to samples of stuttered speech, it was discovered that stutter was much more likely to occur with words that are used *in*frequently.

Early Sentence Position

This descriptor refers to the first three words in sentences, a straightforward designation of readily identified items. However, this apparent simplicity is belied in the analysis of this factor, which reveals its involvement with several other variables.

ANALYSES OF THE "LANGUAGE FACTORS"

Because words are the common substantive reference for all the "language factors," it is appropriate to begin these analyses by addressing the matter of word categories. As noted earlier, the essential significance of word types (grammatical classes) relative to stuttering is in terms of the broad categories of "content" words and "function" words, discussed in Chapter 11. The content–function distinction is focal to the "language factors" involvement in stuttering; the other "factors" actually represent some facet(s) of this distinction.

GRAMMATICAL CATEGORIES

The reader should recall, from Chapter 11, that the categories of content words and function words are not mutually exclusive and that, in connected speech, almost all words have some semantic value. This qualification has special relevance to the claim that stutter occurs much more on content words because they are the important words. The claim that content words carry the meaning of an utterance and, at least by implication that function words do not, flatly ignores certain clear lines of evidence that function words also are quite important to meaning. In fact, many times words clearly identified as function words are critical to the meaning of an utterance. For instance, in a sentence such as "The woman ran _____ the man," clearly different meanings result from whatever function word fills the blank (e.g., *to, from, with*, etc). Another especially pertinent corroboration that function words are often crucial to meaning is that success with certain tasks in intelligence testing require insertion of a proper function word at appropriate points in test sentences.[10] In addition, one will find many instances of errant newspaper headlines that support this point. Examples of such headlines, most of them humorous, are published regularly in "The Lower Case," a section of the *Columbia Journalism Review*. For example, the statement "Grover man receives jail sentence, fine for sex acts" is rendered ambiguous through use of a comma in place of the function word "and" in proper position. Note particularly that with "and" in place, the prosody of the statement is clearly different, becoming appropriate to the intended meaning. Many of these error headlines, although containing no anomaly of punctuation, word selection, or word order, are nonetheless ambiguous. In such instances, the ambiguity, or incorrect "reading," is quickly resolved through use of the proper prosodic expression; a good example is "Squad helps dog bite victim."[11]

In view of the questionable assumption that content words are regularly the more important word type in verbal expression, explaining stutter as reaction to the perceived meaningfulness of words is not very credible. A similar explanatory effort, posited later and couched in the terms of "information load," was at least as unsuccessful.[12] At the same time, as emphasized earlier in the present writing, the content–function distinction is in many respects defensible and useful; these qualities are particularly well reflected in the special value of this distinction for analyses of stutters. However, there is evidence from within the "language factors" research itself that, in respect to stuttering, the content–function connection is less literal, or complete, than much of the relevant writing has indicated.

From a review of several studies[13] addressed to the extent of stutter occurrence with word types of the two major categories, it was discovered that the content–function distinction, relative to the stuttering data reported, contained certain inconsistencies. First, when ranked in terms of measured stutter frequency, word types of the two categories did not separate at a point clearly consistent with the content–function distinction. The rank order of the eight conventional parts of speech, as determined by frequency of stutter associated with each, did show adjectives, nouns, adverbs, and verbs to head the list, in that approximate order.[14] However, the largest difference between any of the ranks occurred between adverbs and verbs, and this difference was over twice as large as that between verbs and the next lower ranked class, pronouns. It also was larger than differences between any of the other ranks. In other words, in terms of rank value based on stutter frequency, verbs were associated more closely with function words than with content words; thus, content words did not separate neatly from function words in terms of stutter extent. Moreover, the amount of stutter varied considerably among subtypes of several word classes; notably among the several types of verb, but also among different kinds of conjunctions and pronouns.

These discoveries indicated that, although stutter is clearly some function of word class, it is not related *categorically* to content–function word types per se, but instead, in some differential way to words of the two categories. The single variable fulfilling this role is linguistic stress, which occurs differentially through words of the various grammatical classes, as reflected in the stress assignment "rules" and word stress patterns presented in Chapter 11.[15] In this respect it is pertinent to note that, in connected speech, the importance of a word to the meaning of an utterance is signaled by an increase in stress.

WORD ACCENT

As noted above, this "factor" is more properly identified as linguistic stress. Stress is a functional aspect of words that, as discussed in Chapter 11, is clearly related to grammatical class. Moreover, linguistic stress turns up as an aspect of all the "language factors."

Brown's (1938) findings regarding the concurrence of stress and stutters, soon replicated by Hahn (1942a,b), were both obtained from subjects reading prose material. Similar findings for spontaneous speech were not reported until 30 years later, during the second era of inquiry (Hejna, 1972).[16] In all three studies, stress was identified by intuitive judgment of the experimenter, a procedure fully justified in view of the fact that the "rules" for stress assignment are part of the intrinsic knowledge of native speakers of the language in expressing its prosody. Some years later attention was directed specifically to the stress–stutter correspondence (Wingate, 1984c) by comparing graphic displays of: (a) a composite of the stutter loci recorded from 35 stutterers speaking a prose passage, to (b) an instrumental record of stress loci in the same material spoken by a carefully selected normal speaker as reference. Curves plotted for the two sets of data showed a clear correspondence. This finding was corroborated in later independent studies (Bergman, 1986; Klouda & Cooper, 1988). A few years later Prins et al. (1991) found, in a similar study, a significant coincidence between stutters and syllabic stress peaks, particularly in polysyllabic words.

It should be kept in mind that, although stress is clearly a principal feature in stutter occurrences in ordinary speech, it is not an independent variable, any more than is any one of the other "factors"—except for syllable-initial position. Certainly one cannot consider stress itself to be the cause of stutters. Several observations contravene such a belief; a simple one is that many stressed syllables are not stuttered. However, an overly literal view of stress (as cause) has emerged in certain recent publications (Prins et al., 1991; Hubbard & Prins, 1994; Hubbard, 1998). A major fault of this research was that stutterers were asked to read contrived prose material that was quite unlike the stress patterns of normal speech.

The role of stress in stutter emerges almost exclusively in normal connected speech. This fact was evident early in the "language factors" research, in the discovery that only minimal amounts of stutter occurred with words said independently, in remarkable contrast to stutter with the same words said in connected speech (Brown, 1938). Importantly, although stress is an intrinsic aspect of words, its significance for speech, and for stutters, emerges in the expression of words in sequence, connected speech, where linguistic stress is the fundamental vehicle of prosody, the "undulating tone" featured in a section of Chapter 11.

WORD LENGTH

This dimension is a structural aspect of words, reflected differentially in the two grammatical categories. As reviewed in Chapter 11, word length is closely related to the content–function distinction, function words being predominantly monosyllabic, whereas content words, varying in length, include many that are of five letters or longer (the distinction introduced by Brown). The variable of word length overlaps the variables of word class, word frequency, and linguistic stress, indicating that they are not separate "factors."

WORD FREQUENCY

A further significance of the content word–function word distinction is that it reflects a substantial difference in frequency of word use. As discussed in Chapter 11, ordinary discourse contains almost as many function words as content words (see Table 11.1), but their usage frequency differs markedly; frequency of word use from the two categories is grossly disproportionate to the numbers of words in each category. The number of content words in one's vocabulary is very large, and varied in references (see Table 11.4) such that most of them are not used frequently. In contrast, one's fund of function words is not only small but consists of words that are used repeatedly. Thereby the two "factors" of word class and word frequency overlap substantially. Also, they relate directly, although differentially, to the dimension of linguistic stress: the frequently occurring function words are most often unstressed in connected speech, whereas the less frequently used content words typically bear stress.

Since usage frequency is so clearly related to grammatical class, one is led to the position that stutter occurrence is some inverse function of the frequency with which words are used; that is, the more often a word is used the less likely it is to be involved in stutter. Other lines of evidence, to be reviewed below, converge on the same deduction. Of course, one must keep in mind that word type (grammatical class) also is intimately involved as an aspect of usage frequency.

The practical effect of these differences must find expression in the processes of word access and production. Generation of a statement hinges principally on pertinent content words that must be selected from a sizable lexicon, and many of those words (even in one's use-vocabulary) are not produced (said) often. Except for the very common ones, content words are then, on the whole, less well "known" for a speaker than are the function words, as well as much less readily accessible. Again, except for the most common content words, their relative infrequency of use means that they are less "rehearsed" by a speaker. In contrast, it seems evident that function words, from a pool of quite limited size, should be accessed much more readily; and, because they are used so often, function words also are well "rehearsed."

Thus, the well-established finding that stutters involve content words dramatically more than function words is in substantial measure an expression of frequency of use. Other important dimensions to the content–function distinction and its connection to stuttering are discussed in following sections.

Frequency and Familiarity

Word frequency and word familiarity are intimately related in that, basically, the familiarity of a word is occasioned by the frequency with which it occurs in a person's experience. That experience is comprised of several sources: originally, and continually, words as heard; then, words as read; and third, words as spoken by the individual. The first two sources, especially the first, are the principal sources of the words an individual understands, identified as one's "recognition vocabulary," which is more extensive than those words known well enough to be used properly (one's "use vocabulary"). The third source of word familiarity, noted above, is the most potent influence, although the range of this influence is narrower than that of the first two sources.

It should be evident that function words are the most familiar of all words—a hallmark of the frequency with which they are used, in all sources. Partly due to their ubiquity, as well as to their unique nature (noted earlier), function words are not even counted in assessments of an individual's vocabulary. Their use-frequency—and, of course, their familiarity and accessibility—are aspects of function words associated with their low incidence in stuttering, as discussed above.

Although word frequency and word familiarity are intimately related, they are not the same. The difference is illustrated by noting words, listed as occurring with comparable frequency, that differ in respect to familiarity. Impressive illustrations of such difference are found in word-frequency lists derived from written materials, such as the widely used list developed by Thorndike and Lorge (1944) and the more recent compilation by Francis and Kucera (1982). The words in each of the following pairs of words, listed in the respective lists as occurring with the same frequency, can be appreciated to differ considerably in familiarity. From the Thorndike–Lorge list: *adverb* and *affiance*, *elastic* and *edifice*, *impossible* and *ibis*, *valueless* and *vacuity*. From the Francis and Kucera list: *ale* and *aficionado*, *daffodil* and *demagogue*, *eyelash* and *edentulous*, *pepperoni* and *palindrome*.

A word-frequency list based on conversational speech provides similar, although less impressive, illustration that involves words of generally greater frequency and familiarity. Berger (1967) obtained recordings of "assorted adult conversations of an informal and unguarded nature ... collected occasionally and irregularly over a period of approximately two years." These conversational samples yielded a total of 25,000 words, containing 2507 different words, of which 2002 were used more than once. Most of these words would be familiar to the average person; in fact, many would be identified as quite common. However, even among these common words, such as *high*, *low*, *table*, *chair*, *dark*, *light* and others included in the Word Association discussion in Chapter 11, the frequency of their use may vary quite a bit, depending upon circumstances.

The prominent associative pairs listed in Table 11.5 can be considered to be equally familiar, in view of the values recording the extent of their association, yet the frequency with which any of the words in Table 11.5 might occur in ordinary conversation will vary, reflecting the circumstances of the conversation. For instance, *king* and *queen* would most likely occur only rarely in conversations sampled in the United States. The occurrence frequency of the other words would depend on more immediate circumstances. Such variability is exemplified in the word frequencies listed by Berger. Some very familiar words were used with comparable frequency: for instance, *old* (12 times) and *new* (15 times); *cold* (8 times) and *hot* (7 times). However, *man* was used notably more often than *woman* (14 times vs. 7); *girl* more than *boy* (31 vs. 20); and *night* more than *day* (33 vs. 20). There were even greater differences: *good* was used 71 times, *bad* only 31; *high* was used 14 times, but no *low* was used in these samples; *big* was used 16 times, but neither an antonym nor a synonym occurred at all.

As could be expected from earlier discussions regarding word types, function words are the most frequently used types in the conversations recorded by Berger, as they would be in any samples of ordinary conversation. Again, the implications for stuttering remain the same. Among the several qualities characteristic of function words (short, unstressed, etc.), they are the words that are the most "rehearsed."

The difference between word familiarity and frequency of word use, which brings into focus the matter of rehearsal (in saying the word), is uniquely relevant to an oddity often reported by stutterers—that they have trouble saying their own name. The typical explanation offered for this phenomenon has been cast in some assumption regarding the individual's self-image, since everyone should certainly know (be familiar with) his own name. However, as remarked by a student in one of my classes, during discussion of word familiarity and frequency: "How often does a person say his (or her) name?" Clearly, one's name is much less rehearsed than even infrequently used content words. The evident significance of rehearsal comes into focus again later in this chapter.

EARLY SENTENCE POSITION

This "factor" too is interwoven with word class, notably so in the language factors research. In written prose—the standard procedural medium in the language factors research—early sentence position overlaps substantially with grammatical class, because the first three words of sentences are predominantly content words.[17] At the same time, the frequency of stutter in early sentence position is not simply an artefact of grammatical class; greater frequency of stutters in that locus may be relatively independent of word type. Still, word type is clearly implicated in the sentence position factor. It must be kept in mind that "early sentence position" does not mean "initial word." Often the first word in a sentence is a function word. However, content words are overly represented among the first three words, which is the original reference for the factor of early sentence position. A series of studies published around the early 1980s, addressed to the issue of early position and word type,[18] led to the conclusion that grammatical class and early sentence position are not separate factors that affect stuttering in some manner unique to each.

Stutter as some function of early sentence position, reported for a substantial number of studies using printed prose, has long been recognized as typical in spontaneous speech. Over many years, reports from numerous sources have noted that stutterers frequently have difficulty "getting started."[19] Interestingly, some of the research addressed to stuttering in early sentence position reported finding, also, that normal speakers tended to evidence normal nonfluencies in similar locus, although always significantly less than is found for stutters. These findings relate pointedly to physiologically based studies of speech production that show a surge of energy in the early stage of utterance, a surge perceived as stress.

In a study bearing directly on this matter of a surge in early utterance position, stutterers and normal speakers were induced to spontaneously say the same series of sentences, which ranged in length from three to five single-syllable words (Shapiro, 1970).[20] An instrumented comparison of these speech samples revealed that, even though the stutterers had spoken without stuttering, their performances departed markedly from the prosodic patterns evidenced by the normal speakers. In the stutterer samples the initial pulses were more vigorous and longer; the overall prosodic patterns were less stable than the patterns of the normal speaker samples, whose contours were consistent with expectation.

Importantly, there is some evidence of an "early position" effect in regard to at least some phrases, although evidence bearing on this phenomenon has been equivocal. In the final analysis, it may well reduce to simply additional evidence of stutter occurring at a "beginning" (see Wingate, 1988, pp. 114ff). In this respect, it is pertinent to note Brown's (1938) comment that sentence beginnings are "a sequence which requires a definite start." (See also the following section on Pause.) The reader should review the graphic display in Figure 11.4 relative to indications of "surge" at phrase initiations following measurable, though brief, pauses.

As revealed in the preceding reviews of what have been considered language factors in stuttering, linguistic stress turns up as related to all of them. In spite of this prominence, stress has been largely ignored in the literature of stuttering. Indifference to the significance of stress has been an oversight comparable to ignoring word/syllable-initial position. In the final analysis, these two features are basic to linguistic dimensions linked with stutter. Syllable-initial position is clearly ubiquitous; linguistic stress continues to emerge as a feature significantly involved in the occurrence of stutter in connected speech.

THE PHONEME–WORD CONNECTION

Throughout the following discussion it is important to bear in mind that syllable-initial position is implicit; that is, the phonemes in reference are word-initial (actually, syllable-initial) phonemes.

As noted earlier, the focus on "speech sounds" led to compilation of a rank order of the relative frequency with which the various phonemes were found to be associated with stutter. The ranking was interpreted as indicating the relative "difficulty" of the various phonemes. It is reproduced as Table 12.1, in which the sounds identified as difficult appear in the left column.

TABLE 12.1   Sound "Difficulty" Ranking, According to Percentage Stuttering*

C	%	V	C	%	V
d	21.7		t	9.1	
z	20.9		hw	8.7	
g	19.8		w	7.6	
tʃ	19.1			6.7	ʒ
dʒ	18.9			6.0	ɛ
v	17.4			5.0	ɪ
k	16.3			4.8	ɔ
θ	15.8			4.7	i
l	15.6			3.8	ou
r	14.6		ð	3.7	ʌ
m	13.6			3.5	eɪ
p	13.0			3.5	aɪ
s	12.4			3.2	ɔ
b	12.3			2.7	ɥ
ʃ	12.1		h	2.4	
n	12.0			1.8	ɑ
f	11.6			1.6	au
j	11.3			1.3	æ
				0.8	ə

*The "easy" sounds appear in the right-hand columns.

Importantly, this ranking of presumed difficulty provided no support for a phonetic factor. Other than the overall consonant–vowel contrast, the phoneme rank could not be accounted for on the basis of phonetic principles, such as phoneme type, or manner or place of articulation; nor could it be rationalized on the basis of the relevant underlying physiology of the various phonemes. Actually, the full ranking requires some qualification of the general claim that consonants are more difficult than vowels, since it is clear that two consonants rank considerably lower than some vowels, and three other consonants are essentially within the vowel range of "difficulty." Because of their low levels in the ranking, these five consonants (/ð/, /w/, /t/, /h/, and /hw/) came to be known as "the easy consonants." This description is based solely on their positions in this ranking since, as with the supposedly difficult sounds, there is no phonetic, physical, or psychological rationale to explain why these five phonemes should be "easy."

As reviewed, the "difficult–easy" account of phonemes and stuttering has no inherent substantive basis. However, a logical and defensible explanation for all of these findings is afforded through reference to psycholinguistic research, as reviewed in Chapter 11. One principle is based in the phonetic structure of the language, specifically as it pertains to a feature we have had reason to emphasize many times before, namely, word-initial position. Analysis of very large samples of (normal) spontaneous speech reveals that, overall, over 70% of word-initial phonemes are consonants. Therefore, since stuttering is a word-initial phenomenon, considerably more stuttering should be expected to involve consonants simply on the basis of frequency of occurrence, since consonants are the more prevalent word-initial phoneme.

However, there is a potentially vexing inconsistency within this finding, posed by an apparent contradiction regarding word-frequency and phoneme type. As noted earlier, analyses of extensive speech samples reveal that, in something over 70% of all words spoken, a consonant is the initial phoneme. Significantly, the percentage of word-initial consonants increases directly with the frequency with which various words occur. Among "common" words, word-initial consonant percentages increase well beyond eighty. If one considers only the most frequently used words, the consonant-initial occurrences approach, or reach, 100%. Now, prominent among the frequently occurring words having the highest percentages of initial consonant are words that begin with the "easy" consonants. The consonant ranking in Table 12.2 reflects these frequency values clearly—with two exceptions (/s/ and /hw/), which are considered below.

The inconsistency mentioned in the preceding paragraph regarding the connection between stutters, consonants, and initial position is as follows. If consonants are intrinsically difficult, then simply in terms of probability a

TABLE 12.2 Rank Order, Frequency of
Occurrence of Consonants and Vowels
in Word-Initial Position in Ordinary
Spontaneous Speech

Consonants*	Vowels
ð	ə
w	ɪ
t	ɑ
s	aɪ
h	ɛ
b	ɔ
m	ɛ
k	ʌ
d	o
j	a
g	au
f	e
p	i
l	ɔt
n	
r	
hw	
ʃ	
θ	
dʒ	
v	
tʃ	
z	
ʒ	

The "easy" consonants are in bold-face.

disproportionate amount of stutter should occur with those initial consonants
that occur most frequently. Therefore (see Table 12.2), at least /ð/, /w/, /t/ and
/h/ should be the consonants most frequently involved in stutter. However, the
pertinent data show exactly the opposite: these most frequently occurring
initial consonants in ordinary speaking are four of the five *least* stuttered, the
so-called "easy" consonants. The phonemes /s/ and /hw/ are exceptions to the

correspondence just noted. Their exception is occasioned by word type and frequency of occurrence. The phoneme /s/, not one of the "easy" consonants, is the most frequent initial phoneme of all the many words in a vocabulary, most of which are content words. In comparison, /hw/, an "easy" consonant, is the initial phoneme of a much smaller number of words, but among which are ones that are used very often.

One need only reflect briefly on one's own word use to appreciate the unique usage-prominence of the "easy" consonants. Consider how often one says words that begin with these five phonemes. Following is a brief set of such words:

> for /ð/: the, that, this, there, then
> for /h/: how, who, have, here, he, him
> for /w/: we, with, was, will, would, were, one
> for /hw/: what, when, where, why, which
> for /t/: to, too, two, tell, time

These words, and others like them that begin with an "easy" consonant, make up a substantial part of any individual's basic use vocabulary, represented in the central dot of Figure 11.3.

Clear illustration of the foregoing description is contained in the findings of Berger's (1967) study of ordinary conversations, discussed earlier. Only 10% of the different words used in those speech samples had one of these five consonants as their initial phoneme, but those same words made up 25% of the total number of words spoken. Moreover, the majority of words beginning with the "easy" consonants are function words, a fact represented clearly in Berger's findings, wherein 78% of the words beginning with one of these five consonants were function words. These useful words are the most familiar words; they also are predominantly short, almost always unstressed, and used again and again.

So, it now seems clear that the low frequency of stutter with /ð/, /h/, /hw/, /w/, and /t/ lies not in any properties unique to them as consonants, but instead in the fact that they are the onsets of certain very common words that are used with especially great frequency, and are predominantly function words.

It is appropriate to direct attention to highly similar circumstances in the data of Table 12.1 that pertain to vowels. Note that the occurrence frequency of word-initial vowels has an inverse relationship to the "difficulty" ranking of vowels, a relationship expressed in a highly significant negative correlation value of −.61; indicating that the more often the vowel occurrence, the less likely a stutter. The most significant item in the two lists is /ə/, without doubt the most frequently occurring vowel and clearly the phoneme (as part of a word) least frequently associated with stutter. Significantly, its dominant feature—its hallmark—is that it is unstressed wherever it occurs; in fact, /ə/ is the ultimate in vowel-form reduction. Actually, some question has been raised whether the sound routinely transcribed as /ə/ is always an actual (though minimal) vowel, or often simply the basic sound of phonation, unmodified by any supralaryngeal shaping.[21] Most often considered to be a phoneme, /ə/ is often called the "neutral" or "indefinite" vowel because of its nondistinctive nature. For practical purposes, there seems little reason to determine if the sound regularly perceived as the schwa (/ə/) is a "true" vowel or simply the basic sound of phonation. In either case, the essential substance—an unstressed vocal pulse—is present. Transcribing either of them as /ə/ is defensible until some acceptable means of differentiation is devised.

It should be noted that the vowel /æ/ is next lowest in the ranking of association with stutter. Significantly, /æ/ is the initial phoneme of several short words that are among those most frequently used: "and," "at," and "as,"—which also are almost always unstressed in ordinary discourse.

Overall it seems clear that there are no substantial grounds whatever for positing a "phonetic factor," in the sense that certain phonemes contribute importantly to stutter occurrence. The apparent connection between stutters and phones (specifically *consonants*) disappears into the variable of word/syllable-initial position. The "grammatical factor," certainly in regard to any significant influence of words from any individual grammatical classes, also fades away. The essence of the grammatical factor reduces to the content word–function word distinction. Frequency of word use emerges as the salient dimension of this distinction, with linguistic stress and word length as intimately related features. As such, the content–function distinction becomes useful as a convenient and reliable shorthand reference that represents these qualities of various words.

The foregoing analysis reveals that the two primary "language factors" (type of phoneme, and grammatical class of words) converge in the routinely ignored variable of word-initial position and, furthermore, that they reduce to a common dimension of usage frequency. Thereby, their significance emerges in the form of evidence that stutter occurrence must be some inverse function of the frequency with which words are used, and the prosodic requirements that their typical use entails. In brief, stuttering is least likely to occur with words that are said often and with reduced stress.

PAUSE

The phenomenon of pause in relation to stuttering has received only intermittent, and minimal, attention. Interestingly, pause received fleeting consideration in one of the original studies from which the "language factors" emerged. Brown (1938) mentioned (silent) pause in terms of its relevance to sentence-initial position. His comments regarding pause were not based on samples of stuttered speech but on reports regarding "performance" speech of normal speakers, obtained in earlier studies of stage speech and of formal readings. He pointed out that, in those reports, pauses between sentences were found to be much longer than the average length of all other pauses in the selections. Brown called attention to these findings to emphasize the matter of sentence beginnings, as "a sequence which requires a definite start." He noted that the lengthier inter-sentence pauses might present "demands that the stutterer's speech mechanism is unable always to meet." However, he clearly favored his interpretation that early sentence position constitutes a (perceptual) "prominence" for stutterers, a conjecture founded in the theme that stuttering represents a psychological reaction of apprehension. Nonetheless, drawing attention to notable pause in those locations does point up the matter of "a definite start," in which certain features of speech production typically are emphasized. The deduction of "excessive demand on speech production" is the more plausible explanation (see analysis of Early Sentence Position, below).

Evidently, a report by Robbins (1935) contains the earliest notation of pause differences in the speech of stutterers compared to normal speakers. He reported that in the oral reading of a short selection, and of 12 unrelated sentences, the average pause length between words was 0.12 seconds for the normal speakers but 3.6 times as long for "bad stammerers." Robbins' report aroused little interest, and not until relatively recent times was research addressed specifically to comparison of (silent) pause in normal and stuttered speech. Watson and Love (1965) reported that, in contrast to normal speech samples, pause distributions in samples from stutterers showed unusually high numbers of brief silent periods of 0.1 to 0.5 seconds, silent periods that could not be attributed to stutter occurrences. These findings—high frequency of brief silent intervals in *non-stuttered* speech samples of stutterers—were corroborated by Love and Jeffress (1971), then by Few and Lingwall (1972) and by Zerbin (1973).

The matter of filled pause has received even less attention than silent pause, perhaps because of the commonness of /ə/ in association with stutter, as reported in Sheehan's lengthy review (1974), noted in Chapter 3. Importantly, there are varieties of filled pause, and various loci in which they occur. The careful analyses of speech samples presented in Chapter 10 were based on various features intrinsic to assessment of fluency, among which were four types of filled pause that had been differentiated in previous study. In the mid-1980s, research making use of these pause types was addressed specifically to the immediate contexts in which both filled and silent pauses occur in spontaneous speech samples of stutterers and normal speakers (Wingate, 1984a, 1988). Stutterers were found to differ significantly from normal speakers on several of the dimensions analyzed. First, stutterers' speech samples contained more of both types of pause. Also, as could be expected, iterative filled pauses were found in only the stutterer samples. Stutterer and normal samples were comparable in respect to certain sequences involving silent pauses and filled pause variants, but differed markedly in certain others. In particular, stutterer samples were characterized by the sequence: SP — FP — SP. The stutterers' pause pattern suggested less effective word retrieval and generally less efficient utterance planning.

RATE

Stutterers' speech rate is discussed here within the topic of Pause since, as discussed in Chapters 10 and 11, pause is a major determinant of speech rate.

The immediately preceding paragraphs noted reviews of a number of literature sources in which the non-stuttered speech of stutterers is revealed to contain an inordinate number of brief (silent) pauses—pauses that are not associated with evident stutter. In other words, there is considerable evidence of many imperceptible silent intervals in the seemingly fluent speech of stutterers. Interestingly, these findings regarding pause have a direct counterpart in data bearing on stutterers' speech rate.

Many comparisons of overall[22] speech rate of stutterers and normal speakers have been reported for samples of spontaneous speech and of oral reading (e.g., Bloodstein, 1944; Johnson, 1961; Minifie & Cooker, 1964; Burke, 1972; Wingate, 1988, pp. 213–226). In these studies the spontaneous speech samples of the two groups were comparable in content, such as from describing the same pictures, or telling a story based on the same picture, or telling of vocational aspirations. Oral reading samples used the same, or similar, prose material. Whether in spontaneous speech or oral reading, the speaking rate of the stutterers was consistently found to be something less than three-fourths the rate of the normal speakers. These findings are consistent with those, noted above, that reveal high levels of brief silent pause in the speech of stutterers.

These routinely found differences in rate are not likely to reflect phonetic, articulatory, or motor abilities. As found so uniformly in research on speech rate in normal speakers, rate is predominantly a matter of (largely silent) pause. It is, then, especially pertinent to recall the statement by Lenneberg, noted in Chapter 10, that, in respect to ordinary spontaneous speech, rate is limited by "the cognitive aspects of language," rather than simply by physical ability to articulate.[23] The "cognitive aspects" of speaking involve planning, word choice, and word accessibility. This description should apply to the speech of stutterers as well, although one might suspect that the extensive brief silent pauses in stutterers' speech, noted above, may have other significance as well.

The mutually reinforcing data regarding silent pause and speech rate indicate anomaly in speech production of stutterers other than, and more fundamental than, the obvious anomalies occurring as stutters.

PROPOSITIONALITY

The first section of Chapter 11, addressed initially to emphasizing that ordinary spontaneous speech is not automatic, moved naturally to discussion of propositionality, which succinctly characterizes the substance of normal speech. The reader should review, there, the source and rationale for the concept of propositional speech, and its contrast to automatic speech.

The concept of propositionality has received little direct attention in the literature of stuttering, even though certain frequent observations clearly raise the issue of propositionality. For instance, it is often reported that stutterers can curse without stuttering or, similarly, that they do not stutter in exclamations of pain, fear, joy, etc. Emissions of this kind also are regularly observed in the speech of aphasics, wherein they are identified as "automatic"—that is, non-propositional. Such emissions are thereby not properly identified as speech, since they lack the essential character of true speech, that it be propositional.

CONNECTED SPEECH

Stutterers are known to also speak certain referential (true) words, and word sequences, without stuttering, such as common expressions of greeting and salutation. Such expressions are phatic utterances, described in Chapter 11; they are utterances having low propositional substance, and are said very often. Many sources have reported that no stuttering occurs in recitative speaking at various assemblages, such as in certain church rituals. In effect, such performance is choral speaking (see Chapter 4). Stutter also is said to not be evident in even solo performances of, for instance, the Lord's Prayer, or the Pledge of Allegiance. Regarding this latter group of examples, it should be clear that the propositional value of such expressions is minimal, and that rehearsal and practice must play a crucial role.

Stutterers frequently report that they stutter little, if at all, in talking to pets, or small children. One should immediately reflect on the kinds of things likely to be said to a pet, or an infant—that is, what the propositional level of such utterances is likely to be. So much of what one says in these circumstances is not "newly generated"; in fact, it is likely to have been said many times before. Such expressions also are most likely to be simple, brief, and follow a particular format. Further, the manner of speaking also is typically altered, see below. In sum, this kind of speech approaches the level of phatic utterance.

Speech addressed to a young child (ages 3 to 5) is likely to have more substance, but it is still not comparable to speaking to adults, or even older children. Extensive research (in several languages) investigating this matter reveals that the nature of speech addressed to young children differs considerably in several respects from the speech, of the same individuals, to older persons. In speaking to young children, speakers make certain important adjustments in the structure of their speech, in implicit recognition of the child's verbal and cognitive immaturity.[24] Evidently, the adjustments are made without conscious intent. Research in this area finds consistently that speech to young children is simpler than usual, contains a smaller and more basic vocabulary, is slower, is expressed in short sentences with clear intervening pauses, and is redundant.

It has long been reported by stutterers that they do not stutter when alone. Reservations regarding this claim should begin by recognizing it as not only subjective but retrospective as well. One also should wonder about the kinds of things a person is likely to say when alone, for instance, the length of utterances, whether they are grammatically complete, the vocabulary used, and the manner in which the utterances are expressed. Such considerations should raise serious doubts that this kind of talking is like ordinary speech. Moreover, objective evidence has accrued that seriously contradicts this claim. Several studies,[25] reviewed in Chapter 5, yielded evidence that, although some individuals may stutter less while speaking (oral reading) when alone, their speech is not without stutter.

The claims reviewed above, and others like them, taken at face value, have routinely been explained in terms that invoke presumed psychological reactions of stutterers, namely, that in such circumstances they are less anxious about their speech and for that reason do not stutter. The most compelling of such claims is the representation that stutterers can fulfill a role in a play without stuttering. The standard explanation for this observation is that, under such circumstances, the stutterer is no longer himself; that he has assumed the (non-stuttering) persona of the character he portrays. This appealing, and evidently quite persuasive, account completely overlooks the fact that the required preparation for acting in a play is to learn one's "lines," and that this memorization is consolidated through many rehearsals. The stutterer-actor is thus speaking "lines" he has not only memorized but has practiced over and over. The lines spoken in a thespian role are thus of a very low level of propositionality. Special note should be made that the lines encompass all dimensions of the message: the sounds and words in sequence, and the pertinent prosody—the rehearsal is "full."

The earliest suggestion that stuttering involves higher levels of the speech production process was made 70 years ago by Samuel Orton, a neurologist with whom Travis worked in his neurophysiological research. Orton, who surely was familiar with the works of Hughlings Jackson, expressed his deduction as follows:

> The emotional element has received much attention in stuttering and has long been popular as an explanation of its occurrence. It is, of course, true that stuttering is not only more frequent but more severe in embarrassing situations and that it rarely occurs in singing or in repetition of material learned by rote. This immediately suggests for us that the difference here is related to the plane of the speech effort rather than to the emotional content of the speech. This brings into relief the propositional element of speech and with one exception this seems to be the plane at which stuttering is most severe and most frequent, and it is often of course in embarrassing and strange situations that the propositional effort is most stressed.[26] (1929, p. 1047)

It is appropriate to note, 70 years after this insightful analysis of observations about stuttering, that so many sources concerned with stuttering are still wedded to, in Orton's words, "the emotional element."

As noted in Chapter 11, the reading aloud of prose material lacks certain important criteria of full propositional speech, and one must keep in mind the often reported finding that more stuttering occurs in spontaneous speech than in reading aloud. Nonetheless, prose material does have appreciable propositional qualities; in fact, various levels of propositionality may be constructed for experimental purposes. Most of the inquiry into linguistic dimensions of stuttering has used prose reading, largely because of the advantages of design and controls that this practice affords. Much of the evidence regarding linguistic dimensions in stuttering has been obtained through prose reading. Importantly, this evidence is consistent with findings obtained through study of stuttering in spontaneous speech.

From the "Language Factors"

Although the research in this area has not dealt directly with the matter of propositionality per se, there is much within those inquiries that is pertinent to the concept. Bases for deducing the significance of propositionality in stuttering emerged very early in this line of inquiry, and also received coincidental support from work having a different research interest.

The first indication in the "language factors" research that stutter occurrence is principally a function of connected speech resulted from Brown's reappraisal of the "difficult sounds" effort. That review led him to posit the "grammatical factor," namely, the content word-function word distinction. In fact, the remarkable difference between the amount of stutter in connected speech (oral reading) and saying individual words (read from a list) was first described by him in terms of the influence of "context." However, the matter of context was soon, and thereafter, ignored under the swell of attention given to the more concrete features of words and phonemes, reviewed earlier. Evidently, the focus on words and sounds had more interpretive appeal, and fit better into preconceptions.

The markedly greater amount of stutter in oral reading of prose as compared to aloud reading of individual words, has been reported a number of times, from various sources. Moreover, the dramatic influence of context also has been revealed coincidentally in other research; for example, findings that if a stutterer reads prose material aloud in the usual manner, and then reads the same material backward, the latter performance yields results comparable to saying the words as a list. In retrospect, this finding might well be expected since there is likely to be as little context in reading something backward as there is in reading a disconnected list of words.

A clear relationship between stutter, grammatical class, and propositionality was revealed in a study done in the early era of interest in linguistic features. That study assessed stutter frequency with content words and function words at three levels of propositionality: a word list, a nonsense passage, and a meaningful passage (Eisenson & Horowitz, 1945). The amount of stutter with function words remained at the same low frequency over all three levels. In marked contrast, stutter with content words increased markedly over the three levels. Stutter involving content words was almost twice that of function words for the word list, increased to over twice as much in the nonsense passage, and then expanded to over four times as much in the meaningful paragraph. These results showed not only the effect of context but that the influence, especially of meaningful context, is expressed through content words. Evidently, whatever underlies the greater incidence of stutter with content words is compounded by their use in propositional utterance. As reviewed in Chapter 11, words in connected utterance are influenced by several dimensions of the context in which they occur. Examples given there illustrated how certain words are pronounced differently in context than in isolation, a difference reflecting coarticulatory variation induced by changes in stress pattern—prosodic influence.

The likelihood of stutter occurrence at various propositional levels is represented in Table 12.3, which indicates the probability of stutter under various speaking circumstances. As noted earlier, most of the inquiry into linguistic dimensions of stuttering has been implemented through the reading of prose material. This procedure lacks some major features of fully propositional speech; in particular, the fundamental process of message generation that involves activities of word selection and their sequential arrangement and, as well, the necessary adjustments of word stress patterns into the larger prosodic line. Thereby, certain fundamental aspects in the task of producing a message in spontaneous speech are bypassed in oral reading. At the same time, oral reading requires the speaker to make adjustments to a range of speech production plans already set forth. He will have a generalized familiarity with the whole process and certain of its dimensions. Most likely he will have only an abstracted appreciation of the basic overall plan of the message, but he will at least sense, empathically, that it *has* a plan. He should have a good grasp of the tone groups within the overall plan, through two important avenues: (1) his experiential, interiorized, and thoroughly practiced knowledge of word stress rules, which include as a basic feature that content words receive stress and function words typically do not; and (2) the presence of graphic prosodic cues in the written material (capital letters, colons, semicolons, commas, and periods) that instruct where to pause, for how long, and something about what the intonation contour should be.

Within the prose material that is to be read aloud, those words that are within the speaker's vocabulary should have readily accessible plans. The

TABLE 12.3 Probability of Stutter at Varying "Levels" of Utterance

Probability	Spontaneous speech	Oral Reading
100%	Important explanations, etc.	
	Ordinary conversation	
	"Small talk"	
		Ordinary prose
	Talking to small children	Altered prose
	Talking to pets	word order changed
	Recitative speaking	nonsense passage
	"Asides"	passage backward
	Phatic statements	Word list
	Curses	
0%	Exclamations	

most likely potential obstacle to the average speaker would be presented by an unfamiliar (content) word whose pronunciation he would have to guess, making use of his abstracted knowledge of sound pattern and stress pattern rules for words in the language, as reviewed in Chapter 11.

The fidelity with which all these plans are executed may be affected by a number of circumstances, some from influences external to the task but also some from within the system itself—as revealed in the speech error samples presented in Chapter 11.

FROM THE "ADAPTATION" EFFECT

This phenomenon, the decrease in stutter upon repetition of the same material, was discussed in Chapter 6. The principal reason for presenting adaptation in this section on propositionality is in regard to an important consideration hardly ever mentioned, namely, that the propositional value of something said repeatedly, especially in immediate sequence, progressively diminishes, a phenomenon known as "verbal satiation."[27] Corroboration of this relationship, from a different angle, is contained in findings that (silent) practice with the meaning of sentences directly facilitates overt production (MacKay & Bowman, 1969). Propositionality is linked intimately with rehearsal, although the extent of that relationship is not evident in adaptation studies. In my awareness, only one adaptation study contains data bearing directly on this matter. That study (Bardrick & Sheehan, 1956) included an adaptation sequence in which subjects reread the same sets of numbers. Even the initial reading of this highly non-propositional material took less than half the time for reading ordinary prose of comparable length. However, of particular significance for the present discussion, the amount of stutter decrease changed little over the five sequential readings; rehearsal of such material produced little evident benefit.

Several "adaptation" studies have yielded findings pertinent to important dimensions that underlie the evident benefit of rehearsal, as embodied in the adaptation effect. For some while during the era of active interest in the adaptation effect, it had seemed to me that rehearsal with the prosody of a reading selection was likely to make a major contribution to the evident benefit of an adaptation sequence. This led to a study (Wingate, 1966a) designed to explore that hypothesis. A reading passage was created in which the punctuation could be altered at many points, which made it possible to prepare a number of differing versions of the same passage, each of which still maintained essentially the same statement regarding the same topic. Each version of the passage had the same words (and therefore the same phonemes) in the same sequence, but the altered punctuation of each version required a somewhat different prosodic expression. Stutterers reading the same version of the passage five times in succession (the standard adaptation procedure) evidenced the usual decrease in stutter.[28] However, when the same subjects read, sequentially, the five prosodically altered versions of the passage, the decrease in stutter was temporarily reversed and, overall, severely reduced. The typical "adaptation effect," improvement in performance, was disrupted by reducing literal ("full") rehearsal. The results are displayed in Figure 12.2a.

These results indicate that the typical decrease in stutter found in the standard adaptation procedure is not a function of reaction to words or to phones, either as stimuli or as cues, since the sequence of words and phones remained the same in the prosodically altered versions of the passage. Instead, the progressive decrease in stutter (or, improvement in the reading) in the standard "adaptation" sequence evidently results from saying the same thing over and over in essentially the same way. The usual decrease of stutter in the "adaptation effect" is explained more credibly as due to rehearsal of the material being spoken—like the early period of learning one's lines for a play.

Very similar findings resulted from an adaptation study undertaken from a quite different orientation (Gould & Sheehan, 1967). That work was couched in a belief that silence is stressful for stutterers, that it increases stutterers' anxiety about speaking, which results in more stuttering. Accordingly, it was predicted that interposing 5 minutes of enforced silence, after the second reading in an adaptation sequence, would result in increased stutter. It was further predicted that the amount of stutter would increase proportionally with three separate interposed conditions that were presumed to pose increasing levels of stressful silence.

The results are shown as Figure 12.2b. Clearly, reading the passage five times in immediate succession yielded the typical decrease in stutter (curve D). In contrast, interrupting the consecutive sequence of readings for 5 minutes markedly disrupted a decrease in stutter—interfered with speech improvement. Moreover, the effect was the same for all three conditions of presumably differential emotional stress. Then, in all three conditions, improvement resumed after the imposed silence was lifted, although some of the early gain was lost during the period of silence. The interference with rehearsal in this procedure, although different in kind from that in the foregoing study, had the same effect—disrupting a progressive decrease in stutter (or, improvement in speech).

Some years later Bruce and Adams (1978) assessed the influence of whispered readings on the outcome of an adaptation series. It was found that

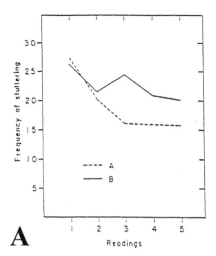

FIGURE 12.2a   Stuttering adaptation under usual condition (five immediately sequential readings of a passage) (curve A), and on sequential reading of five prosodically altered versions of that passage (curve B) Reprinted with permission from Wingate (1966).

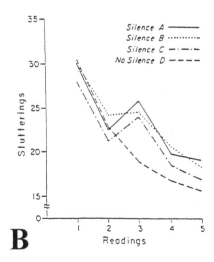

FIGURE 12.2b   Stuttering adaptation under usual condition (five immediately sequential readings) (curve D), and under three conditions in which a silent interval was interposed after the second reading (curves A, B, and C). Reprinted with permission from Gould & Sheehan (1967).

whispered readings did not contribute to adaptation, that practice in reading aloud was superior to whispered practice in effecting stuttering adaptation; the benefits of practice require the full activity. It is significant that the vocal dimension of the speech signal evidently was critical for the improvement effected.

Along similar lines, Brenner *et al.* (1972) had stutterers recite sentences from memory after either silent, lipped, whispered, or aloud rehearsal. Aloud rehearsal resulted in fewer stutters than any of the other conditions. Again, the vocal dimension evidently was critical to improvement.

Most recently, Max and Caruso (1998) reported finding, in an adaptation series with eight stutterers, an increase in articulation rate, a decrease in vowel and word duration, and a decrease in the extent of consonant–vowel transition. The authors describe these changes as consistent with those that occur during skill improvement for non-speech activities, that is, improvement due to practice or rehearsal. However, the improvement should not be construed simply in terms of motor acts, including the several dimensions of motor coordination required in speaking. It is more aptly expressed in the rationale of the "fault line" concept (Wingate, 1988). That concept, described later in this chapter, is supported by the findings of Prins and Hubbard (1990), additional evidence that stuttering adaptation occurs not as a function of changes in surface parameters (motor acts) but because repeated readings of a passage reduce demands upon central motor-linguistic processes, reflecting the broader, more comprehensive aspects of speech production.

One should keep in mind that speech production requires marvelous organization. Rehearsal of any speech sequence undoubtedly enhances the process in its entirety. Pertinent evidence for this deduction is found in research in which the variable of interest was the amount of hesitation in repeated spontaneous speech. Goldman-Eisler (1968) employed two procedures utilizing wordless action cartoons. Subjects were first asked to simply describe the cartoons—repeatedly. The second procedure required interpreting the cartoons—again, repeatedly. As might be expected, the amount of hesitation was considerably greater for the interpretation task. The findings regarding rehearsal revealed progressive decrease in number of hesitations for both conditions, remarkably so for the repeated interpretations.

With repeated speaking of the same substance, the overall demands of speech production lessen. The propositionality of the material diminishes as the benefits of practice accrue, and all processes involved become less novel, more routinized, partly from increasing familiarity but principally through rehearsal.

LEXICAL ACCESS

WORD ASSOCIATION AND WORD-FLUENCY

Research employing each of these procedures with stutterers has yielded evidence of less facile word-retrieval capability.

Word Association

Research in this vein has been pursued along two somewhat differing lines of inquiry. One has been mounted essentially as exploratory; the other was undertaken in reference to revealing possible emotional variables (a frequent use of word-association procedure). The exploratory studies used established "stimulus" word lists; the emotionally oriented line employed lists that were modified or specially created for the purpose.

Results from these varied studies can be summarized briefly in two common findings: stutterers took longer to produce associations, or they gave more "uncommon" or "individual" associations.

Word Fluency

Several studies employing this procedure, with children and adults,[29] have consistently found stutterers to function considerably less well than normal speakers. In one study (Wingate, 1988, chap. 8) subjects' word lists were further analyzed to assess the extent of "alliterative assonance," the number of words in sequence that also had the same vowel as the syllable nucleus of the word (of its first syllable if a polysyllabic word). Examples include: "seat, seem, season, seal," and, for consonant clusters, "spin, spit, spill." On this special measure, too, the normal speakers scored significantly higher than the stutterers.

The measure of alliterative assonance was included because of its relevance to the "fault line"concept, with its focus on the latent separateness of initial consonant(ism) and syllable nucleus. It was my supposition that word access by normal speakers would show more evidence of syllable integrity, as reflected in the syllable nucleus becoming part of an associative base—that is, that among normal speakers, the search for "s"-words would more often incorporate the syllable nucleus as well.

TOTAL "DISFLUENCIES"

Another, independent line of inquiry also yields substantial evidence that stutterers' word retrieval skills are less efficient that those of normal speakers. Over many years, an extensive range of research, involving both children and adults, has compared the total amount of "disfluency" (stutters plus "normal nonfluencies") recorded in the speech of stutterers and of normal speakers. Throughout this research, regardless of the size of the study populations,[30] the findings have consistently revealed stutterers to evidence substantially more total "disfluency" than normal speakers. The total, of course, includes stutters, which properly should be discounted in such comparisons. However, the bias thereby introduced is negligible. The critical dimension of these findings is that, in all comparisons, the speech of stutterers contains substantially more "normal nonfluencies" than does the speech of normal speakers.

As emphasized in Chapter 10, the term *hesitation phenomena* correctly identifies what have been called, improperly, "normal nonfluencies" in the literature of stuttering. Psycholinguistic study of normal speech has revealed these events to be regular aspects of (normal) fluency. Moreover, that same research has found evidence to propose, as reviewed in Chapter 11, that certain forms of hesitation phenomena, especially (but not limited to) pause types, seem clearly to be overt indices of speech production planning. As discussed earlier, making appropriate word choices is a crucial dimension of such planning. The compelling evidence that the speech of stutterers contains so many hesitation phenomena concurs with other evidence, just reviewed, of inefficient word retrieval capability among stutterers. The findings regarding the extensive brief silent intervals in the speech of stutterers would seem pertinent to the matter of word retrieval.

Inquiry addressed to a range of verbal dimensions in stuttering (Wingate, 1988, chaps. 7, 8) yielded several findings especially pertinent to the subject of lexical access and word use. One such finding deserves mention here. The stutterer and normal subjects in the study reported there were matched for their achievement on a recognition vocabulary test, a measure of word knowledge that does not require a defining statement. A second vocabulary test, which required giving definitions (in this instance, in writing), was also administered. On this second measure, the stutterers used more words in their definition efforts, yet scored lower than the normal speakers. Since the two groups had evidenced the same level of vocabulary knowledge on the recognition measure, the lower achievement of the stutterers in definition (expressive) vocabulary indicated less efficient word access and use. Similar evidence emerged in certain other comparisons made in that research.

Problems in word access and retrieval are compounded by the demands of incorporating the word(s) into the prosodic line of the intended utterance. The word(s), in essential form (phoneme constituents and stress pattern), should be available at the right time to contribute to and fit into the prosodic line, which develops in regard to the individual words and their role in the intended utterance. Evidently the initial phone is the initial access feature, but certainly the rime must play a critical, even determinant, role; its major element, the syllable nucleus, is the dimension that underlies creation of the prosodic line. The findings from study of speech errors, reviewed in Chapter 11, clearly support this assessment.

Additionally, the speaker is confronted with the matter of initiation, making another beginning, whether of a new sequence or of resuming wherever one had stopped (or was stopped). Such beginnings require processes incident to producing the "new" syllable/word, whose initial portion, in view of syllable asymmetry (see Chapter 11) presents an inherent obstacle. A major dimension of the obstacle, contained in the syllable structure itself, inheres in the latent potential separation of the initial consonant(ism) from the vowel nucleus, as expressed in the syllable structure hypothesis and illustrated in the speech error findings exemplified in Chapter 11. Significantly, linguistic stress is most often an aspect of the obstacle posed by initiation, and throughout, proper timing in the patterning of sequential syllables is critical.

TRANSITION

Consonants (in word-initial position) have long been identified as the salient feature of stutter occurrences.[31] However, as typically expressed, this observation describes stutter as occurring *on* (initial) consonants, which is a misperception. In some stutters, the initial consonant seems to be maintained as a posture. More often, however, the initial consonant (or blend or cluster) actually is produced; in fact, production is overdone, being expressed either as iteration or extension. Whatever its actual form, the aberration is manifest as a classic clonic or tonic feature that marks the stutter *event*. It follows, then, that the "block" represents principally what should follow in the normal production sequence, namely, the vowel form, the syllable nucleus—the crucial element in the prosodic line.

The "block" epitomizes what I have referred to as the stutter *event*: the inability to move on, to develop the essence of the syllable. Most often the "block" occurs relative to an impending stressed syllable. A frequent accompaniment to these events is "the neutral vowel" (/ə/), or something that sounds like it; in any case, it is clearly a most "reduced" sound, a matter significant in itself. Whatever the actual configuration of that sound, its importance lies in the fact that it reflects the inability to effect the appropriate syllable pulse, to develop the syllable nucleus, to attain the "peak" of the rime. Recall that in ordinary speech, adjustments for production of the nuclear vowel are under way during production of the initial consonant, and that production of the syllable involves ballistic movement that blends consonant and vowel.

I have called the latent separation within the syllable the "fault line" (Wingate, 1988), in analogy to geologic structures in which a surface indication, discernible upon inspection, marks the site where a latent division, which extends far below the surface, may separate.[32] In the case of syllables, the latent division is at the juncture of initial consonant(s) and the following vowel, the syllable nucleus. The potential separation is of initial consonant(s) from the rime, a separation that typifies occurrences of stutter.

The following excerpt from *The Structure of Stuttering* (Wingate, 1988) relates the fault-line concept to: (a) the syllable–structure hypothesis, (b) word/syllable-initial position in ordinary speech, (c) a common type of speech error, and (d) stutter:

> Analyses of the syllable from the standpoint of both speech production and linguistic structure point to the special nature of the initial portion of the syllable, and recognize the unique relationship between onset and rime— between initial consonantism and vowel nucleus. At the same time, although the two analyses direct attention to the same locus, and its special features, their characterization of the circumstances at that locus differ considerably. At the linguistic (lexical) level, onset and rime are intrinsically separable; they are interchangeable parts that evidently retain their idealized phonological representation. In contrast, at the level of signal production, onset and rime are "unitized"; speech performance of onset and rime represents an intricate blending of the complex muscle systems involved in the differential production of consonants and vowels, such that the identities of consonant and vowel are merged and blended. This dramatic contrast, which can be said to characterize syllable-initial position, suggests that the relationship of onset to rime can be considered a "fault line" in the complex process of speech production. This fault line, which is the site of many errors in verbal expression—as in "slips of the tongue"— is also evidently vulnerable to the more dramatic breakdown that is represented in the occurrence of stutters.
>
> The inference from this analysis is that breakdown at the fault line is the critical feature, the crux, of a stutter event. It appears to be no coincidence that the focal language features involved in a stutter event are precisely those that are highlighted in the analyses of syllabic structure. Also, although the stutter event finds expression as a breakdown at the level of

execution, that is, in motor performance, it seems likely that the fault extends from higher levels of the hierarchy of neural organization for language expression, through several stages of the process that extends from the plane of verbal formulation to the level of final motor execution. (p. 184)

It is once again worthwhile to point out that typically, in sequences of normal speech, whether a word is produced as intended *or as a speech error*, the initial consonant(s) and the rime are integral, produced in one continuous blend in which adjustments for the syllable nucleus are under way during production of the initial consonant(s). In stutters, this does not happen. Evidently, the word does not "arrive" as an assembly; the two major syllable constituents identified in the syllable–structure hypothesis (initial consonantism and rime) are not "unitized," and the speaker cannot immediately integrate them properly.

The preceding discussion expresses, somewhat more elaborately, the description of the stutter *event* presented in Chapter 3. Again, as in that description, and in some other places in the book, it is necessary to emphasize that, although certain other phenomena (such as repetition of a word, phrase, etc., or some accessory feature) may occur in the vicinity of the stutter event, the crux of a stutter is revealed in that unique event of *inability to move forward*.

The reader is encouraged to read again the description of stutter from Johnson and Brown, reproduced early in this chapter, and to review the relevant analysis presented in Chapter 3.

SUMMARY

In the traditional, broad sense of the term, "speech" is well understood as an internal (neural) system for generating and producing externally expressible meanings. Stutters reflect a breach in this system. Stutters should not be viewed as phenomena external to the speech process, as is the case when someone intentionally imitates stutter, but as representing disorder within the process itself. Stutters are events within the fabric of speech; they are tears in that fabric, which occur at points of vulnerability.

One of the facts about stuttering, presented in Chapter 4, is that stutters do not occur randomly. Significant influences on stutter occurrence exist within the speech system, centering in the closely interrelated "language factors," which, considered with some care, reduce to attributes of *words*: word type, word structure, early sentence position, and use-frequency, and how words are used, the level of propositionality.

Most often stutters occur early in a tone group and invariably involve syllable-initial position, at the juncture of initial consonant(ism) and syllable nucleus. As noted throughout this book, syllable-initial position is the focal vulnerability. This locus is identifiable as a fault line where a stutter, revealing separation of the two syllable constituents (consonant and vowel), represents a failure of normal transition of the initial consonant(ism) into the syllable nucleus, a failure experienced as inability, which stutterers have referred to as the "block."

In broad perspective, the disordered speech production manifested as stutter seems well described in reference to prosodic expression, occasioned in substantial measure by anomalies in the processes involved in retrieving words and interleaving them smoothly into the prosodic line of an intended verbal sequence.

The evidence reviewed in this chapter augments content covered in Chapter 11 regarding the intimate relationship of speech production and cognitive function. Of particular relevance to stuttering, this relationship has special significance for certain important facts about stuttering, namely, that stuttering is principally a disorder of childhood, and that very substantial remission of stuttering occurs frequently as childhood progresses. These two facts are clearly related to cognitive status and speech capability, both of which improve as the child matures (see again Figure 11.5).

Some content in the present chapter is relevant also to other of the facts about stuttering, notably the ameliorative conditions. Further, there is much that is especially pertinent to matters germane to management, to be considered in the final chapter.

NOTES

1. Particularly in view of its subsequent corruption, by Johnson.
2. As well as use of the word "spasm."
3. The development of this incredibly persuasive viewpoint is the topic of chapter 7 in *Stuttering: A Short History of a Curious Disorder* (Wingate, 1997).
4. Acceptance of such description of stuttering threatens to move the field backward some 50 years.
5. Even by that time, the observation that stutters occur in word-initial position was so widely attested that, in this search for "difficult sounds," the effort was made to create reading material having as many different sounds as possible *in word-initial positions*, since that was where the supposedly difficult sounds would be located.

6. Noted well before the twentieth century (see Wingate, 1997).

7. At least it was grandly ignored.

8. The reader is encouraged to review discussion of this word category distinction in Chapter 11.

9. Analysis of the most frequently used 1000 words from one source (Wingate, 1998) showed that, for each 100-word level, phoneme count is consistently larger than letter count by one unit.

10. For instance, in the Minkus Completion Test: "The streams are dry, _____ there has been little rain."

11. The title of a collection of headline "flubs" compiled by Gloria Cooper (1980).

12. The failure of the "information load" notion, in general as well as for stuttering, is covered in pp. 89–92 of *The Structure of Stuttering* (Wingate, 1988).

13. Including the original Brown reports.

14. As noted earlier, over some time there were repeated (unsuccessful) attempts to discover a "gradient" of stutter occurrence within the content word classes.

15. This matter is considered in detail in *The Structure of Stuttering* (Wingate, 1988, chap. 5).

16. Although the work had been done in 1955 as a dissertation.

17. This feature was especially clear in the passage used by Brown (see Wingate, 1979a).

18. For details of this work see Wingate (1979a,b, 1982).

19. One of Francis Bacon's observations, "Of Stuting," recorded in his book *Sylva Sylvarum* (p. 85, No. 386), published in 1627, included in his description: "they that Stut, doe Stut more in the first offer to speake than in Continuance."

20. Described in Wingate (1982, 1988, pp. 172–174). The study was replicated by Doyle (1981) with similar results.

21. This matter came into focus in Chapter 3.

22. The reader should recall that speech rate varies within a complete utterance.

23. Many years ago, Strother & Kriegman (1943) found that stutterers were as capable as normal speakers in diadochokinesis. These findings have remained unchallenged, in spite of some attempt to present stuttering as an articulatory problem (e.g., Zimmerman, 1980).

24. See Broen (1972), Ferguson (1964), Garnica (1977), Phillips (1973), Sachs *et al.* (1976), Snow (1972), and Snow & Ferguson (1976).

25. See Bryngelson (1955), Hahn (1940), Porter (1939), Razdol'skii (1965).

26. Under greatest pressure.

27. The phenomenon has been recognized for a long time. See, for instance, Bassett & Warne (1919), Osgood (1952), Smith & Raygor (1956).

28. The typical substantial decrease in the second reading is evidently due in part to actual (overall) adaptation to the situation. See Wingate (1972).

29. See Wingate (1988, p. 210).

30. See Wingate (1988, especially chap. 2). Significantly, the large subject populations of the studies reported by Johnson & Associates al. (1959) and Johnson (1961) are included.

31. See Wingate (1997). Moreover, in the "difficult sound/difficult word" contention, arising in this century, these are considered to be the cause of stutter.

32. The San Andreas Fault is a classic example, likely to be known to most readers.

CHAPTER 13

Neural Background

A neurosurgeon very soon gains the impression
that in dealing with the cerebral cortex he is still
at a distance from the highest level of integration.

W. Penfield and T. Rasmussen,
The Cerebral Cortex of Man (1959)

*T*he quotation selected as the epigram for this chapter was chosen because it expresses a matter vital to understanding the operation of the
human brain, especially in regard to its "higher" functions, of which
speech is central. The pertinence of the quotation will become evident as the
content of the chapter develops.

Just as advance in the study of stuttering requires understanding the processes of speech production, it also should include an awareness of what is
currently known regarding the neurologic structures and functions that evidently are relevant to speech production. This chapter presents a brief overview
of the extensive literature regarding central nervous system function relative
to speech production, principally as certain aspects of that information evidently relate to stuttering.

Much of the content to be presented is from a field identified loosely as
"neurolinguistics," in which a very extensive literature embraces many dimensions of inquiry. The scope of this chapter must be limited to consideration of
representative content having relevance to our special interest. However, the
reader is encouraged to become acquainted with the range of substance in this
field. Entry into this literature is provided through citations made throughout
the chapter and selected general reference sources noted at the end of the
chapter. Exploration should lead one to appreciate the daunting task facing
efforts to relate speech to brain processes.

An instructive introduction to current circumstances in the field will be found on pages 189 through 230 in the June 1983 issue of *The Behavioral and Brain Sciences*. Those pages consist of a "Target Article" on cortical mapping, by George Ojemann, followed by 15 peer commentaries on the substance of that article. The information contained in those pages remains current; it is likely to be so for some time to come.

SOME BRAIN BASICS

Knowledge of certain general features of brain structure and apparent functions is basic to matters central to this chapter.

Figure 13.1 presents two left lateral views of the external configuration of the human brain, showing major structures and certain areas important to references in discussion that follows. Part A illustrates the three major "divisions"[1] of the brain: (a) the cerebrum, or cerebral hemispheres, (b) the cerebellum, and (c) the brain stem. The points of reference for the cerebrum include the frontal, parietal, occipital, and temporal "lobes" and the two major visible fissures: the fissure of Rolando, or central fissure, and the fissure of Sylvius, or lateral fissure. A third major fissure, the longitudinal fissure, separates the two (left and right) hemispheres.

The term "lobes" of the cerebrum has been written with quotation marks in this initial reference because, in general, the boundaries of the lobes are ill-defined, except for the delineations posed by the central and lateral fissures. The term "fissure" also must be understood figuratively, since the cortical surface is largely continuous.

In this part of Figure 13.1, the "ghost" illustration of the higher brain stem shows the position of that structure relative to the cerebrum. Chief among the important nuclei in the higher brain stem is the thalamus, a body that figures prominently in later discussions. Other subcortical structures, particularly the limbic system, also are mentioned in regard to speech production. The limbic system, sometimes even called the limbic "lobe," refers to a ring of structures at the level of the thalamus that are known to be instrumental in several functions vital to the organism, particularly, for our interest, as the source of activation. The reader is reminded here of discussion in Chapter 11 regarding the role of motivation in the generation and production of speech.

It seems appropriate to note here the substantial evidence that the thalamus is importantly involved in the generation of, and disturbances in, speech production. Some of the findings that bear pointedly on the evidently critical thalamic role in speech are presented later in this chapter. The reader will find

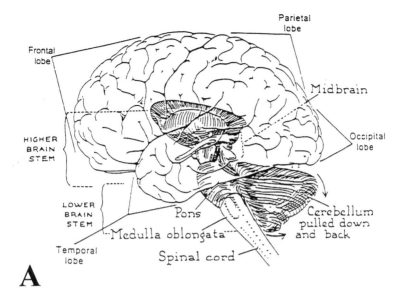

A

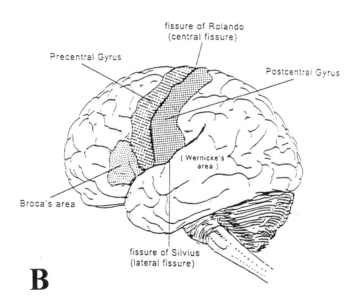

B

FIGURE 13.1   Left lateral view of the brain. (A) Gross anatomy, showing location of brain stem structures. The higher brain stem includes the thalamus and certain other integrative structures. (B) External features focal in text discussion. Reprinted with permission from Penfield & Roberts (1959, fig. II.1).

discussion of other pertinent findings in Chapter 9 of *The Structure of Stuttering* (Wingate, 1988).

Part B of Figure 13.1 emphasizes several other features of the cerebrum that are particularly relevant to discussions later in this chapter regarding speech production, and stutter.

THE CORTEX

Traditionally, the cerebrum has received the greatest amount of attention; in fact, it is often spoken of as "the brain." This special status has arisen from study of the neuronal surface of the cerebrum, the cortex.[2] Findings yielded by this extensive study have occasioned a view that equates the cortex with the "higher" functions of the brain. In fact, one frequently finds, in discussions of brain function, statements that speak of the cortex as containing "the higher centers." It is of particular interest that this image rests heavily on the fact that speech was discovered, quite dramatically, to be clearly related to certain areas of the cortical surface.[3]

The cortex is a continuous sheet of tissue composed of neurons (ganglion cells) and the physical substance that supports them (glial cells). The number of ganglion cells is estimated to be upwards of 10 billion. Each cell has a principal axon, which has varying numbers of branches whose terminals make synaptic contact with the multiple dendrites of other neurons. The number of synaptic connections made by a neuron are measured from hundreds to tens of thousands. These truly astronomical figures should be kept in mind when attempting to conceive of the complexity of neuronal patterns that must underlie all voluntary activity, including, of course, even the simplest features of speech production.

The continuous sheet of cortex is "rumpled" into convolutions, called gyri (singular, gyrus), which are delineated to some extent by the infoldings, called sulci (singular, sulcus). The sulci are simply indentations in the cortical surface, not literal defining limits. However, they are aids to reference for location of the gyri they outline. Certain of the gyri, grossly identifiable and reasonably similar in locus and configuration over different individuals,[4] are given names for purposes of reference. Although the gyri thereby assume a certain unique identity, one should keep in mind that the cortex is a continuous sheet, a condition that has special relevance to the matter of "areas" of the cortex. At the same time, the cellular structure of the several layers of the cortex differ in various areas. Some discussion of cortical areas is introduced later.

Two readily identified gyri are positioned on either side of the fissure of Rolando, or central fissure, the latter term providing the reference for the names of these gyri: the precentral gyrus is the gyrus just forward of the central fissure; the postcentral gyrus is the one just rearward of that fissure. The precentral gyrus is closely associated with motor functions of the body, and is often referred to as "the motor strip." The postcentral gyrus is closely associated with sensory functions; understandably, it is often called "the sensory strip."

Both gyri are identified here largely because they are routinely discussed as a parallel pair. However, our interest will focus on the precentral gyrus, principally because portions of it are clearly involved in speech production. Moreover, certain findings involving the precentral gyrus are pointedly relevant to stutter. These matters will be discussed in the section addressed to localization.

"Lower" Is More Likely Higher

As mentioned above, the higher human functions, of which speech is paramount, have been understood traditionally to be functions of the cerebral cortex. "Higher," in the sense just expressed, is a psychological reference, which has been applied somewhat analogically to the brain. However, certain fundamentals of nervous system structure seriously qualify that image. Phylogenetically (repeated in ontogeny), the central nervous system is basically a tube of neural tissue that, over evolutionary time, began to swell at its rostral (forward) end, the swellings gradually ballooning into the superstructure that became identifiable as the cerebral hemispheres. Actually, then, the cortex is an extensive panoply of end neurons from nuclei that constitute the subcortical structures.

Among these nuclei, the thalamus is especially significant. The central importance of the thalamus, and its neuronal radiations, is reflected in the massive thalamic peduncles, three of which are shown in Figure 13.2. A fourth peduncle, the inferior thalamic peduncle, also substantial, is not shown. These peduncles are huge neuron bundles consisting of thousands of neurons that link thalamic nuclei with the cortical surface. The crucial role of the thalamus has been recognized for many years, and continuing research has increased appreciation of its significance (Sherman & Guillery, 2000). The thalamus is the center of information processing in the brain, acting as a relay and controlling information within the brain, including between different cortical areas.

Consistent with the epigram for this chapter, much that has been learned from investigations into cortical localization corroborates the inference, drawn from the history of neurological development, that the purportedly "higher" centers are actually subordinate to certain of the structures that usually have been considered as "lower" levels of the central nervous system. This matter

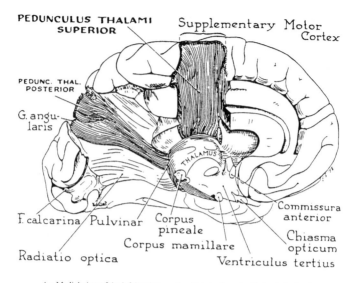

A – Medial view of the left hemisphere, in which the Superior Thalamic Peduncle and the Posterior Thalamic Peduncle are featured in partial sagittal section

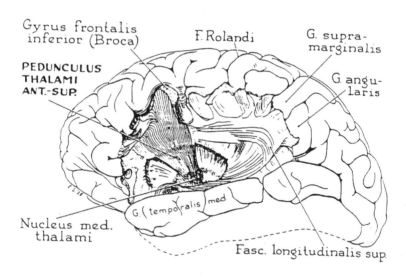

B – Medial view of the right hemisphere, in which the Anterior-Superior Thalamic Peduncle is featured in partial sagittal section

FIGURE 13.2   Three of the thalamic peduncles. Reprinted with permission from Penfield & Roberts (1959, figs. X.20 and X.22).

has special pertinence to conceptions of speech production, and will be discussed in a later section.

ASYMMETRY

We are accustomed to perceiving ourselves, each other, and other animal forms as symmetrical, that is, with each side of the body mirroring the other side. This organization is assumed readily in respect to evidently paired features—arms, hands, legs, eyes, ears, etc. The perception is accurate in the gross sense of paired units. However, typically, we are unaware of the extent of asymmetry within those seemingly mirrored pairs. Inspection of the extremities will reveal many deviations from mirror imaging. For instance, the pattern of veining on the backs of one's hands are not mirror images. Fingerprints of the two hands do not mirror each other. Similar differences will be found for other body parts.

Undoubtedly, the most impressive evidence of bodily asymmetry is found in the structure we observe most often: the face. Vernacular testimony to facial asymmetry finds expression in the thespian's wish to be viewed from "my best side." Dramatic illustration of such asymmetry has been produced as follows. A full-face picture of an individual is cut vertically at the facial midline; a reversed (mirror image) copy is then made of each half; then combination full-face pictures are created by joining each mirrored half with its original half. Comparison of these two constructed images with each other and with the original full-face photograph is most impressive, sometimes startling. Often one can discern a sort of "family resemblance" among the three images, but sometimes a similarity is difficult to perceive. However, most often a resemblance is noted between the original photograph and one of the constructed images. In these instances, the facial half that combined with its mirrored form most resembles the original photograph is recognized to have the features that determine the usual perception of the individual. That half of the face is considered to be the determining, or "dominant" half.[5] Samples of these images will be found in Kolb and Wishaw (1980), Sackheim et al. (1978), and Wolff (1943).

The examples of bodily asymmetry presented above are only partial evidence of the fact that, contrary to routine perception of the body as symmetrical, body asymmetry is the rule. Departures from symmetry are evident in internal structures as well; particularly, for our interest, in asymmetry of the brain. The left and right cerebral hemispheres are not, overall, mirror images of each other. The ubiquitous complication occasioned by variation among individuals has posed difficulties for measurements, yet clear differences in certain physical features of the hemispheres have been determined by many investigators. Anatomical differences may suggest functional differences, which are of greatest interest, for they indicate something about internal organization. One anatomic difference that is particularly relevant to our interests relates to the temporal lobes. The most obvious aspect is the length and angle of the Sylvian fissures of the two hemispheres, being longer and less slanted on the left. Plausibly related functional differences will be noted in the section dealing with cortical areas.

LATERALITY

Compelling evidence of asymmetry in cerebral functions emerges from a range of inquiries into hemispheric specialization. The reader should become acquainted with these findings, presented in sources such as *Left Brain, Right Brain*, by Springer and Deutsch (1998). However, even behavioral observation tells something significant about asymmetry of function. The most obvious indication is "handedness." This universally recognized evidence of asymmetry in function is, however, only one dimension of the lateral preferences an individual may express. For instance, persons also typically show a leg preference for kicking, or in putting on lower-body clothing, and the like. Assessments of laterality often reveal mixed dominance, or crossed dominance.[6] Further, a person's handedness may vary relative to the type of activity undertaken; such as writing left-handed, but eating with the right hand. Handedness may shift in those bimanual activities in which one side "leads," such as in batting a ball. And then there are the "switch-hitters," who are able to bat from either side. In view of the vagaries in expression of lateral preference, these phenomena should be viewed it terms of "sidedness." Although hand preference, typically for writing, is most often the accepted indicator of cerebral asymmetry, the matter is not that simple.

The expression "lateral preference" is misleading, since there is no reason to consider that laterality is a matter of choice. The great bulk of evidence indicates that laterality is not acquired, but that it is inherent in the individual. The distribution of handedness in populations is a compelling aspect of the phenomenon: left-handedness occurs in less than 10% of populations; most likely it is as low as 6%.[7] If handedness were a matter of chance, or effected by various external influences, one should expect a population distribution closer to half and half. Additional evidence that left-handedness is unique is found in both research and clinical findings that point to greater bilaterality among left-handers.

The phenomenon of lateral preference supported the concept of cerebral dominance, the idea that one of the cerebral hemispheres determines the expression of lateral preferences. It was noted in Chapter 4 that, in the early decades of the twentieth century, a persuasive hypothesis regarding the nature of stuttering explained it in reference to the cerebral dominance concept. The essence of that account is that, (a) since speech involves action of midline structures, proper activation requires appropriate controls from each hemisphere, and (b) one hemisphere should therefore be dominant so that effective coordination of the midline structures can be effected.

Explanation of stuttering in terms of cerebral dominance evidently was precipitated, and for some time supported, by reports of: (a) stutter associated with forced change of handedness, and (b) a higher incidence of left-handedness among stutterers. The results of relevant research, pursued during that era, were mixed, and interest in cerebral dominance waned, due in large measure to the burgeoning persuasion that stuttering is a psychological problem. The issue of more left-handedness among stutterers is still not resolved. As illustration, opposing statements regarding the matter are made by Calvin and Ojemann (1980) and by Springer and Deutsch (1998). The role of laterality in stuttering remains undetermined. However, although the matter is seldom discussed in recent works, some sources continue to find reason to consider that laterality is involved somehow in stuttering.[8]

In application to stuttering, the cerebral dominance concept accounted for the disorder essentially in terms of motor function. More important, the hypothesized struggle for cerebral dominance carried the assumption that the two hemispheres are essentially equal participants in the struggle, and that therefore either hemisphere could attain the dominant role. In contrast, stuttering as anomaly of speech production, the position adopted in this book, looks to processes beyond motor activation and control. Moreover, it does not conceive the two hemispheres to be generally equivalent, nor as being in matched competition. At the same time, it acknowledges that whatever conditions underlie the evident differences in function of the two hemispheres, including laterality, they are likely to be involved in speech production—and in stuttering.

Although certain areas of the two hemispheres evidently do function equivalently—for instance, the "motor strips" (see below)—there is now considerable evidence that various functions of the hemispheres differ in certain important respects. A wide range of evidence has led to summary characterization of left-hemisphere function in terms such as "serial," "sequential," "analytic," and the like, in contrast to description of the right hemisphere's mode as "parallel," "configurational," "synthetic," and so on. A representative set of these dichotomies it presented in Springer and Deutsch (1998). Although all of such distinctions are not accepted uniformly by all workers in the field, there is general agreement regarding functional differences of the two hemispheres, largely along the lines reflected in the above descriptions. It is now quite well established that most functions basic to speech are related predominantly to the left hemisphere. For that reason, a lateral view of the left hemisphere is always shown when speech is discussed in reference to central nervous system functions (as in Figure 13.1). The difference in functional "style" of the two hemispheres, especially in contexts addressed to speech, is cast in terms of the left hemisphere being more attuned to processes that are essentially verbal, and the right hemisphere to processes largely visuospatial in nature.

A review of findings regarding the range and extent of hemispheric differences in function is beyond the scope of the present work. Students should read at least chapters 2 through 5 of *Cerebral Lateralization* (Geschwind & Galaburda, 1987), and explore other sources such as the book by Springer and Deutsch (1998), noted earlier. However, certain findings within the available extensive research and clinical reports are especially relevant to our interest and should be brought into discussion here. Of particular pertinence is the substantial evidence that speech is represented predominantly, although not exclusively, in the left hemisphere; a reasonable estimate, in reference to many sources, would be close to 90%. Notably, the fact that speech can be described as serial and sequential has been the principal basis for having characterized the left hemisphere in the terms used in the dichotomies mentioned above.

SPEECH AND HANDEDNESS

It seems that most often, left-hemisphere representation of speech is associated with right-handedness. However, the apparently substantial cerebral asymmetry regarding hemisphere of speech representation and its relation to handedness is not an absolute, invariant property of cerebral organization. In particular: (a) in some right-handed individuals speech is represented in the right hemisphere, and (b) among the left-handed, speech may have major representation in either hemisphere. A more general basis for qualification regarding hemisphere of speech representation is contained in evidence that the right hemisphere routinely participates in speech production. Although the nature and extent of its participation are not clear, there is reason to believe that a major right-hemisphere contribution involves prosodic dimensions.

GENDER VARIABLES

The sex of an individual is related in some significant way(s) to hemispheric specialization, to laterality, and, of course, to stuttering, although the interconnections are obscure. As noted in Chapter 4, the incidence of stuttering among males is dramatically higher than among females. Other relevant differences between males and females are not as compelling, yet evidence for such differences is reported frequently.

Over many years evidence has accrued that, in general, females have greater verbal facility than males. This acknowledged difference is enhanced by findings that females perform better with tasks involving verbal function and memory, and that, in contrast, males do better with visuospatial tasks. These findings indicate gender-conditioned differences in capabilities associated with the left-hemisphere versus right-hemisphere functional modes noted earlier.

The foregoing findings articulate well with a range of pertinent evidence, obtained from diverse avenues of investigation that, overall, males are more lateralized than females both for verbal abilities (left hemisphere) and spatial skills (right hemisphere). To phrase these findings alternatively, females show greater bilateral representation for both types of function.

Quite recently, investigations by Gur et al. (1999) found that proportional differences in grey matter to white matter[9] in the left versus right hemispheres of males compared to females provide a credible rationale for the observed differences in performance of the sexes on tasks that apparently reflect differential hemisphere functions.

LOCALIZATION OF FUNCTION

The idea that various human "faculties" are linked specifically with certain locales of the brain was first proposed in the conjectures of phrenology, a set of assumptions proposed early in the nineteenth century regarding where various human faculties "reside" in the brain. The superficiality of this conception is well reflected in the central belief of that system, namely, that the presumed sites of the various faculties were revealed externally in related prominences on the surface of the skull, which were therefore evident to external inspection (see Spurzheim, 1908/1833).[10] The doctrine of phrenology was debated actively during much of the nineteenth century; however, the debate was largely between supporters of phrenology and persons who believed that the brain acted as a whole. The essential notions of phrenology, especially regarding identification of human faculties by palpating bumps on the skull, became passe following discoveries from investigation of actual brain tissue.

REVELATIONS FROM TRAUMA

Significantly, it was defect of speech that, early in the second half of the nineteenth century (1861), led to the first evidence of cerebral localization of function in humans. The speech defect was dramatic—complete loss of speech, subsequently called aphasia, that occurred in a patient of a French surgeon, Paul Broca. Autopsy of this patient, and then of subsequent patients with similar speech defect, revealed a lesion in "the posterior portion of the third frontal convolution" of the left cerebral hemisphere. This location, subsequently known as "Broca's area," is indicated in part B of Figure 13.1. Then, in 1874, a German neurologist, Karl Wernicke, described patients who were unable to understand speech, although their speech production appeared to be intact. Autopsy revealed that the anatomical area associated with such defect also was in the left hemisphere, but in the temporal lobe, in the approximate position indicated in part B of Figure 13.1. Circumscription of Wernicke's area is not rendered in Figure 13.1 because of much uncertainty about the extent of this area; an uncertainty well documented by Bogen and Bogen (1976). Actually, a substantial, but not well-defined, temporal–parietal area subsequently has been linked to overall speech processes, not simply to speech perception. Further, another cortical region, to be called the "supplementary speech area," was identified in the frontal lobe just anterior to the upper range of the precentral gyrus, and lapping over into the longitudinal fissure (its outline is discernible in the two displays of Figure 13.4).

Beginning with Pierre Marie's careful review of Broca's results, in 1906, many reservations, qualifications, and criticisms were expressed in regard to the early reports of localization, and to ongoing research as well. Gradually it was recognized that the symptomatologies of Broca's area and of Wernicke's area, as originally described, required considerable revision. Still, a double-aspect conception of "expressive aphasia" (Broca's area) and "receptive aphasia" (Wernicke's area) persisted. Not unexpectedly, in view of the largely connectionist ambience in which these views developed, the concept of "conduction aphasia" described possible connections between what were considered to be the two primary speech areas, a concept supported by later discovery of the arcuate fasciculus, a bundle of nerve fibers extending between the two regions.

In addition to locales identified as Broca's area and Wernicke's area, certain anatomical differences between the left and right hemispheres are suggestive of functional differentiation. For instance, the more prominent Sylvian fissure of the left hemisphere, noted earlier in this chapter, is associated with certain plausibly speech-related differences between the two hemispheres. The planum temporale (temporal plane), an area on the surface of the temporal lobe lying within the Sylvian fissure, is considerably larger in the left hemisphere. The inferable significance for speech is that this surface is close to Wernicke's area, and also to the inner surface of the temporal lobe,[11] an area now widely accepted as playing an important role in memory. However, before imputing any speech-specific functions to the left planum temporale, one should keep in mind that, in the great apes too, the left hemisphere planum is larger than the comparable area on the right hemisphere.

It is impossible to briefly summarize the historical sequences regarding these concepts and relevant findings.[12] However, one should note that the tendency to conceive of various speech processes in terms of focal "centers" has persisted. As with the several linguistic models of speech production noted early in Chapter 11, the prevailing neurological conceptions of this marvelous process reflect the influence of familiar images of systems having various parts. Ongoing exploration continues to be couched in this orientation, abetted, understandably, by continued description of various "loci" of certain speech-related functions, even though, as noted below, the reference to "speech areas" is somewhat misleading. Although there is compelling evidence that certain regions of the brain somehow participate importantly in high-level functions—such as speaking—one should treat circumspectly the idea that specific locales are "responsible for" special operations. Importantly, the matter of verbal organization, critical in respect to words, let alone connected speech, remains obscure. More profoundly, the ultimate mysteries of formulation, propositionality, and meaning continue to be especially recondite.

Discovery through Stimulation

Identification of loci of function based on autopsy of stroke victims and other brain injury, such as war wounds,[13] faces many limitations, not the least of which is that the extent of tissue involvement is unclear. Substantial improvement in localization study attended the seminal work in cortical "mapping" that was initiated during the second quarter of the twentieth century by Wilder Penfield and his co-workers, particularly Theodore Rasmussen and Lamar Roberts.

Since cerebral tissues have no sensation, cortical localization in humans[14] is made possible through direct stimulation of exposed cortex of live, conscious patients whose speech capability, evidently intact, enables them to participate in the investigation. The opportunity to conduct cortical mapping emerged as an aspect of the effort to treat epilepsy surgically. Subsequent explorations, undertaken by other surgeons, have always proceeded on the same grounds, that is, as an opportunity presented by surgical exposure of the brain for some medical condition, principally epilepsy. Consequently, the point has been raised that stimulation data are not obtained from truly normal brains. Another qualification mentioned in regard to this work is that data obtained from stimulation, though perhaps similar to those from injury effects, are not the same. It should also be noted that, predominantly, the obtained data do not include children, largely because, among other considerations, they cannot be expected to fully participate in the process, which requires following certain instructions and giving introspective reports.

The procedures involved in cortical mapping via electrical stimulation are described well in Penfield and Rasmussen (1955) and Penfield and Roberts (1959). Other procedures are described in Toga and Mazziotta (2000a).

Exploration of the cortical surface by electrical stimulation refined, and added substantially to, identification of "speech areas" of the brain revealed through trauma. Significantly, in the many series of cortical exploration that have been conducted over many years, electrical stimulation of the cortex has never caused speech to occur. The stimulation either does not affect speech or interferes with it. The "speech areas" have been located only negatively, that is, by disrupting ongoing speech. Moreover, the whole matter of "speech areas" faces substantial qualification in view of the frequently reported evidence that excision of even Broca's area has resulted in only transitory aphasia (Zangwill, 1975).

It is especially remarkable, then, that only electrical stimulation in the thalamus has elicited some speech: words and phrases, reported by Schaltenbrand (1965) and by Schaltenbrand and colleagues (1971). Here again it is pertinent to recall this chapter's epigram—namely, that the cerebral cortex is still at a distance from the highest level of neurologic integration.

Cortical mapping also has identified the location of areas representing other functions. Various areas of the human cerebral cortex, notably on the precentral and postcentral gyri, have been identified as involved with, sometimes as "essential to," certain other bodily functions, motor or sensory. The sequence of areas on the precentral gyrus ("motor strip") of both hemispheres is displayed in Figure 13.3. This figure, representing the precentral gyrus of both hemispheres, was constructed to illustrate that the functions depicted evidently are comparable on the two hemispheres. Sensory areas corresponding to the motor sequence are located on the postcentral gyrus; the sensory areas are not illustrated in Figure 13.3.

Note that the representation of body areas is inverted.[15] In certain sources, these illustrations of area sequences on the precentral gyrus are accompanied by a "homunculus," an inverted body-image cartoon in which exaggerated drawing of various parts of the body image emphasize the considerable variation in neural representation of body areas. The variations in body area representations are indicated in Figure 13.3 by the lengths of the bars associated with each area, drawn at the periphery of each side of the figure. Note that the bars representing areas involved in vocalization are drawn outside the peripheries of the figure.

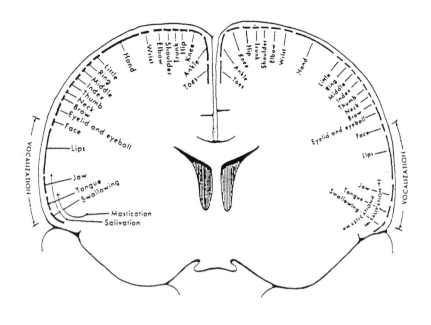

FIGURE 13.3   Graphic representation of cerebral cross-section along the precentral gyrus ("motor strip"), showing the sequences of actions elicited by electrical stimulation of cortical sites. The lengths of the solid bars at the periphery represent an estimate of the average relative cortical areas from which the actions indicated were elicited. Adapted with permission from Penfield & Rasmussen (1955, figs. 9 and 22).

Penfield and Roberts (1959, p. 25) described the motor cortex as an "arrival and departure platform" whose function is "to transmit, and possibly to transmute ... the patterned stream of impulses which arises in the centrencephalic system and passes on out to the target in voluntary muscles." Penfield's concept of the "centrencephalic system" was created to denote an integrating organization within the higher brain stem, which includes the thalamus on both sides.

In contrast to results obtained from the "speech areas," electrical stimulations along the sequences of the "motor strip" do elicit actions of the structures represented.[16] Significantly, the actions elicited are never skilled or dexterous; most are simple movements, no more complicated that those of a newborn infant. One partial exception is vocalization. Compared to other elicited motor actions, vocalization is complicated, involving innervation of abdominal muscles, pharynx, larynx and tongue. This vocalization is "a sustained or interrupted vowel cry, which at times may have a consonant component" (Penfield & Roberts, 1959, p. 120). However, it involves less than the coordination and sequential activation of the pertinent structures in the form intrinsic to speech, particularly the imbrications that produce syllables and their margin.

Importantly, stimulation-elicited movements of some of the structures employed in speech, the jaw and tongue, were found to occur bilaterally. In comparison, movements of the lips, and face, were mostly contralateral, occasionally bilateral. Movements of the eyes, eyelids, and eyebrow, and pupil dilation, often occurred with elicited movements of lips and jaw. Such concurring movements are of special interest relative to accessory features in stuttering, as discussed in Chapter 3.

Note that vocalization is elicited over a substantial area, from either hemisphere. The extent of representation for vocalization is remarkable: fully twice as great as for either of the next lengthier representations (lips, and hand). The area for vocalization extends over representations for lips, tongue, and jaw—all integral to speech. Vocalization also is elicited by stimulation in what is called the supplementary speech area, noted earlier, located just forward of the precentral gyrus on the coronal surface of the cerebrum. That area is discernible in Figure 13.4.

At this point, it is pertinent to note that midbrain structures also are importantly involved in vocalization. Significantly, it has been well established that the emotions arise from within the same structures, notably the limbic system and the thalamus. This concurrence carries profound implications regarding the role of motivation in speaking and, as well, the well-known effect of emotional arousal on speech—and on stuttering.

The preeminence of vocalization, and the extent of locales from which it can be elicited, speaks clearly to the importance of this function. Readers should recall the discussion developed in Chapter 11 regarding vocalization as the essential foundation of speech.

DISRUPTED SPEECH

Electrical stimulation of certain cortical areas can disrupt ongoing speech in several ways. It has resulted in: hesitation and slurring; distortion and repetition of words; confusion of numbers while counting; misnaming, in some areas with perseveration, at other sites without this effect; inability to name, with retained ability to speak; and, most dramatic, complete arrest of speaking.

Speech arrest has particular import for stuttering, which is addressed below. Speech arrest bears on the matter of lexical access, which is important for our interests, as noted in Chapters 11 and 12; therefore, the topic merits some attention here.

Inability to Name

Inability to give the name of some object, a limitation called "anomia," is a curious phenomenon, variously reported for some aphasic disturbances. The patient is asked to name an actual or pictured familiar object, such as a watch, hat, key, or nickel. Often, while unable to give its name, the patient can illustrate, or even describe, the use of the unnamed item. Particularly remarkable are those instances in which a patient will use the word appropriately in an immediately sequential spontaneous utterance.

Occasionally, during ordinary discourse, most normal speakers will be unable to immediately recall a particular word. Often the word will "come to mind" within a short time, although sometimes not until much later. In either case, during the period in which the word cannot be recalled, the speaker often will have some fairly accurate sense of certain of the word's structural features, notably its initial phone or number of syllables—the TOT (Tip of the Tongue) phenomenon, discussed in Chapter 11.

"Inability to name" (anomia), although perhaps seemingly akin to the TOT phenomenon, is substantially different in certain important respects. Giving the name for some actual or pictured object has been characterized as "naming on confrontation" and recognized, for some time, as different from word-finding in connected speech (Oldfield, 1966; Geschwind, 1967). For instance, in the naming task, the words sought are almost exclusively nouns, which are to be produced with no supporting context. Also, in anomia the patient evidently has no awareness of any features of the sought word. Further, a patient may give another, unrelated word, sometimes repeatedly, even though recognizing that the repeated word is incorrect.

Penfield and Roberts (1959) gave several examples of anomic phenomena resulting from cortical stimulation. The following examples are quite typical of instances found in aphasic patients. With the electrode touching his cortex, one patient was unable to name the picture of a foot, but said, "What you put in your shoes." Another patient could not name a (real) comb, but said, "I comb my hair."

Although presently of uncertain significance, it bears mention that, in the latter example, the "same" word, inaccessible as a noun, was produced spontaneously as a verb. However, grammatical class, per se, may not be a critical factor. In both of the foregoing examples, the pragmatic description given by the patient clearly would seem to involve visuospatial representation, which

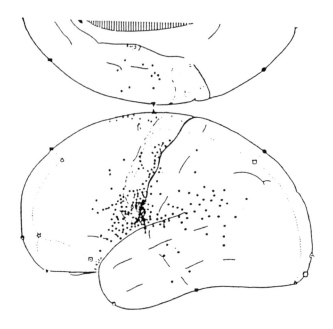

Left Hemisphere

FIGURE 13.4   Areas on the cortex where mild electric stimulation caused arrest of ongoing connected speech, in 35 different operations. In all cases, the left hemisphere was recorded as dominant, from the individual's handedness. Note that arrest was produced on each hemisphere, although from more loci and over a wider area, on the left. Reprinted with permission from Penfield & Roberts (1959, figs. VIII.4 and VIII.12).

brings to mind the matter of right hemisphere contribution to verbal expression, noted earlier.

Speech Arrest

Speech arrest has most direct relevance to stutter, because the critical fault in stutter is inability to move forward, to be "blocked," to find one's speech arrested. Comparable phenomena occurring in the course of cortical stimulation procedure are instructive.

Figure 13.4, from Penfield and Roberts (1959), shows the cortical areas where electrical stimulation resulted in complete arrest of speech. Note that

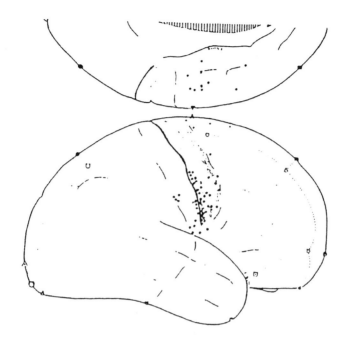

Right Hemisphere

the effect is obtained on both hemispheres and that the heaviest concentration is in the precentral gyrus. It is of particular interest that the position and extent of loci resulting in speech arrest correspond with the region in which vocalization is elicited.

In two-thirds of the cases of speech arrest reported in the Penfield studies, the patient simply stopped talking. In other cases, speech arrest was accompanied by simple movements of the lips, mouth, or the eyes and eyebrow. Occurrences of these accompanying events are especially relevant to the matter of accessory features in stutter, discussed at length in Chapter 3. Particularly notable are the accompanying actions involving the eyes: the reader should recall that such phenomena figured prominently in the several studies addressed specifically to cataloging accessory features of stutter.

Exemplary direct observations, reported for some occurrences of speech arrest, are of special note. In several instances, actual slight stutter was observed, reported as such by the investigators. In other instances, stutter was represented in such description as "clonic movement of the mouth while continuing to try to say the word."

Patients were routinely aware that their speech was arrested. Often they subsequently reported simply that they had been unable to speak during the stimulation. However, some described their experience. One patient reported having felt "like stuttering." Others gave specific descriptions, for example, "difficulty in making my lips say 'yes,'" or "I couldn't say 'five.'" Such descriptions are clearly reminiscent of complaints made by many stutterers; often expressed in a general statement that they know what they want to say but can't say it.[17]

Of special interest are findings that speech arrest has resulted from electrical stimulation of certain subcortical areas. Ojemann (1983) reported complete speech arrest from stimulation of the lateral aspect of either the left or the right ventrolateral thalamus.[18] In addition, a particularly notable finding was that stimulation anteriorly in the medial central thalamus evoked two types of speech error not previously described. One kind of error was of speaking the same wrong word each time some other word was expected; such occurrence duplicates a form of perseveration frequently reported to occur in aphasic patients. The other unique error, especially pertinent to our interest, was perseveration on the first syllable of the word attempted—a kind of occurrence that duplicates one of the two classic features of stutter, protraction (the other being iteration), discussed in Chapter 3.

Findings from another source are consistent with the latter finding. Abe *et al.* (1993) reported a patient with a subcortical lesion whose speech was characterized by repetitions of word-initial syllables. The area they identified was the same area reported by Ojemann. Abe *et al.* described these occurrences as "stuttering-like repetitions," considering them distinguishable from true stuttering. This report, aside from its pertinence to neurologic factors in stuttering, is especially relevant to the matter of identification of stuttering. The phenomenon reported by Abe *et al.* resembled the other classic feature of stutter (iteration) but did not duplicate it, a distinction recognized as such by those authors. One should note that this matter bears pointedly on issues of stutter identification—not only in regard to claims that question the reliability of stutter identification but, in particular, matters like SLDs (Stutter-Like Disfluencies), and "within-word disfluencies," discussed in Chapter 7. Regarding the latter issues, note that the phenomena observed by Abe *et al.* are, by description, much more stutter-like than are repetitions of single syllable words, yet these authors still did not consider them to be stuttering.

An article by Bhatnager and Andy (1989) is pertinent to this discussion. These authors report a patient whose stuttering was relieved following electrical stimulation in the thalamus.

"Spasms of the Glottis"

It is relevant to include here some discussion of this concept, which was expressed quite often during the nineteenth century. The description of stutters as "spasms of the glottis" represents a deduction that stuttering is more an anomaly of producing sound than in executing any particular segments (phones). Since the "glottis" is the opening between the vocal folds, this description really refers to action of the folds.

The conception has a certain credibility in view of several pertinent observations—namely, (1) that sound making for speech is generated at the larynx, (2) that stuttering is interruption in sound making, and (3) that stutter typically has an oscillatory dimension (clonus), which suggested "spasms."

Attention to the larynx as the site of stuttering also was mentioned several times during the first half of the twentieth century. Eventually, Wyke (1970) offered the plausible hypothesis that stuttering is a manifestation of *phonatory ataxia*, which results "from temporal dysfunction in the operations of the voluntary and/or reflex mechanisms that continuously regulate the tone[19] of the phonatory musculature during speech." It is well to keep in mind that laryngeal function is subject to both voluntary and reflex control; in fact, the latter has priority, in that the primary glottal function is to prevent matter from entering the (trachea and) lungs. Still, although aberrant laryngeal reflexes may play some role in stutter, laryngeal involvement does not seem to be simply a matter of phonation itself, but rather phonation as elaborated into speech. One reason for this reservation is that simple phonation, in the form of the neutral vowel (/ə/), often occurs as an evident adjustment to a nascent stutter. Also, often the sound is used intentionally as a "starter" to resolve the block. In fact, using /ə/ in this way has been recommended as a technique by many sources.

There are other reasons to consider that stutter is not appropriately described in terms of phonation per se. Not the least of these are the findings regarding variation in stutter occurrences as some function of the propositional level of utterances, and the closely related matter of rehearsal. Even more compelling reasons are found in the dramatic reduction in stutter occasioned by the ameliorative conditions, principally: singing, rhythm, auditory masking, and delayed auditory feedback (DAF), in all of which phonation is basic, but, more importantly, modulated. The value of these conditions in working with stuttering is discussed later.

Although the foregoing discussion gives reason to doubt that stuttering may be a *phonatory* ataxia, the concept of ataxia in regard to stuttering does retain some appeal.

OTHER NEUROLOGIC INVESTIGATION

NEUROLOGIC STUDY OF STUTTERING

Neurologically oriented study of stuttering was pursued briefly during the fourth decade of the twentieth century. This interest was encouraged substantially by the research of Lee Travis and his colleagues, and influenced in part by the concept of cerebral dominance. However, investigation along these lines was soon eclipsed by the burgeoning preoccupation with psychologically oriented exploration. In fact, substantial efforts were made to interpret the results of existing neurologic, and physiologic, studies in terms of emotional reaction (e.g., Hill, 1944a,b). Neurologic investigation of stuttering has remained overshadowed by psychological persuasions.[20] Still, expressions of interest in the neurologic basis of stuttering gradually have emerged again, especially since the 1970s. It is of particular interest, in view of the earlier attention to laterality and cerebral dominance, that much of the revived neurological study has been mounted in respect to differential function of the cerebral hemispheres.

A review of the resurgent neurological exploration of stuttering, extending into the early 1980s, is presented in Moore (1984), a source recommended to the student. Much of the more recent study has employed a variety of noninvasive procedures (that is, not involving surgery). In addition to electroencephalography, which also was employed earlier, modern methods of investigation have included computerized tomography, magnetic resonance imaging, regional blood flow, and photoemission scanning. Such procedures are generally preferred over electrical stimulation because they cover wider areas; also because they are viewed, realistically, as "logically formidable." Studies employing the noninvasive procedures were reviewed recently by Watson and Freeman (1997). Investigation along this line continues, as found in two very recent reports. In one (De Nil et al., 2000), PET scans suggested some anomaly of speech-related function in stutterers, possibly related to laterality; in the other (Ingham et al., 2000), stuttering was reported to be linked to blood flow changes in several cortical areas.

Use of these noninvasive procedures is frankly exploratory, and casts a wide net. The various procedures are not equivalent in value; their specialized measurements often lack adequate resolution in one or another dimension. Even though certain findings suggest approximate locales of possible anomalous activity, these procedures remain rather crude measures in spite of their advanced technology, especially in regard to intricacies of neural function (Thatcher, 1994). Further, the significance of their findings is qualified by such procedural matters as whether or not the subject is speaking, and the extent of verbal expression at the time. It is relevant to note the comment by Grabowski and Damasio (2000) that, in spite of the extent of imaging work currently being done, "understanding the functional anatomy of language is still framed by the results of lesion studies."

In general, the yield from noninvasive procedures adds to earlier evidence that, among stutterers, there are anomalies in central nervous system function that involve more than motor processing. However, it seems that the technological refinements afforded by these esoteric procedures have been invested with a promise they are unlikely to fulfill. They have contributed little more than corroboration of previous indications, and it is questionable whether the findings represent much progress in understanding the essential nature of stuttering. Overall, the findings from modern procedures, taken as evidence that stuttering reflects anomalies of neural processes are, as summarized by Watson and Freeman (1997, p. 162), "not fundamentally different from that voiced by Hartley, Combe, and Kussmaul in the eighteenth and nineteenth centuries." It is especially noteworthy that the deductions of those early writers were based simply on direct, unassisted observation.

ACQUIRED STUTTERING

Sources discussing various neurological disorders occasionally observe phenomena that are reminiscent of stutter. In these sources, the anomalous speech phenomena typically are described either as only resembling stutter, or as different from "true" stuttering. It is pertinent to note that these descriptions are directly relevant to the matter of identification of stuttering, inasmuch as they state a clear differentiation of stutter from similar phenomena.

One description of special interest along this line is contained in a report by Luria (1970). He noted that certain patients had difficulty in word-finding in connected speech, but, in contrast to the anomia often seen in aphasia, they had no difficulty in naming actual or pictured objects. He described the disordered speech of these patients as "effortful and lacking in fluency," and that it was somewhat reminiscent of stuttering in respect to the patients' "tendency to repeat syllables, words, sometimes phrases."

Other sources give descriptions that are more suggestive of stutter, which has led to the designation "acquired stuttering." Still, in these sources too the phenomena are identified as only resembling stuttering. Acquired stuttering has been reported for a wide variety of neurologic disorders, arising from disease or trauma, and affecting various areas of the brain. As such, acquired stuttering is recognized as not likely to reflect a uniform condition.

The most notable single account regarding acquired stuttering is contained in a report by Market *et al.* (1990), which presents relevant data regarding 81 cases, obtained from a carefully prepared survey of 100 speech clinicians throughout the United States.[21] The findings reported from those sources indicated that acquired stuttering differs from actual stuttering on several significant dimensions. Most important: in acquired stuttering the events that resemble the cardinal features of stutter (iterations and protractions) are not limited to initial syllables, a clear contrast to a criterial dimension of actual stutters, which, the reader should recall, involve predominantly word-initial but not word-final position. These sources also reported that the phenomena they observed differed from typical stuttering on several other important dimensions. In order of significance, these other dimensions are: (a) the deviations involve function words as well as content words, (b) the anomalies are not related to the propositional level of an utterance, (c) accessory features occur rarely, and (d) there is no evident adaptation effect.

A DRUGS COROLLARY

It is appropriate to introduce here some brief discussion of efforts to treat stuttering with drugs.[22] Like the noninvasive technologies reviewed above, the use of drugs for stuttering also is exploratory, and in certain respects as unrefined as the noninvasive neurologic procedures. However, in contrast to the latter, drug studies have proceeded in reference to certain presuppositions regarding particular sources of the disorder. These assumptions are reflected in the various drugs tried, that is, in respect to the conditions for which a drug has been prescribed previously. Thus, the medications tried with stuttering have ranged from sedatives to anticonvulsants—the use of sedatives and tranquilizers reflecting the view that stuttering is the result of anxiety, and trial of anticonvulsants arising from an assumption that stuttering is some kind of neurologic spasm.

It is important that the reader have a general appreciation of how drugs are developed and of the process by which their effects are assayed. Many drugs have been developed and prescribed on the basis of considerable knowledge of both mammalian physiology[23] and the chemical composition of certain substances. The objective of this knowledge is to find, in the compounds, properties that will have the desired effect on those aspects of the physiology that are to be "treated." Still, current medicinal use of drugs continues to follow the age-old pragmatic approach to remedies, and throughout there is a considerable amount of trial and error. There remains in the entire undertaking a considerable dimension of inspired guess work and serendipity—the discovery of penicillin, and of tranquilizers, being two good examples. Also, new medicines often are found by seeking compounds similar to ones already known, and some drugs, developed for one condition, may somehow turn out to be more useful for another condition. And then there are those drugs whose eventual use was originally a side effect, such as Propecia and Viagra.

Systemic administration of drugs may be likened to a shotgun discharge at a vaguely outlined, rather amorphous target. Some of the buckshot can be expected to hit the same part of the target, but varying amounts will also strike other things, some close to the target, others at varying distances (the latter representing a drug's "side effects"). For a drug to have any likelihood of producing its anticipated effect, its "target" must be correctly specified and identified.

To date, over 25 different systemic drugs have been tried for stuttering; many, being variants of similar compounds, have had the same general objective. As could be expected, decrease in patient anxiety was the common objective of a number of these medications. Another objective frequently sought was to reduce muscular hypertonicity. The one drug tried most often was haloperidol, evidently for its reported effect on both anxiety and hypertonicity. Haloperidol is called a "major tranquilizer," a rather euphemistic equivalent of "antipsychotic drug." This drug has been used most often in the effort to reduce symptoms of serious mental illness, especially schizophrenia, but also has been prescribed for severe behavior disorders and hyperactivity. Of special interest, it has been reported to alleviate tics and symptoms of Tourette's syndrome, which is undoubtedly the reason for trying it for stuttering. In addition to its generally poor results with stuttering, haloperidol has several unpleasant side-effects, which most of the stutterer recipients have not been willing to tolerate.[24]

None of these drugs has yielded more than a minimal effect on stuttering. As could be expected, certain tranquilizers have induced relaxation and improvement in attitude. However, regarding those few reports claiming some success with stuttering, the effect is largely limited to some reduction in accessory features. There is no evidence, from either experimental or clinical work, that any drugs affect stuttering per se, undoubtedly because they do not address the critical feature of the disorder—the speech arrest, the "block," the inability to move on.

For stuttering, the real "target" is an inability to proceed in connected speech at certain loci in the speech sequence, an inability revealed by one or both of two unique markers, which sometimes are accompanied by accessory features (Chapter 3). Further, stutters occur neither regularly nor randomly; their occurrences are some function of variables inherent in the speech production process (Chapter 12). Thus, for stuttering, it is inordinately difficult to specify a drug to aim at the shifting real target. It is not surprising, then, that the best result, of only a few drugs, is to have hit a few "things nearby," namely, those accessory features that are most like tics.

Within the past decade, an unusual nonsystemic drug trial for stuttering has been to inject laryngeal musculature with botulinum toxin (a deadly poison if taken internally). Local injection of small doses of botulinum had been found useful in the treatment of certain movement disorders in which abnormal contraction or tremor is the prominent symptom (Hallett, 1997, 1999; Ludlow, 1993; Schnider et al., 1997). Evidently, trial of this procedure for stuttering was prompted by its prior use for spasmodic dysphonia (Cook & Lewin, 1994; Dunne et al., 1993), and based on a presumption that stuttering too might be due to hypertonicity of the laryngeal musculature. However, the result of botulinum injection did little to encourage this notion. In a few stutterers an effect was said to be only "short term," and that subjects were disturbed by the side effects.

The botulism experiment may well have been abetted by recollection of the view that stuttering is "spasms of the glottis," described earlier. It is worth noting that the concept was an important influence that led Dieffenbach to perform his infamous lingual surgeries to cure stuttering (see Wingate, 1976, 1997). The issue of laryngeal function in stuttering is considered in the next chapter.

SUMMARY

Neurologic findings most relevant to stuttering have emerged in the course of neurologic investigation concerned with speech. The most pertinent findings have resulted from electrical stimulation of both cortical and subcortical loci, in regions also found to be involved in speech production. Electrical stimulation of several areas of the brain has elicited the following phenomena that are much like what occurs in stutter: speech arrest, repetition in word-initial syllables, and protraction of word-initial syllables.

Modern noninvasive procedures for cerebral exploration are not sufficiently sensitive to yield the level of detail obtainable even from electrical stimulation technique. Although these findings generally support previous evidence of anomalies in neurologic function among stutterers, they add little that is of value to understanding the nature of stutter. Moreover, it is doubtful that such broad exploratory procedures will reveal—as is evidently assumed—some locale(s) responsible for stuttering; it seems unlikely that the cause of the disorder is localized in some cortical area.

Stuttering is best conceived, and investigated, as unique events within the processes of speech production; the nature of those processes themselves remain well beyond present-day neurologic inquiry. It follows that the neurologic origins of stuttering are at least as obscure as those intrinsic to speech production, and are likely to remain so as long as the neurology of speech production itself is not understood.

Study of the central nervous system has revealed that certain areas of the brain are importantly involved in—sometimes are indispensable to—certain functions. However, there is considerable variation in regard to those functions that evidently can be localized and, as well, to aspects of their locales. Localization is evident for certain basic sensory and motor functions, but higher levels of function are by no means as identifiable. For instance, "Wernicke's area" is rather shapeless, especially relative to early accounts, and "Broca's area" too is not as well delineated as typically described. Moreover, substantial amounts of tissue in Broca's area has been removed without permanent impairment of "motor speech" function.

The conception of cerebral function in terms of relatively autonomous areas responsible for certain operations is supported by evidence that certain areas of the brain clearly are important to certain basic functions. This conception corresponds to our familiarity with other systems made up of parts, including the human body, that evidently function in that way. Moreover, the conception seems to have been enhanced by awareness of modern-day achievements with electronic apparatus: computers, robotics, and the work in "artificial intelligence." However, we should not be unduly impressed, or conceptually swayed, by the remarkable achievements in such modern technology, which clearly is based on parts and interconnections. Even persons sophisticated about computers appreciate the limitations of those astounding machines, which, moreover, are created by humans and also always are activated and controlled by humans. It remains questionable if the "separate parts" conception[25] is adequate to account for the system that must underlie the marvelously complex and intricate functions evidently involved in speaking. Speech would seem to be poorly analogized to machine models. Dresher and Hornstein (1976) point out that writings in the area of Artificial Intelligence reveal a rather cavalier naivete in regard to speech processes and the mind. They emphasize that an adequate explanation of human speech awaits "the elaboration of unanticipated theories of great complexity." Their remarks are relevant also to extant models of speech production, as discussed briefly in Chapter 11.

At this time, it seems that an adequate and accurate description of ordinary spontaneous speech in neurologic terms is a phantasm projected only vaguely in the far distant future. It may well be that a full understanding of the neurology of speech production faces the insurmountable limit of "necessary fallibility" in science, described by Gorovitz and MacIntyre (1976). Quite likely, then, speech production is a process befitted as *ein ding an sich*, a description from philosopher Immanuel Kant that refers to something beyond discernment and understanding. Still, the subject remains worthy of carefully reasoned inquiry.

At the same time, pessimism relative to clearly identifying the neurological substrate of stutter need not carry pessimism in respect to management of the disorder. First, it is difficult to see how even a reliable identification of a neurological "source" of stutter might be translated into effective management of the disorder, other than through medical or surgical means. Second, at least reasonably effective management procedures have been, and are currently, available. These methods can be improved through better understanding and application of underlying principles of speech production.

SOURCES FOR EXPLORATION

Students seriously interested in neurologic research concerned with speech production, and stuttering, will find pertinent reports to appear most frequently in the journals listed below. In addition to the references cited in this chapter, reports in the following journals will expand one's avenues of inquiry:

Archives of Neurology
Archives of Neurology and Psychiatry
Brain
Brain and Language
Neuropsychologia

NOTES

1. I am reluctant to speak of divisions of the brain, even in a superficial sense. Although "parts" are evident, even more so upon dissections, one must keep in mind the extent of their neuronal interconnections. This reservation comes to mind in speaking of the "lobes" of the cerebrum.

2. "The external layer of an internal organ." Actually, the cerebral cortex is covered by protective membranes.

3. It is relevant to note that support for this image has been contributed, unwittingly, by the mundane fact that the cortex is closest to the top of the human form—that is, it is literally "higher."

4. The first of many qualifications that speak to individual differences.

5. Several hypotheses have been offered for these asymmetries, for instance, as reflecting personality types (Wolff, 1943), or as principal avenue for emotional expression (Sackheim, 1978).

6. Assessments of eye preference and ear preference enlarge the possibilities.

7. Moreover, this very low incidence must have existed over a long time. The Latin word meaning "left" is "sinister," a matter reflecting the fact that for centuries left-handedness was sufficiently odd that it was viewed as an omen portending evil. (See "sinistral," and compare to "dextral.")

8. See Blood (1985), Records et al. (1977), Sussman & MacNeilage (1975), Webster (1986), and Wingate (1988).

9. Grey matter indicates ganglion cells and their dendrites; white matter indicates connective neurons sheathed in myelin.

10. Originally published in 1833, the 1908 republication should be available in, or through, many libraries.

11. Of both hemispheres.

12. The interested reader is referred to the first two chapters in Toga & Mazziotta (2000b).

13. Many brain-injured soldiers of the two world wars, from both sides.

14. Study of other animal forms has contributed substantially to localization knowledge. For an informative review, see Gibson (1962).

15. Something of an irony relative to "higher" and "lower," a matter that arose earlier.

16. On the contralateral side, naturally, for structures unilaterally controlled.

17. An aspect incorporated into the World Health Organization description of stutter.

18. He also reported several other speech-specific effects of stimulation in this area.

19. Here meaning muscle tone.

20. The interested reader is referred to chapter 6 in *Stuttering: A Short History of a Curious Disorder* (Wingate, 1997).

21. The extent to which acquired stuttering occurs, overall, in neurologic disorders is not known. Physicians with whom I have discussed the matter indicate that the percentage is low.

22. Brady (1991) gives a recent review.

23. Due to physiological similarities over many mammalian species, drugs intended for human use are developed, and tested, on nonhuman species.

24. Haloperidol also has been described as a dangerous drug, likely to induce any of several different defects or disorders.

25. Henry Head (1926) decried this conception as "diagram making." Freud too (see Freud, 1953) rejected the conception of discrete "centers." The reader is reminded that analogous reservations were expressed in Chapter 11 regarding extant models of speech production.

PART **IV**

Denouement

CHAPTER 14

Derivations

His treatment, according to Kingsley, was "naturally" and without dodge or trick, to teach the patient to speak consciously, as other men speak unconsciously.

Klingbeil (1939)
(said of James Hunt, 1870)

This final chapter is concerned primarily with a rationale, and related approach, for dealing with stuttering. It presents an orientation to the disorder based predominantly on the substance of preceding chapters and principles derived from that substance.

A defining attribute of this orientation is that it is *atheoretical*—specifically, that no account will be made of what have been accepted as "theories" of stuttering. The field of stuttering has been too much absorbed in theories, with their presumptions of cause, in spite of the fact that none of those ventures is supportable. The pertinent issues have been drawn in Chapters 1, 2, and 6.

Ordinarily one could expect that the last chapter in a book of this kind would focus on procedures for stuttering "management." Matters of that sort will be addressed, but from a point of departure having a rationale quite different from the usual themes of stuttering management. Before presenting this new departure, it seems pertinent to offer a brief historical review as background for the orientation expressed in this chapter.

MANAGEMENT: A BRIEF HISTORY

In the past half century, discussions of stuttering management typically have been presented in terms of: (a) therapy, and (b) counseling. The use of these two terms is actually quite new in the history of speech disorders, a circumstance reflecting the prominent twentieth century influence of psychology. In particular, the connotation of "counseling" has shifted considerably, in the past half century, from its traditional meaning of imparting information and advice, to a sense engendered within the field of mental health. A major influence in this shift was the writings of Carl Rogers, initially from his book *Counseling and Psychotherapy*, published in 1942, and extended in subsequent writings, especially *Client-Centered Therapy* in 1951.

Isolated efforts to treat stuttering have been made for centuries, mostly within medicine, with the extent of interest increasing substantially in the nineteenth century.[1] This special interest was concurrent with an expanding general interest in speaking well, pressed by educated "men of letters." Undoubtedly, the remarkable discoveries regarding aphasia, beginning in the late nineteenth century, contributed to the growing interest in speech and speech disorder, such that by the early years of the twentieth century speech education and concurrent attention to speech problems were being incorporated into public education in the United States and certain European countries.

A Shift in Identity

In the early decades of the twentieth century, efforts to deal with speech problems were described as "speech correction," and personnel pursuing this activity were identified as "speech correctionists." Accordingly, the original name of the professional association in the United States was *The American Academy of Speech Correction*, established in 1925. "Speech correction," and derivative terms, continued to be widely used for many years. References to "correction" of speech problems appeared regularly in various professional literature sources, including the official organ of the association, the *Journal of Speech Disorders*, publication of which began in 1936. For more than a decade that journal, and other sources, contained many references to "correction" of speech disorders,[2] and the use of certain other words of similar reference, such as "re-education," "instruction," "remedial," and "training." Some references to "speech *pathologist*" and "treatment" are found only infrequently during this period, and regularly in a medical context. In the late 1940s, the word "therapy" entered the literature of speech disorders. Although this word, too, appeared originally in medical contexts, the shift in identity that it reflected was under way, and use of the word increased steadily. Then, in 1955 the terms "Speech Pathology" and "Speech Therapy" appeared as index categories in what was by then the *Journal of Speech and Hearing Disorders*,[3] and continued throughout subsequent expansions of that publication.

Therapy

Significantly, references regarding stuttering were in the forefront of the increasing use of the word "therapy," and those references openly reflected the expanding influence of psychology. The following citations from the *Journal of Speech Disorders* illustrate this trend. The 1946 volume contained an article titled "Hypnosis in a System of Therapy for Stutterers" (Moore, 1946). Then in 1950 (by then the *Journal of Speech and Hearing Disorders*), there appeared "Two Aspects of Stuttering Therapy" (Villarreal, 1950), in which one of the two aspects was the psychological one. Four years later, in "An Integration of Psychotherapy and Speech Therapy through a Conflict Theory of Stuttering" (Sheehan, 1954), the psychological dimension was clearly dominant.

The "therapy" of speech disorders, especially in regard to stuttering, was being submerged into a preoccupation with possible emotional factors. By 1957, Lee Travis, a prominent figure[4] in the profession for many years, had reason to write that "Speech pathologists have manifested in both practice and research an ever-quickening interest in psychotherapy" (Travis, 1957, p. 965). That interest would continue to expand, especially in the area of stuttering, which it enveloped. The persuasion remains prominent among current writings in professional, semiprofessional, and lay sources.

Counseling

For some time the term "counseling" appeared only sporadically in the literature of speech disorders, and principally in respect to parents. However, from the beginning its use extended beyond its essential meaning of "mutual exchange of ideas, opinions, etc; discussion and deliberation."[5] In 1959, the *Journal of Speech and Hearing Disorders* carried an article titled "Counseling Parents of Stuttering Children" (Sander, 1959). The "counseling" recommended in that article departed from counseling in its traditional sense of giving advice. Sander contended that parents should be led "to fully appreciate the part they play in the development or prevention of stuttering." Although that theory-driven belief remains a conjecture, it has been restated often, well into current times. A few years later the *Journal* carried an article titled "Parent Counseling by Speech Pathologists and Audiologists" (Webster, 1966) that emphasized the emerging specialized sense of "counseling." Webster's statement repeated the position espoused in a contemporary publication in which a distinction was made between "guidance," wherein the objective is to give information and make recommendations, and "counseling," in which the focus is addressed to the emotional dimensions of the situation.[6] It is in this sense that the "counseling" of stutterers has been directed primarily at the range of feelings they might have, or are presumed to have, especially in regard to their stuttering.

Of course, the feelings a stutterer may have regarding his stuttering should be addressed, yet it must be recognized that individual stutterer's feelings vary considerably in this respect. Not all stutterers have the extent of negative reactions to their stuttering that are routinely presumed by clinicians who want to offer "counseling," in its specialized sense.

BASIS OF MANAGEMENT

Routinely, management of a disorder is based on knowledge of the disorder acquired from careful study, and typically with special reference to the relevant normal condition. Being knowledgeable about the nature of speech and the structure of stutter is essential for dealing effectively with the disorder, for this knowledge supplies the rationale for the direct assistance undertaken and the counsel offered.

Ethical considerations alone require that anyone acting in the capacity of a speech professional should apprise the stutterer and, where appropriate, his parents as well as others concerned with his welfare, of what can honestly and defensibly be reported regarding the disorder. This requirement clearly implies its inverse—namely, that stutterers and other concerned persons should not be told things that are not soundly supportable in reference to objective, rationally based findings. The classic violation of this requirement is Wendell Johnson's "Open Letter to the Mother of a Stuttering Child," a fabrication disseminated widely between 1938 and 1983,[7] and popularly subscribed at least during that period. Some reflection of its substance has continued to appear, and the conjecture underlying that unconscionable statement has found expression in many ways. A fairly recent full reproduction of the conjecture appears in Selmar (1991), in a booklet specifically addressed to parents. Other vestiges persist; for instance, the search for some anomaly in parent–child interaction continues, in spite of extensive contradictory evidence.[8]

Professionally responsible counsel for parents should recognize the full extent of the unfortunate persisting influences attributable to Wendell Johnson and his coterie of the "Iowa school." A synoptic review of those excesses is presented as Chapters 7 and 8 of *Stuttering: A Short History of a Curious Disorder* (Wingate, 1997); certain of those distortions are addressed briefly in earlier chapters of this book.

My immediate concern is with the most reprehensible of his distortions, the "evaluation hypothesis," namely, the conjecture that stuttering arises in the child because parents react to the child's normal irregularities in fluency as abnormal, and call them "stuttering." This contention, often inappropriately called a "theory," is entirely conjecture. It is a thoroughly unscientific supposition that lacks any credible support; moreover, even data presented as support clearly contradict it (see discussion in Chapter 4 regarding Johnson's major effort in this vein, *The Onset of Stuttering*). Even more than simply conjecture, it is a fabrication built upon Johnson's obsession with his stuttering as an intolerable blemish on his desired image of being a superior normal person.[9]

The "evaluation" conjecture impugns parents, especially mother, as the cause of stuttering, a contention audaciously expressed in Johnson's "Open Letter." The substance of that letter, then as ever since, has had no visible means of support, although such impression was conveyed in its bold authoritative assertions. The calumny of that letter, and perpetuation of the shallow "theory" behind it, must be shared by those persons in the profession who not only have failed to raise sensible question but have actively abetted the supposition in various ways.

Very recently the *San Jose Mercury News* published a report (Dyer, 2001) revealing that Johnson had pressed his obsession beyond the limits of ethical principles. The report tells how Johnson undertook to test his "theory" by taking advantage of twenty-two children in an Iowa orphanage. Johnson persuaded a graduate student, under the guise of providing speech therapy, to persistently and intensely harass these "experimental subjects" for any irregularity of fluency. Reportedly six (n.b.!) of the twenty-two children so treated were said to have "developed" stuttering; a claim, in the report, grounded largely on the featured testimony of one victim, who described how the experiment had ruined her life. In most respects, however, the report lacks the kind and extent of detail necessary to properly assess the findings. The design and procedure of the "experiment" seem to have been quite haphazard, and it is by no means clear that the resulting speech anomalies were really stuttering. However, even if they were, only six out of twenty-two is hardly support for the "theory," as claimed. Moreover, even the "theory" doesn't propose that children receive the kind of correction embodied in this intense assault. (And, even if the speech anomalies were not stutters, the whole "experiment" was truly an assault on trusting children.) A notable error in Dyer's investigation is that professional commentary evidently was obtained only from individuals associated with the University of Iowa. These persons were most likely the source of such statements as: "ground-breaking theory," which the "experiment" supposedly supported; as well as the insupportable conclusion that the "theory improved treatment and understanding of stuttering"; and the indefensible claim regarding its supposed benefit to untold numbers of stutterers.[10] There is no evidence, anywhere, that a youngster's stuttering has been alleviated by ignoring it, or through persuading parents that it's all very normal. Claims in this vein are little more than suppositions riding along on the fact of remission, which traditionally is ignored by proponents of such orientation. The same disclaimer is applicable to the claimed efficacy of the currently-in-favor "early intervention strategies." None of these assumptions have been subjected to adequate investigation.

CONTENT FOR COUNSEL

The content of the following three sections is abstracted from preceding chapters, where adequate supporting documentation was incorporated in the discussions. These summary reviews present the major topics that concerned parties should come to understand.

During the course of working with stutterers and, where appropriate, parents and other concerned persons, they should be familiarized with the character of stuttering and, as well, the nature of normal speech. Accordingly, it is appropriate to include here: (a) a brief review of the nature of ordinary speech, abstracted from the content of Chapter 11, and (b) a synopsis of the character of stutter, drawn from Chapters 3 and 12. In addition, there is (c) the substantial body of information about stuttering that is so important for gaining the breadth of perspective necessary for one to view the disorder realistically. This information is presented, in itemized form, in a following section.

SUMMARY OF NORMAL SPEECH

Our intuitive sense of speech is that it consists essentially of words, which convey meaning. Words are the focus of our attention as we listen to speech—which is, basically, how we have acquired them for our own use. Our intuition about our own speaking consists largely of awareness of the intent to convey a certain meaning, which then emerges in overt expression in a form ordinarily perceived as a sequence of words having a somewhat amorphous acoustic structure.

The structure of speech in overt expression consists of sound generated at the larynx (phonation), which is modulated by adjustments of the larynx and the vocal folds within it (vocalization), elaborated and refined by resonances in the supralaryngeal cavities (vowel forms), and set into the basic units of speech (syllables) by the effect of various constrictions (consonants) in the supralaryngeal cavities.[11] The consonant constrictions create syllables by briefly obstructing or impeding vocalization, such that it occurs in pulses, bearing individual vowel-form qualities—the syllable nuclei (depicted in Figure 11.4).

A speaker is quite unaware of how his intended meaning becomes transformed into overt expression, since those neural processes are not perceivable. However, pertinent research, with relevant deductions, indicates that this process proceeds in subconscious planning, basically in terms of words and word groupings. Ordinarily, the speaker also is largely unaware of the processes integral to the structure of overt speech, outlined above. Although these aspects of verbal expression are observable introspectively, they are regularly so imbricated and merged as to be obscure. Fortunately for purposes of correction, persons can be helped to recognize, and control, these processes.

As noted above, we conceive speech to consist of words. We listen to speech in terms of words. Words also are paramount in our thinking; in our cognition and planning of what we intend to say; and in our awareness of what we actually do say. However, *we speak in syllables*—the basic units of speech, produced in tone groups and organized as undulating tone—the prosodic line.

Most syllables have a standard structure: (a) initiating gesture (consonantal) and (b) "all that follows"—the latter containing always a nucleus (vowel form) and usually a consonantal termination. The nuclei are the critical segments (phones) of the syllable; in connected speech they are the substance of the undulating tone (voicing, prosody), organized into tone groups as determined by the stress patterns of the words in the utterance and the overall intended meaning. The tone groups that follow one another are interspersed with silent intervals of varying duration; most of these intervals are intrinsic to the message being conveyed, and listeners are rarely aware of them.

It is important to remember that, although the constituent phones of any syllable can be transcribed as individual segments, they are not separate entities in the syllable as spoken.[12] Instead, syllables are produced ballistically, the phones merged into each other. Evidently this structural form is especially distinctive of the transition of syllable-initial consonant into the vowel-form nucleus of the syllable.

Synopsis of Stuttering

Stuttering is manifestly a disorder of speech, a distinctive anomaly characterized by two unique markers of a stutter *event*. Often an occurrence of stutter is described as a "block," a term that clearly identifies the nature of the stutter *event*—inability to continue speaking. Further analysis leads to recognition that stuttering is an intra-syllabic phenomenon, an event that involves the early portion of a syllable.

Careful study has revealed consistently that stutters involve syllable-initial position. Over many years, this occurrence was believed due to consonants being more difficult (to execute) than vowels. However, through realization of how syllables are produced normally, the fault is seen to lie in a failure of transition into the vowel nucleus. In stutter, the normal integrity of the syllable is fractured. Since the initiating consonant, or its (silent) "posture," is regularly attained, the evident inability to continue involves principally the syllable nucleus, the segment that carries the vocalization, the undulating tone.

Important Substantive Findings

The items below, which encapsulate a range of findings presented in more detail in earlier chapters, contain important information regarding the disorder that can defensibly be reported to stutterers and parents. These items constitute a broad evidential base for a comprehensive perspective of stuttering.

1. Stuttering is a disorder in the production of speech, as described previously. It is not something that overlays speaking, like some kind of foreign matter with which the individual's (normal) speech has been contaminated. It is not something "removable"; it is a defect within the speech process of certain individuals.

2. Stutters do not fall within the purview of normal speech. Although identification of all occurrences of stutter may not be absolute, they are, for the most part, discriminable from ordinary irregularities that occur in normal speech.

3. Stuttering is largely a disorder of childhood. Most stuttering occurs in children under the age of 8.

4. Stuttering does not "develop." Further, no observable *anlage* have been identified that might indicate children who are "at risk" to "develop" stuttering. Stuttering rarely gets worse, and most often does not even persist at the same level as the child grows. (See next item.)

5. Remission/recovery:

   a. In the majority of young children, stuttering subsides spontaneously.

   b. For cases in which spontaneous remission does not occur, recovery can be achieved through personal effort.

   c. Cases of remission/recovery are likely to evidence some residual tendency to stutter.

6. No reliable prognostic signs have yet been identified. Even prospects for remission can be stated only in terms of approximate percentage.

7. There is no known cure for the disorder, although substantial improvement is possible. The results of treatment efforts are generally uncertain, and variable; improvement is an individual matter.

8. The cause of stuttering is not known. (Nonetheless, many conjectures of cause have been offered, most of which have centered on complaints or observations that invoke some psychological/emotional source.)

9. Stuttering is not a psychological problem.

   a. No typical personality, nor characteristic personality variables have been identified, from adequate study.

   b. Although environmental circumstances may influence occurrences of stutter, there is no evidence that such factors are its source.

   c. Fear and anxiety have been overstated as sources of stuttering. There are many people who evidence anxiety about speaking but do not stutter; most notable are certain individuals whose marked anxiety about speaking has led to a special category designation—namely, "Reticents."

10. Parental policies cannot be held accountable for the disorder, on any of the grounds contended, such as:

    a. general policies of child management,

    b. parental speech, as a model,

    c. style and manner of parental speech in child interaction,

    d. parental attitudes about speech, speaking or stuttering,

    e. untutored parental efforts to deal with the stuttering.

11. There is no evidence, nor plausible rationale to claim, that stuttering can be prevented.

12. Most likely the disorder has a genetic basis.

    a. This is strongly suggested by relevant research, which has extended many existing casual reports.

    b. Speech is a function of the central nervous system. Individual differences, clearly evident in other human capacities, are certainly present for speech—in other words, a matter of individual constitution.

    c. An organic basis is supported directly by items 5 and 13, and indirectly by items 14 and 15.

    d. Family history of stuttering is, so far, the only potential source for an "at-risk" factor.

13. Stuttering is clearly gender-related.

    a. Stuttering appears at least four times more often in males than in females.

    b. The difference is chromosomal, not behavioral (i.e., not a matter of masculinity vs. femininity). Males are physiologically the more vulnerable sex.

14. Stuttering is found all around the world; that is, it occurs in widely differing cultures, with their varying practices in child-rearing, demands on the individual, etc.

15. Stuttering is an ancient disorder. Again, varying cultures, etc. It is relevant that stuttering occurs in various social classes; certain famous and important people have stuttered, ranging from kings to commoners of varying "stations." Also, in current times, many highly successful, though not famous, persons stutter.

16. There are certain conditions of oral expression under which no, or minimal, stuttering occurs. The effect is most dramatic in the following conditions: singing, speaking to rhythm, speaking with auditory masking, and delayed auditory feedback. There are other conditions that also have been found to have a considerable beneficial effect. Among them, ones of particular note are: choral speaking, speaking in monotone, speaking in a stereotyped dialect.[13]

CONSIDERATIONS IN DIRECT MANAGEMENT

In spite of the various "theories" of stuttering, therapies for the disorder are essentially pragmatic; that is, treatment methods are not derived from theories but, rather, are practically based efforts. Although the rationale for what is done typically makes reference to some point of view regarding a presumed cause, or determining influences, what is done always involves adjustments of speaking. Moreover, the adjustments typically engage principles as illuminated above, even though these principles are seldom recognized and some other rationale is offered for the improvement achieved.

THE AMELIORATIVE CONDITIONS

These conditions were reviewed at some length in Chapter 4. They serve as a primary focus for discussion with stutterers, and concerned others (1) because of their dramatic effect on stuttering, an effect that induces speech which is seemingly normal, and (2) because of the evident dimensions of effect that these several conditions have in common. The two most readily identified dimensions of effect are (a) slowing down and (b) emphasis on voicing—which turn out to be essentially facets of the same effect. Both of these dimensions emerge as salient features of various approaches to treatment, although one or the other may be the one in focus—whether recognized or inadvertent. It should be noted that "slowing down" has been advocated, and used, many times in the history of stuttering (recommended by Mather, 1724, and by Warren, 1837),[14] although it was routinely dismissed by speech professionals in the twentieth century.

RECENT APPLICATION

The substance of both effects described above (slowing down and emphasis on vocalization) have emerged in a number of recent therapy efforts, although evidently not recognized as such. Slowing down, seemingly the more evident of the two dimensions effected via the ameliorative conditions, has figured prominently in these recent efforts.[15] Sometimes a procedure is described openly as "slowing down," but others emphasize "stretched" speech, "smooth" speech, or similar descriptors that are essentially other ways of talking about slowing down. One also finds, in this literature, occasional reference to "prolongation," a treatment procedure whose use has waxed and waned over a long period of time. Prolongation was employed by practitioners of the nineteenth century, and recurrently during the twentieth century, during which time it evidently was not recognized to epitomize slowing down. Actually, prolongation represents the original "stretched" speech.

It is crucial to recognize that the slowing of speech induced by the ameliorative conditions, and by the variously named therapy procedures noted above, is not simply a reduction in rate. The "slowing down" in focus here is of a special form. As reported in Chapter 10, variations in rate of ordinary speech are due primarily to differences in the amount of (silent) pauses, predominantly very brief pauses. In full contrast to a slower rate due to silences, the slowing down induced by the special conditions being reviewed here is occasioned by extending the sound of speech.

Now, extending the sound of speech is implemented almost exclusively through its vowel-forms. Actually, only vowel-forms (those phones whose substance embodies vocal fold vibration) are technically classifiable as *sounds*.[16] Thus, extending the sound of speaking is effected essentially via the syllable nuclei—vowel-forms, the true *sounds* of speech.

Discussion of prolongation brings a ready association to another procedure having a similar history—easy onset. This procedure was also used extensively during (at least) the nineteenth century and into contemporary times. In fact, the two procedures very often have been used together.[17]

Significantly, *easy onset* and *prolongation* address the critical syllable constituents: easy onset focuses on syllable initiation with transition into the "peak" of the syllable nucleus; prolongation enhances this function through emphasizing the (vowel) nucleus. Together, the two procedures interface neatly with what evidently needs attention in working with stutters; rather like a mold and its casting. They address the features critical to the integrity of the syllable.

In addition to the current therapies noted above, another category of treatment approach deserves mention. In the latter, considerable emphasis is placed on respiration and breath control. Advocates of this kind of approach would do well to study the methods employed by Hermann Klencke, a German physician, during the latter half of the nineteenth century and well into the twentieth. His methods, characterized by him as "a medico-pedagogic system of speech gymnastics," was reported by respectable sources to be eminently successful. It is of great interest that, although he addressed considerable attention to muscular actions controlling breath, these activities were, overall, subsidiary to tone formation and control of voicing. Also, significantly, the ultimate exercises in his system concentrated on slowing down, assisted directly through the use of rhythm.

DEVICES

Appliances for stuttering have a long history, and anyone seriously interested in the disorder should become knowledgeable about them.[18]

Many oral appliances appeared during the nineteenth century and well into the twentieth; a U.S. patent having been awarded as late as 1959. The appliances created during that lengthy era are generally referred to as "oral devices," since most of them were designed to be held in the mouth. It is of particular interest that these appliances were developed in reference to what was thought to cause stuttering. Analyses of the evident role of these instruments (Wingate, 1976, 1997) indicate that their effect turns out to be similar to that induced by the ameliorative conditions.

Late in the twentieth century, a new type of appliance appeared, made possible by the development of miniaturized electronic gadgetry. These electronic devices are unique not only in respect to their substance but also in terms of the rationale for their creation. These instruments were developed from a much more pragmatic base than the oral devices; simply, that they afforded a portable means for inducing three of the most effective ameliorative conditions—rhythm, auditory masking, and delayed auditory feedback. An electronic metronome was the first to be developed; then a device that generated masking noise; and subsequently an instrument to delay hearing one's own speech.

The most recent electronic appliances go directly to the objective: the sound-producing system, the vibrating vocal folds in the larynx. The objective of these devices, identifiable as "voice enhancers," is to provide special feedback of voicing, achieved through tactile transmission of laryngeal vibrations. Of particular interest, prospective users of these devices are given training in their use—significantly, the training focuses on speaking slowly and deliberately. Relative to their feedback value, one stutterer (Weiss, 1992) noted that the same effect can be achieved more simply by holding one's hand next to an ear. Actually, a more direct means of sensing laryngeal vibrations is to place thumb and forefinger to one's throat where the larynx is palpable. This maneuver also allows one to sense vertical movements of the larynx.

Use of Devices

Oral devices were routinely dismissed or ridiculed by speech and hearing professionals, at least in the United States. It seems that the electronic appliances have been regarded more tolerantly. However, the prevailing attitude regarding appliances is that they are "crutches"—which, of course, they are.

But that is no reason to ignore or denigrate them. One should consider that real crutches, and many other assistive appliances, are used widely, and with acceptance and support, by persons having a range of other handicaps. Corrective lenses or a hearing aid are so common that they are hardly considered to be appliances. Other assistive devices, such as a wheelchair, braces, or a cane, are more likely to be recognized as such, but their use does not evoke negative attitudes; in fact, quite the contrary. A relevant consideration is that, typically, such aids are used only as long as the person needs them; some may be needed lifelong, others only temporarily. There is no good reason to disparage stutterers' use of an assistive device. Some stutterers may find them useful indefinitely; others may need them only over a short term. A particularly unique aspect of stutterer appliances is that they can be used as instructional support.

The real problem underlying a negative attitude toward appliances for stuttering is the implicit, but potent, denial that stuttering is a *real* handicap. This denial is the other face of the belief that stuttering is "something psychological," some kind of "a bad habit," an unfortunate environmental influence, a fleeting exaggeration of something that is essentially normal. Such ideas reflect the behaviorist conception of stuttering as "a problem" in which the individual's normal speech is overlaid with unnecessary acts, which constitute stuttering. This belief, still active and disseminated, originated in the contention stated often by Wendell Johnson that "Stuttering is not something that happens, but something you *do*." In other words, stuttering does not reflect a condition inherent in the individual, a true handicap; it is simply superfluous activity that the individual has acquired, somehow. This behaviorist position about stuttering, in maintaining that there is nothing essentially different about the individual who stutters, incorporates a presumption that the person thereby has at least some responsibility for the occurrences of his stutter.

In view of the foregoing, it is of interest that, among relatively recent publications in the field, there are surprisingly frequent statements purporting stutterers' "feelings of guilt and shame"—which, moreover, are implied to be a standard condition. One must wonder if these are feelings genuinely expressed by stutterers themselves, and how frequently they may be reported spontaneously. Over many years of working with stutterers, I found the very rare expressions along this line to be typically cast more in terms of being a disappointment to some person, not a prevailing attitude. I am inclined to view the reports of "guilt and shame" more as theory-driven suggestion rather than spontaneous testimony. That pair of terms emerged as a special formulation by Joseph Sheehan, introduced into the field years ago (Sheehan, 1958a) and repeated intermittently since then, although still without substantive support.

Guilt and shame are emotions that typically arise from an awareness, or belief, of having done something wrong, either intentionally or from erroneous or inadequate performance, or actual dereliction. In my experience with physically handicapped persons, guilt and shame may be expressed by those who are responsible for their condition; otherwise, the emotions are of a quite different order. The issue being drawn here is that, if any number of stutterers really do experience guilt and shame for their stuttering, they must have come to feel somehow responsible for it. It would seem that psychological accounts of stuttering provide the underpinning. If a stutterer is allowed to believe, or is in some fashion led to believe, that stuttering is something in the nature of a bad habit, or a pattern of reactions, or a set of beliefs, or other explanation of that sort, a burden of responsibility is laid on the individual, from which guilt could then arise.

DIRECT EFFORT WITH STUTTERING

It was not intended that this book should include extended discussion of special management procedures.[19] However, it seems appropriate to present an overview of management strategy. Overall, one must accept that, for stutterers of any age, change must come from the individual. The essential policy is to provide relevant instruction where appropriate, in a context of support and patience. The latter, in fact, is all that may be necessary in the case of many young stutterers. Where direct management is indicated, the following orientation seems most supportable.

Working with the individual stutterer is realistically conceived as analogous to coaching, an endeavor that involves teaching of principles and related knowledge, demonstration and direct instruction of methods and techniques, and supervision of their implementation. These dimensions of the process are employed as needed over the course of progress toward the goal; and sometimes there is need to review "the basics." The objective of coaching, in general, is to help the individual develop and apply skills that are pertinent to the goal. With stuttering the objective is similar; in this case, the goal of the effort is to acquire skills needed to speak better.

The important principles regarding speaking and stutter are discussed above. Of course, explication of these principles should be adjusted to the individual's level of comprehension. With appropriate illustration and demonstration, modes of instruction appropriate to grade levels are feasible with youngsters of school age. Actually, the essential principles, properly presented, are grasped readily by children in the early grades. Younger children can be engaged in activities that implement various ameliorative conditions, selected as appropriate to circumstances, through which they can be brought to appreciate the essentials of the instruction. Actually, the simplest procedure to illustrate, explain, implement, and rehearse is slowing down, of the form emphasized earlier. In the case of children below school age, and even of ones in early grades, parents can be the major, even the sole, source of assistance and guidance.

An impressive introduction to instruction is afforded by demonstrating the use of an electronic larynx. The demonstration allows clear illustration of the dimensions of speech process, especially the central dimension of sound production. Although recent versions of this instrument have added volume and pitch controls, these should be ignored because they confound the desired illustration. For the purpose intended here, one is interested only in the instrument's basic function of generating vibration at the laryngeal site, which produces sound that can be shaped into quite intelligible speech. However, the quality of this speech will be monotone, a matter that must be emphasized, to contrast it with ordinary speech. Speech produced by using an electronic larynx does not have the undulating tone that is the hallmark of ordinary, normal speech. One should then explicate how changes in air pressure and laryngeal adjustments effect the modulations of basic sound generation that are characteristic of normal speech. To this end, demonstration and pertinent explanation should be extended to the real larynx, of the instructor and of the student, through "feedback" of laryngeal activities obtained by placing thumb and forefinger at the appropriate site.

Introduction of the ameliorative conditions follows naturally in the instruction. They provide an almost casual, yet unique, source for implementing a direct effort with the individual. Their effect is uniformly impressive, and they interface so neatly with what evidently needs attention in correcting stutter. Each of these conditions can be shown to elicit essentially the same effect, whose dimensions should be described carefully, and the individual's attention directed to sensing them. In these exercises the individual can be helped to sense the nature of speech production, to appreciate what evidently goes wrong in stutters, and what needs to be done to effect change.[20]

It seems evident that the improvement wrought through *easy onset* and *prolongation* can be related readily to the effects induced by the ameliorative conditions. In making use of easy onset and prolongation, care should be taken to ensure that the individual understands the features of each, how they relate to each other and to the objective of their employment.

SOME PERSPECTIVE

Certain vignettes from experiences with stutterers have unique value for a comprehensive outlook regarding the disorder. The following describe a range of view offering a breadth of perspective that should support a rational attitude regarding management.

Earl S., about 26 years of age, was an easy-going fellow, neither shy nor forward. His stutter was rather mild, but stable and obvious, usually a combination of clonic and tonic features. In his typical good humor he reported the following.

For several years he had coached the Little League baseball team of his general neighborhood, an activity that was satisfying to him and evidently also to his young players. Sometime during his second season, a "new kid" moved into the area and joined the team. All went as usual for a couple of weeks until, during a practice, the "new kid" mocked Earl's stutter. The boy was immediately upbraided by one of the "veteran" players, who said, "You let him alone. He can't help it; he was born that way." Over subsequent years the membership of the team gradually changed, but no similar episode occurred.

It seems most likely that Earl's stutter had been a subject of discussion in his defender's home, where it was explained to him that stuttering is a (*true*) handicap.

Earl's experience illuminates several important matters in regard to attitudes toward stuttering. One of these pertains to the issue of teasing. Certainly teasing does occur, and parents, teachers, and concerned others should make efforts to at least minimize it. But teasing is not routinely malicious, and many times the mild teasing that does occur is intermittent, transient, and appears in a general context of acceptance. Moreover, there are numerous instances in which the child is well-liked and popular—an outstanding example being Wendell Johnson himself (see Wingate, 1997, p. 113). Of course, if a child is concerned about teasing, the matter must be dealt with directly.

Scott D., about 28 years old, was a regular member of a young adult treatment group. He was personable and well-liked by the others, even though a suggestion he made intermittently was not well-received by all. His suggestion was to "bring it out in the open," by which he meant that one should verbally acknowledge his stutter to others, and let likely conversation about it develop. His major point was that stuttering is obvious, cannot really be hidden, so why try to cover it up? Also, he said, trying to hide it takes too much effort, and besides, it usually doesn't work anyway.

Members of the group eventually came to realize that efforts to obscure, or even appear to disregard, one's stutters implies that the listener(s) also are expected to not notice them—to which listeners typically accede. This unspoken collusion establishes an awkward situation that creates at least some tension for both parties; both are caught up in pretending that nothing unusual is happening. "Bringing it out in the open" punctures the pretense and allows a more relaxed interchange. In addition, a more satisfyingly casual atmosphere often develops when the auditor(s) thereupon feel free to explore their curiosity about the disorder. Stutterers can be helped to appreciate such conditions by presenting them with the analogy of circumstances one might (or has) encounter with a person having some obvious physical handicap.

Brian F. was a 21-year-old college junior, describable as "an all-American boy." Bright, personable, animated and having a delightful sense of humor, he was socially active, popular, and a better-than-average student. In the course of our lengthy professional relationship, he disclosed several personal ventures that reflected impish enterprise. Brian lived in enviable circumstances, which he enjoyed and appreciated. He came for help because he aspired to be in Naval ROTC but was not accepted because of his stutter, which was mild and predominantly clonic.

The crux of this vignette involves Brian vis-à-vis his father. I had occasion to speak several times with the father, who initiated our contacts largely out of curiosity regarding my opinion and the management efforts being attempted. The father was a kindly man, gentle in manner and speech, who had retired early from a very successful career. He told of having stuttered himself, "much more severely than Brian," until well into his twenties. He had overcome his stuttering after many years of applying various techniques, some of which were obtained via speech therapists. He reported that Brian had stuttered from preschool age, that the stuttering probably had shown some slow improvement over the years, but seemed by then to have remained much the same for some time. Brian had received speech therapy throughout much of his schooling, but it did not seem to help very much.

Father said that, in regard to overall capability and personality, he was sure Brian would do well in whatever he undertook—with the reservation that it was not likely to be a career in the Navy. He believed that Brian's interest in the Navy was sincere, but doubted that it was sufficiently strong to lead him to correct his stuttering. He remarked that, in contrast to his own struggle with the disorder, "Brian's stuttering isn't bad enough to really bother him." It was an opinion acknowledged by Brian, and though he spoke frequently to the issue of applying himself, he showed little improvement during a full academic year and part of the following summer. Eventually he (smilingly) mused that probably he had better start thinking about finding another career choice.

Colleen W. was already well-recovered by the time I first knew her, when she was a graduate student. It was not until years later that I learned she had "stuttered badly" as a child and had worked, through her own creative efforts, to gradually attain her admirable level of fluency, readily regarded as normal in quality.

Her most poignant recollection of her early stuttering was that she could not read aloud in early-grade classes. She would "get stuck on the first word," and after some abortive efforts would have to return to her desk. She also recalled being embarrassed about being excused to go to speech therapy, which was not helpful—she "got no direction or suggestions."

She began to work at the problem herself. A major change came about when she got a part in a children's theater play. Although still unable to read aloud independently, her parents helped her learn her lines. The success gave her feelings of achievement and confidence. Subsequently, "memorization was the thing," which she extended to memorizing paragraphs from school books while walking home. She remained active in theater throughout middle school, gaining confidence and developing a sense of what continuous speech was like. Sometime around her sophomore year she discovered she could even speak fairly rapidly by making the effort to speak in phrases. From other experiences she also arrived at some realization of a connection between singing and speaking.

Gradually she came to realize that "voicing undergirds everything." Although she also "became good at" word substitutions, and at using "starters," ranging from "uh" to a number of pet phrases, she had found the essential principles of connected speech, and worked continuously to use them in the way they are expressed in ordinary speaking.

Over the time I have known her, she has been characteristically personable, outgoing, evidently self-assured, and personally confident. Clearly very bright intellectually as well as personally, she converses easily and with animation. She has been eminently successful professionally, having held several positions of high responsibility that require extensive speaking. She acknowledges that a stutter still occurs, rarely, but she is not troubled by it. Her achievement is an admirable model of commitment and perseverance of which all stutterers should be made aware.

NOTES

1. Essentially in reference to the Western world. Extended coverage of the important historical material noted in this section is presented in Part II of *Stuttering: A Short History of a Curious Disorder* (Wingate, 1997).

2. Note Van Riper's widely used text, *Speech Correction*, published through several revisions from 1939 to 1963.

3. In 1948 (Vol. 13), "*and Hearing*" was added to the title of this publication.

4. Travis was the first person to be intentionally educated as a speech and hearing scientist at the doctoral level (Seashore, 1942, p. 134; see Wingate, 1997, p. 71).

5. *Webster's New World Dictionary of the American Language*.

6. The references of that article are weighed heavily with citations centering in the writings of Carl Rogers.

7. For a brief critique, see Wingate (1997, pp. 124–125).

8. See extensive literature review by Nippold & Rudzinski (1995).

9. Johnson was obsessed that he not be "only a stutterer, an inferior person. The thought of that was always detestable" (1930, p. 80).

10. A particularly distressing feature in these professional commentaries is the readiness to excuse Johnson's unconscionable act in terms of "the culture of the time." Are heinous acts to be written off through reference to some vague temporal ambience?

11. Attempting to include reference to the glottal stop /ʔ/ in this description proved too cumbersome, since it is technically laryngeal. However, its effect is identical to that of other stops.

12. See "The Literacy Complication" in Chapter 9.

13. These conditions, and certain other circumstances, are discussed in Wingate (1984a).

14. The recommendation by Cotton Mather, in 1724, is reported in Bormann (1969). Warren (1837) discusses the matter more broadly. Slowing down is discussed extensively in Wingate (1976).

15. See, for example, contributions published in Curlee (1993).

16. Most consonants are properly identified as *noises*. Excepting syllabic consonants, of course; their resonances constitute (unstressed) syllable nuclei.

17. See Chapter 4 in Wingate (1997).

18. Oral devices are discussed in Katz (1977), Wingate (1976, pp. 279ff), and Wingate (1997, pp. 39ff). Electronic devices are discussed in Wingate (1997, pp. 188ff).

19. A fund of pertinent procedures is discussed in Wingate (1984a).

20. Of the four ameliorative conditions featured here, three require some kind of instrumental assistance, but only delayed auditory feedback requires special equipment. Rhythm is produced easily by a variety of simple means; for auditory masking, a cassette tape of "white noise" should be available from any speech and hearing center. Wearable units for all three effects are available for purchase.

References

Abe, K., Yokoyama, S. Y., & Yorifuji, S. (1993). Repetitive speech disorder resulting from infarcts in the paramedian thalami and midbrain. *Journal of Neurology, Neurosurgery and Psychiatry, 56*, 1024–1026.

Adams, S. (1932). A study of the growth of language between two and four years. *Journal of Juvenile Research, 16*, 269–277.

Alfonso, P. J. (1990). Subject definition and selection criteria for stuttering research in adult subjects. In *Research needs in stuttering: Roadblocks and future directions*. Rockville, MD: ASHA.

Anderson, N. S. (1965). Word associations to individual letters. *Journal of Verbal Learning and Verbal Behavior, 4*, 541–545.

Andreski, S. (1972). *Social science as sorcery*. New York: St. Martin's Press.

Andrews, G., Craig, A., Feyer, A.-M., Hoddinott, S., Howie, P., & Neilson, M. (1983). Stuttering: A review of research findings and theories circa 1982. *Journal of Speech and Hearing Disorders, 48*, 226–246.

Andrews, G., Morris-Yates, A., Howie, P., & Martin, N. (1991). Genetic factors in stuttering confirmed. *Archives of General Psychiatry, 48*, 1034–1035.

Aron, M. L. (1967). The relationship between measurements of stuttering behavior. *Journal of the South African Logopedic Society, 14*, 15–34.

Au-Yeung, J., & Howell, P. (1998). Lexical and syntactic context in stuttering. *Clinical Linguistics and Phonetics, 12*, 67–78.

Au-Yeung, J., Howell, P., & Pilgrim, L. (1998). Phonological words and stuttering on function words. *Journal of Speech and Hearing Research, 41*, 1019–1030.

Ayres, J., & Hopf, T. (1993). *Coping with speech anxiety*. Norwood, NJ: Ablex.

Bacon, F. (1651). *Sylva Sylvarum: or, a natural history of ten centuries.* London: W. Rawley.

Ball, G. F., & Hulse, S. H. (1998). Birdsong. *American Psychologist, 53*(1), 37–58.

Barber, V. (1939a). Studies in the psychology of stuttering, XV: Chorus reading as a distraction in stuttering. *Journal of Speech Disorders, 4,* 371–383.

Barber, V. (1939b). Studies in the psychology of stuttering, XVI: Rhythm as a distraction in stuttering. *Journal of Speech Disorders, 5,* 29–42.

Bardrick, R. A., & Sheehan, J. G. (1956). Emotional loading as a source of conflict in stuttering. *American Psychologist, 11,* 391.

Barr, H. (1940). A quantitative study of the specific phenomena observed in stuttering. *Journal of Speech Disorders, 5,* 277–280.

Bassett, M. F., & Warne, G. J. (1919). On the lapse of verbal meaning with repetition. *American Journal of Psychology, 30,* 415–418.

Beers, C. W. (1945). *A mind that found itself.* Garden City, NY: Doubleday.

Bender, J. F. (1943). The prophylaxis of stuttering. *Nervous Child, 2,* 181–198.

Bennett, J. C., & Plum, F. (1996). *Cecil textbook of medicine.* Philadelphia: Saunders.

Berger, K. (1967). The most common words used in conversation. *Journal of Communication Disorders, 1,* 201–214.

Bergmann, G. (1986). Studies in stuttering as a prosodic disturbance. *Journal of Speech and Hearing Research, 29,* 290–300.

Beveridge, W. I. B. ((1961). *The art of scientific investigation.* New York: Vintage Books.

Bhatnager, S., & Andy, O. (1989). Alleviation of stuttering with human centremedian thalamic stimulation. *Journal of Neurosurgery and Psychiatry, 52,* 1182–1184.

Blankenship, J., & Kay, C. (1964). Hesitation phenomena in English speech: A study in distribution. *Word, 20,* 360–373.

Blood, G. W. (1985). Laterality differences in child stutterers: Heterogeneity, severity levels, and statistical treatments. *Journal of Speech and Hearing Disorders, 50,* 66–72.

Bloodstein, O. (1944). Studies in the psychology of stuttering, XIX: The relationship between oral reading rate and severity of stuttering. *Journal of Speech Disorders, 9,* 161–173.

Bloodstein, O. (1958). Stuttering as an anticipatory struggle reaction. In J. Eisenson (Ed.), *Stuttering: A Symposium.* New York: Harper & Row.

Bloodstein, O. (1960). The development of stuttering, II: Developmental phases. *Journal of Speech and Hearing Disorders, 25,* 336–376.

Bloodstein, O. (1969). *A handbook on stuttering.* Chicago: National Easter Seal Society.

Bloodstein, O. (1970). Stuttering and normal nonfluency: a continuity hypothesis. *British Journal of Communication Disorders, 5,* 30–39.

Bloodstein, O. (1984). Stuttering as an anticipatory struggle reaction. Chapter 9 in R. F. Curlee & W. H. Perkins (Eds.), *Nature and treatment of stuttering: New directions.* San Diego: College-Hill Press.

Bloodstein, O. (1990). On pluttering, skivering and floggering: A commentary. *Journal of Speech and Hearing Disorders, 55,* 392–393.

Bloodstein, O. (1993). *Stuttering: The search for a cause and a cure.* Boston: Allyn & Bacon.

Bloodstein, O. (1995). *A handbook on stuttering* (5th ed.). San Diego: Singular.

Bloodstein, O. (1997). Stuttering as an anticipatory struggle reaction. Chapter 8 in R. F. Curlee & G. M. Siegel (Eds.), *Nature and treatment of stuttering: New directions.* Boston: Allyn & Bacon.

Bloodstein, O. (1999). Altered auditory feedback and stuttering: A postscript to Armson and Stuart (1998). *Journal of Speech, Language, and Hearing Research, 42,* 910–911.

Bluemel, C. S. (1913). *Stammering and cognate defects of speech.* New York: G. E. Stechert & Co.

Bluemel, C. S. (1932). Primary and secondary stammering. In *Proceedings of the American Society for the Study of Speech Disorders* (pp. 91–102). (Also in *Quarterly Journal of Speech, 18,* 187–200.)

Bobrick, B. (1995). *Knotted tongues: Stuttering in history and the quest for a cure.* New York: Simon & Schuster.

Bogen, J. E., & Bogen, G. M. (1976). Wernicke's region—where is it? *Annals of the New York Academy of Sciences, 280,* 834–843.

Boomer, D. S., & Dittman, A. T. (1962). Hesitation pauses and juncture pauses in speech. *Language and Speech, 5,* 215–220.

Boomsliter, P. C., Hastings Jr., G. S., & Creel, W. (1971). The "instant" of the syllable. *Journal of the Acoustical Society of America, 49,* 104.

Boomsliter, P. C., Creel, W., & Hastings Jr., G. S. (1973). Perception and English poetic meter. *Publications of the Modern Language Association of America, 88,* 200–208.

Bormann, E. G. (1969). Ephphatha, or some advice to stammerers. *Journal of Speech and Hearing Research, 12,* 453–461.

Brady, J. P. (1991). The pharmacology of stuttering: A critical review. *American Journal of Psychiatry, 148,* 1309–1316.

Brady, J. P., & Berson, J. (1975). Stuttering, dichotic listening, and cerebral dominance. *Archives of General Psychiatry, 32,* 1449–1452.

Brandenburg, G. C. (1918). Psychological aspects of language. *The Journal of Educational Psychology, 9,* 313–332.

Breitenfeldt, D. (1996). [Personal commentary] *Letting Go* (October/November issue). Anaheim Hills, CA: National Stuttering Association.

Brenner, N. E., Perkins, W. H., & Soderberg, G. A. (1972). The effect of rehearsal on frequency of stuttering. *Journal of Speech and Hearing Research, 15,* 474–482.

Brigance, W. N. (1936). How fast do we talk. *Quarterly Journal of Speech, 18,* 337–342.

Broen, P. A. (1972). *The verbal environment of the language learning child.* American Speech and Hearing Association Monograph No. 17 (December).

Brown, A. S. (1991). A review of the tip-of-the-tongue experience. *Psychological Bulletin, 109,* 204–233.

Brown, R. (1973). *A first language: The early stages.* Cambridge: Harvard University Press.

Brown, R., & McNeill, D. (1966). The "tip of the tongue" phenomenon. *Journal of Verbal Learning and Verbal Behavior, 5*, 325–337.

Brown, S. F. (1938). The theoretical importance of certain factors influencing the incidence of stuttering. *Journal of Speech Disorders, 3*, 112–120.

Brown, S. F. (1945). The loci of stutterings in the speech sequence. *Journal of Speech Disorders, 10*, 181–192.

Brown, S. F., & Moren, A. (1942). The frequency of stuttering with relation to word length during oral reading. *Journal of Speech Disorders, 7*, 153–159.

Bruce, M. C., & Adams, M. R. (1978). Effects of two types of motor practice on stuttering adaptation. *Journal of Speech and Hearing Research, 21*, 421–428.

Bruno, F. J. (1992). *Family encyclopedia of child psychology and development.* New York: Wiley.

Brutten, E., & Shumaker, D. (1967). *The modification of stuttering.* Englewood Cliffs, NJ: Prentice-Hall.

Brutten, G. J., Bakker, K., Janssen, P., & Van Der Meulen, S. (1984). Eye movements of stuttering and nonstuttering children during silent reading. *Journal of Speech and Hearing Research, 27*, 562–566.

Bryant, F. (1917). Influence of heredity on stammering. *Journal of Heredity, 8*, 46–47.

Bryngelson, B. (1938). Prognosis in stuttering. *Journal of Speech Disorders, 3*, 121–123.

Bryngelson, B. (1955). A study of the speech difficulties of thirteen stutterers. Chapter 36 in W. Johnson (Ed.), *Stuttering in children and adults.* Minneapolis: University of Minnesota Press.

Burke, B. D. (1972). Variables affecting stutterers' initial reactions to delayed auditory feedback. *Journal of Communication Disorders, 8*, 141–155

Butterworth, B. L. (1980). Some constraints on models of language production. In B. L. Butterworth (Ed.), *Language production,* Vol. 1: *Speech and talk.* London: Academic Press.

Butterworth, B. L. (1982). Speech errors: old data in search of new theories. In A. Cutler (Ed.), *Slips of the tongue and language production* (pp. 73–108). New York: Mouton.

Byrne, M. E. (1931). A follow-up study of one thousand cases of stutterers from the Minneapolis Public Schools. In *Proceedings of the American Society for the Study of Disorders of Speech.*

Cabañas, R. (1954). Some findings in speech and voice therapy among mentally deficient children. *Folia Phoniatrica, 6*, 34–39.

Calvin, W. H., & Ojemann, G. A. (1980). *Inside the brain.* New York: New American Library.

Campbell, J. H., & Hill, D. G. (1987). *Systematic disfluency analysis.* Evanston, IL: Northwestern University Press.

Carrell, J. A., & Tiffany, W. R. (1977). *Phonetics: Theory and application.* New York: McGraw-Hill.

Carroll, L. (1876). *The hunting of the snark.* London.

Chomsky, N. (1957). *Syntactic structures.* The Hague: Mouton.

Chomsky, N. (1959). Review of Skinner's *Verbal behavior*. *Language, 35*, 26–58.

Chomsky, N. (1965). *Aspects of the theory of syntax*. Cambridge: MIT Press.

Chomsky, N. (1970). The case against B. F. Skinner. *New York Review of Books, 30* (December), 18–24.

Chomsky, N., & Halle, M. (1968). *The sound pattern of english*. New York: Harper & Row.

Christenfeld, N. (1996). Effects of a metronome on the filled pauses of fluent speakers. *Journal of Speech and Hearing Research, 39*, 1232–1238.

Conture, E. G. (1990). *Stuttering* (2nd ed.). Englewood Cliffs, NJ: Prentice-Hall.

Conture, E. G., & Kelly, E. M. (1991). Young stutterers' nonspeech behaviors during stuttering. *Journal of Speech and Hearing Research, 34*, 1041–1056.

Conwell, R. (1890). *Acres of diamonds*. Philadelphia: Inter-Ocean.

Cook, M. J., & Lewin, J. S. (1994). Spasmodic dysphonia: New diagnosis and treatment opportunities. *Nurse Practitioner, 19*, 67–68, 70, 72–73.

Cooper, G. (1980). *Squad helps dog bite victim*. New York: Doubleday.

Cordes, A. K., & Ingham, R. J. (1995). Stuttering includes both within-word and between-word disfluencies. *Journal of Speech and Hearing Research, 38*, 382–386.

Coriat, I. (1958). In E. F. Hahn (Ed.), *Stuttering: Significant theories and therapies*. Stanford: Stanford University Press.

Cotton, J. (1936). Syllabic rate: a new concept in the study of speech rate variation. *Speech Monographs, 3*, 112–117.

Crystal, D. (1976). Developmental intonology. In W. von Raffler-Engel & Y. Lebrun (Eds.), *Baby talk and infant speech*. Amsterdam: Swets and Zeitlinger.

Cullinan, W. L., Prather, E. M., & Williams, D. E. (1963). Comparison of procedures for scaling the severity of stuttering. *Journal of Speech and Hearing Research, 6*, 187–194.

Curlee, R. F. (1993). *Stuttering and related disorders of fluency*. New York: Thieme Medical Publishers.

Cutler, A. (1982). *Slips of the tongue and language production*. New York: Mouton.

Daly, J. A., McCroskey, J. C., Ayres, J., Hopf, T., & Ayres, D. M. (1997). *Avoiding communication: Shyness, reticence and communication apprehension*. Cresskill, NJ: Hampton Press.

David, E. E., & Denes, P. B. (Eds.) (1972). *Human communication: A unified view*. New York: McGraw-Hill.

Dechert, H. W., & Raupach, M. (Eds.) (1987). *Temporal variables in speech*. The Hague: Mouton.

Delattre, P. (1963). Comparing the prosodic features of English, German, Spanish and French. *International Review of Applied Linguistics, 1*(3), 193–210.

De Nil, L. F., Kroll, R. M., Kapur, S., & Houle, S. (2000). A positron emission tomography study of silent and oral single word reading in stuttering and nonstuttering adults. *Journal of Speech, Language, and Hearing Research, 43*, 1038–1053.

Denes, P. B., & Pinson, E. N. (1993). *The speech chain*. New York: W. H. Freeman.

de Saussure, F. (1964). *Course in general linguistics.* Trans. Wade Baskin. New York: The Philosophical Library. (Originally published 1915.)

Diehl, C. F. (1968). Stuttering: What are we talking about? *CEC, Division for Children Communication Disorders, 4,* 7–9.

Dillon, J. (1983). Cognitive complexity and duration of classroom speech. *Instructional Science, 12,* 57–66.

Doll, E. A. (1953). *The measurement of social competence.* Circle Pines, MN: American Guidance Service.

Dollard, J., & Miller, N. E. (1950). *Personality and psychotherapy.* New York: McGraw-Hill.

Doran, E. W. (1907). A study of vocabularies. *Pedagogical Seminars, 14,* 401–438.

Doyle, J. A. (1981). *Phrasal stress patterns in the fluent speech of stutterers and nonstutterers: A replication.* Unpublished master's thesis, Washington State University.

Dresher, B. E., & Hornstein, N. (1976). On some supported contributions of artificial intelligence to the scientific study of language. *Cognition, 4,* 321–398.

Drever, J. (1915–16). A study of children's vocabularies, I, II, III. *Journal of Experimental Pedagogy, 3,* 34–43, 96–103, 182–188.

Dunne, J., Hayes, M., & Cameron, D. (1993). Botulinum toxin A for cricopharyngeal dystonia. *Lancet, 342,* 559.

Dyer, J. (2001). Ethics and orphans: The "monster study". *San Jose Mercury News,* June 10, p. 1.

Eisenson, J. (Ed.) (1958). *Stuttering: A symposium.* New York: Harper & Row.

Eisenson, J. (1975). Stuttering as perseverative behavior. In J. Eisenson (Ed.), *Stuttering: A second symposium* (pp. 401–452). New York: Harper & Row.

Eisenson, J., & Horowits, E. (1945). The influence of propositionality on stuttering. *Journal of Speech Disorders, 10,* 193–197.

Ervin-Tripp, S. M. (1961). Changes with age in the verbal determinants of word-association. *American Journal of Psychology, 74,* 361–372.

Evan, B. (1960). *The natural history of nonsense.* New York: Vintage Books.

Fahn, S. (1982). The clinical spectrum of motor tics. *Advances in Neurology, 35,* 341–344.

Fairbanks, G. (1960). *Voice and articulation drillbook.* New York: Harper & Row.

Fairbanks, H. (1944). The quantitative differentiation of samples of spoken language. *Psychological Monographs, 56,* 19–38.

Ferguson, C. A. (1964). Baby talk in six languages. In J. Gumperz & D. Hymes (Eds.), *The ethnography of communication. American Anthropologist, 66(6),* Pt. 2.

Few, L. R., & Lingwall, J. B. (1972). A further analysis of fluency within stuttered speech. *Journal of Speech and Hearing Research, 15,* 356–363.

Finn, P. (1997). Adults recovered from stuttering without formal treatment: Perceptual assessment of speech normalcy. *Journal of Speech, Language, and Hearing Research, 40,* 821–831.

Fletcher, J. H. (1928). *The problem of stuttering.* New York: Longmans, Green.

Fletcher, J. H. (1958). In E. F. Hahn (Ed.), *Stuttering: Significant theories and therapies*. Stanford: Stanford University Press.

Fonagy, I. (1966). Electrophysiological and acoustic correlates of stress and stress perception. *Journal of Speech and Hearing Research, 9,* 231–244.

Fournie, M. (1887). *Essai de psychologie*. Paris. [Cited in Lashley (1951).]

Francis, W. N., & Kucera, H. (1982). *Frequency analysis of english usage: Lexicon and grammar*. Boston: Houghton Mifflin.

Frasier, J. (1955). An exploration of stutterers' theories of their own stuttering. In W. Johnson & R. R. Leutenegger (Eds.), *Stuttering in children and adults*. Minneapolis: University of Minnesota Press.

French, N. R., Carter, C. W., & Koenig, W. (1930). The words and sounds of telephone conversations. *Bell System Technical Journal, 9,* 290–324.

Freud, S. (1914). Slips of the tongue. Chapter 5 in *The psychopathology of everyday life*. New York: Macmillan.

Freud, S. (1936). *The problem of anxiety*. New York: Norton.

Freud, S. (1953). *On aphasia: A critical study*. New York: International Universities Press.

Fries, C. C., & Traver, A. A. (1950). *English word lists*. Ann Arbor: George Wahr.

Froeschels, E. (1915). Stuttering and nystagmus. *Monatschrift für Orenheil, 49,* 161–167.

Froeschels, E. (1921). A study of the symptomatology of stuttering. *Monatschrift für Orenheil, 55,* 1109–1112.

Froeschels, E. (1956). Theory–therapy. In E. F. Hahn (Ed.), *Stuttering: Significant theories and therapies* (pp. 41–47). Stanford: Stanford University Press.

Froeschels, E. (1961). New viewpoints on stuttering. *Folia Phoniatrica, 13,* 187–201.

Fromkin, V. (1971). The nonanomalous nature of anomalous utterances. *Language, 47*(1), 27–52.

Gale, M. C., & Gale, H. (1902). Vocabularies of three children of one family at two and three years of age. *Pedagogical Seminars, 9,* 422–435.

Galton, F. (1833). *Inquiries into human faculty and its development*. London: Macmillan.

Ganong, W. F. (1997). *Review of medical physiology*. Los Altos, CA: Lange Medical Publications.

Garnica, O. K. (1977). Some prosodic and paralinguistic features of speech to young children. In C. E. Snow & C. A. Ferguson (Eds.). *Talking to children: Language input and acquisition*. Cambridge: Cambridge University Press.

Gerken, L. A., & McGregor, K. (1998). An overview of prosody and its role in normal and disordered child language. *American Journal of Speech–Language Pathology, 7,* 38–48.

Geschwind, N. (1967). The varieties of naming errors. *Cortex, 3,* 97–112.

Geschwind, N., & Galaburda, A. M. (1987). *Cerebral lateralization*. Cambridge: MIT Press.

Gibson, W. (1962). Pioneers in localization of brain function. *Journal of the American Medical Association, 180,* 944–951.

Gifford, M. F. (1958). In E. F. Hahn (Ed.), Stuttering: Significant theories and therapies. Stanford: Stanford University Press.

Gilger, J. W. (1995). Behavior genetics: Concepts for research and practice in language development and disorders. Journal of Speech and Hearing Research, 38, 1126–1142.

Glass, A. (Ed.) (1987). Individual differences in hemispheric specialization. New York: Plenum.

Goldman-Eisler, F. (1952). Individual differences between interviewers and their effects on interviewee's conversational behavior. Journal of Mental Science, 98, 660–671.

Goldman-Eisler, F. (1957). Speech production and language statistics. Nature, 180, 1497.

Goldman-Eisler, F. (1968). Psycholinguistics: Experiments in spontaneous speech. New York: Academic Press.

Goldstein, K. (1948). Language and language disturbances. New York: Grune and Stratton

Goodell, E. W., & Studdert-Kennedy, M. (1995). Acoustic evidence for the development of gestural coordination in the speech of 2-year-olds. Journal of Speech and Hearing Research, 36, 707–727.

Goodstein, L. D. (1958). Functional speech disorders and personality: A survey of the research. Journal of Speech and Hearing Research, 1, 358–377.

Gorovitz, S., & MacIntyre, A. (1976). Toward a theory of medical fallibility. Journal of Medical Philosophy, 1, 51–71.

Gould, E., & Sheehan, J. G. (1967). Effect of silence on stuttering. Journal of Abnormal Psychology, 72, 441–445.

Grabowski, T. J., & Damasio, A. R. (2000). Investigating language with functional neuroimaging. Chapter 14 in A. W. Toga & J. C. Mazziotta (Eds.), Brain mapping: The systems. San Diego: Academic Press.

Gray, M. (1940). The "X" family: A clinical and laboratory study of a "stuttering" family. Journal of Speech Disorders, 5, 343–348.

Gregory, H., & Hill, D. (1993). Differential evaluation and differential therapy for stuttering children. Chapter 2 in R. F. Curlee (Ed.), Stuttering and related disorders of fluency. New York: Thieme Medical Publishers.

Gur, R. C., Turetsky, B. I., Matsui, M., Yan, M., Bilker, W., Hughlett, P., & Gur, R. E. (1999). Sex differences in gray and white matter in healthy young adults: Correlations with cognitive performance. Journal of Neuroscience, 19, 4064–4072.

Hahn, E. F. (1940). A study of the relationship between the social complexity of the oral reading situation and the severity of stuttering. Journal of Speech Disorders, 5, 1–14.

Hahn, E. F. (1942a). A study of the relationship between stuttering occurrence and phonetic factors in oral reading. Journal of Speech Disorders, 7, 143–151.

Hahn, E. F. (1942b). A study of the relationship between stuttering occurrence and grammatical factors in oral reading. Journal of Speech Disorders, 7, 329–335.

Halle, M., & Vergnaud, J. R. (1980). Three-dimensional phonology. Journal of Linguistic Research, 1, 83–105.

Hallett, M. (1997). Utility and physiology of botulism toxin for involuntary movement disorders. U.S. Department of Health and Human Services, National Institutes of Health, Institute of Neurological Disorders and Stroke.

Hallett, M. (1999). One man's poison—clinical applications of botulinum toxin. *New England Journal of Medicine, 341,* 118–120.

Halliday, M. A. K. (1967). *Intonation and grammar in British English.* Janua Linguarum, Series Practica, 48. The Hague: Mouton.

Halliday, M. A. K. (1975). *Learning how to mean: Explorations in the development of language.* London: Arnold.

Hamre, C. E. (1992). Stuttering prevention, I: Primacy of identification. *Journal of Fluency Disorders, 17,* 3–23.

Hargreaves, W. S., & Starkweather, J. A. (1959). Collection of temporal data with the duration tabulator. *Journal of the Experimental analysis of Behavior, 2,* 179–183.

Harris, R. A. (1993). *The linguistics wars.* New York: Oxford University Press.

Head, H. (1926). *Aphasia and kindred disorders of speech.* London: Cambridge University Press.

Hejna, R. F. (1972). The relationship between stress or accent and stuttering during spontaneous speech. *Asha, 14,* 479 [abstr.].

Helm, A., Butler, R., & Benson, D. (1978). Acquired stuttering. *Neurology, 28,* 1159–1165.

Hill, H. (1944a). Stuttering, I: A critical review and evaluation of biochemical investigations. *Journal of Speech Disorders, 9,* 245–261.

Hill, H. (1944b). Stuttering, II: A review and integration of physiological data. *Journal of Speech Disorders, 9,* 289–324.

Hockett, C. P. (1967). Where the tongue slips, there slip I. *Janua Linguarum, 32,* 910–936.

Horn, M. D. (1926). The thousand and three words most frequently used by kindergarten children. *Childhood Education, 3,* 118–122.

Horsley, I. A., & FitzGibbon, C. T. (1987). Stuttering children: Investigation of a stereotype. *British Journal of Disorders of Communication, 22,* 19–35.

Howell, P., & Williams, M. (1988). The contribution of the excitatory source to the perception of neutral vowels in stuttered speech. *Journal of the Acoustical Society of America, 84,* 80–89.

Howes, D. J., & Geschwind, N. (1969). Quantitative studies of aphasic language. Chapter 16 in D. M. Rioch & E. A. Weinstein (Eds.), *Disorders of communication* (pp. 229–244). New York: Hafner.

Hubbard, C. P. (1998). Stuttering, stressed syllables and word onsets. *Journal of Speech, Language and Hearing Research, 41,* 802–808.

Hubbard, C. P., & Prins, D. (1994). Word familiarity, syllabic stress pattern, and stuttering. *Journal of Speech and Hearing Research, 37,* 564–571.

Hubbard, C. P., & Yairi, E. (1988). Clustering of disfluencies in the speech of stuttering and nonstuttering preschool children. *Journal of Speech and Hearing Research, 31,* 228–233.

Hubble, E. (1954). The nature of science. In C. P. Haskins (Ed.), *The search for understanding.* Cambridge: MIT Press. (Originally published in E. Hubble, *The nature of science and other essays* [University of California: Huntington Library, 1954].)

Hudson, R. (1984). *Word grammar.* Oxford: Basil Blackwell.

Hunt, J. (1860). *Stammering and stuttering, their nature and treatment.* Hastings, England: Ore House. (Reprinted by Hafner Publishing, London, 1967.)

Ingham, R. J., Fox, P. T., Ingham, J. C., Zamarripa, F., Martin, C., Jerabek, P., & Cotton, J. (1996). Functional lesion investigation of developmental stuttering with positron emission tomography. *Journal of Speech and Hearing Research, 39,* 1208–1227.

Ingham, R. J., Fox, P. T., Ingham, J. C., & Zamarripa, F. (2000). Is overt stuttered speech a prerequisite for the neural activity associated with chronic developmental stuttering? *Brain and Language, 75,* 163–194.

Jagger, J., Prusoff, B. A., Cohen, D. J., Kidd, K. K., Carbonari, C. M., & Joh, K. (1982). The epidemiology of Tourette's syndrome: A pilot study. *Schizophrenia Bulletin, 8,* 267–278.

James, W. (1890). *The principles of psychology,* Vol. 1. New York: Holt.

Jasper, H. H., & Murray, E. (1932). A study of the eye-movements of stutterers during oral reading. *Journal of Experimental Psychology, 15,* 528–538.

Johnson, W. (1930). *Because I stutter.* New York: Appleton.

Johnson, W. (1934). *Stuttering in the preschool child.* State University of Iowa, Child Welfare Pamphlet #37.

Johnson, W. (1946). *People in quandaries: The semantics of personal adjustment.* New York: Harper.

Johnson, W. (1948). Stuttering. Chapter 5 in W. Johnson & D. Moeller (Eds.), *Speech handicapped school children.* New York: Harper.

Johnson, W. (1949). An open letter to the mother of a stuttering child. *Journal of Speech and Hearing Disorders, 14,* 3–8.

Johnson, W. (1955). A study of the onset and development of stuttering. Chapter 3 in W. Johnson & R. R. Leutenegger (Eds.), *Stuttering in children and adults.* Minneapolis: University of Minnesota Press.

Johnson, W. (1956). Stuttering. Chapter 5 in W. Johnson & D. Moeller (Eds.), *Speech handicapped school children* (2nd ed.). New York: Harper.

Johnson, W. (1961). Measurements of oral reading and speaking rate and disfluency of adult male and female stutterers and nonstutterers. *Journal of Speech and Hearing Disorders,* Suppl. 7, 1–20.

Johnson, W. (1963). The problem of stuttering. Chapter 9 in D. C. Spriestersbach (Ed.), *Diagnostic methods in speech pathology.* New York: Harper & Row.

Johnson, W. (1967). Stuttering. Chapter 5 in W. Johnson & D. Moeller (Eds.), *Speech handicapped school children* (3rd ed.). New York: Harper.

Johnson, W., & Associates (1959). *The onset of stuttering.* Minneapolis: University of Minnesota Press.

Johnson, W., & Brown, S. F. (1935). Stuttering in relation to various speech sounds. *Quarterly Journal of Speech, 21,* 481–496.

Johnson, W., & Brown, S. F. (1939). Stuttering in relation to various speech sounds: A correction. *Quarterly Journal of Speech, 25,* 20–22.

Johnson, W., & Knott, J. R. (1936). The moment of stuttering. *Journal of Genetic Psychology, 48,* 475–480.

Johnson, W., & Knott, J. R. (1937). Studies in the psychology of stuttering, I: The distribution of moments of stuttering in successive readings of the same material. *Journal of Speech Disorders, 2,* 17–19.

Johnson, W., & Moeller, D. (Eds.) (1948). *Speech handicapped school children.* New York: Harper.

Johnson, W., & Moeller, D. (Eds.) (1956). *Speech handicapped school children* (2nd ed.). New York: Harper.

Johnson, W., & Moeller, D. (Eds.) (1967). *Speech handicapped school children* (3rd ed.). New York: Harper.

Johnson, W., & Rosen, L. (1937). Studies in the psychology of stuttering, VII: Effect of certain changes in speech pattern upon frequency of stuttering. *Journal of Speech Disorders, 2,* 105–110.

Jonas, G. (1977). *Stuttering: The disorder of many theories.* New York: Farrar, Straus and Giroux.

Jones, R. K. (1966). Observations on stammering after localized cerebral injury. *Journal of Neurology, Neurosurgery and Psychiatry, 29,* 192–195.

Joseph, R. (1982). The neurophysiology of development: Hemispheric laterality, limbic language and the origin of thought. *Journal of Clinical Psychology, 38,* 4–33.

Jung, J. H. (1989). *Genetic syndromes in communication disorders.* Boston: Little, Brown.

Karlin, I. W. (1959). Stuttering: Basically an organic disorder. *Logos, 2,* 61–63.

Katz, M. (1977). Survey of patented anti-stuttering devices. In R. W. Rieber (Ed.), *The problem of stuttering: Theory and therapy* (pp. 181–206). New York: Elsevier.

Kavanagh, J. F., & Cutting, J. E. (1975). *The role of speech in language.* Cambridge: MIT Press.

Kehoe, D. (1999). [Personal commentary] *Letting Go* (March issue). Anaheim Hills, CA: National Stuttering Association.

Keppie, E. V. (1952). *Speech improvement through choral speaking* (3rd ed.). Magnolia, MA: Expression.

Kidd, K. K. (1977). A genetic perspective on stuttering. *Journal of Fluency Disorders, 2,* 259–269.

Kidd, K. K. (1980). Genetic models of stuttering. *Journal of Fluency Disorders, 5,* 187–201.

Kidd, K. K. (1983). Recent progress in the genetics of stuttering. In C. L. Ludlow & J. A. Cooper (Eds.), *Genetic aspects of speech and language disorders* (pp. 197–213). New York: Academic Press.

Kidd, K. K. (1984). Stuttering as a genetic disorder. In R. Curlee & W. Perkins (Eds.), *Nature and treatment of stuttering* (pp. 149–169). San Diego: College Hill.)

Kidd, K., Reich, T., & Kessler, S. (1973). A genetic analysis of stuttering suggesting a single major locus. *Genetics, 74*(2), Pt. 2, S137.

Kidd, K., Kidd, J., & Records, M. (1978). The possible causes of the sex ratio in stuttering and its implications. *Journal of Fluency Disorders, 3,* 13–23.

Kidd, K., Heimbuch, R., & Records, M. (1981). Vertical transmission of susceptibility to stuttering with sex-modified expression. *Proceedings of the National Academy of Sciences, 78,* 606–610.

Klingbeil, G. M. (1939). The historical background of the modern speech clinic. *Journal of Speech and Hearing Disorders, 4,* 115–132.

Klouda, G. V., & Cooper, W. E. (1988). Contrastive stress, intonation, and stuttering frequency. *Language and Speech, 31,* 3–20.

Kolb, B., & Wishaw, I. Q. (1980). *Fundamentals of human neuropsychology.* San Francisco: W. H. Freeman.

Kopp, H. E. (1963). Eye movements in reading as related to speech dysfunction in male stutterers. *Speech Monographs, 30,* 248.

Kowalczyk, P. A., & Yairi, E. (1995). *Features of F-2 transitions in fluent speech of children who stutter.* Paper (SA-664) presented at the annual convention of the American Speech Language Hearing Association, Orlando, FL.

Kozhevnikov, V. A., & Chistovich, L. A. (1965). Speech on *Articulation and Perception.* Moscow: Nauka. (Translated by the U.S. Department of Commerce, Joint Publications Research Service, Washington, DC.)

Kucera, H., & Francis, W. N. (1967). *Computational analysis of present-day American English.* Providence: Brown University Press.

Ladefoged, P. (1963). Some physiological parameters in speech. *Language and Speech, 6,* 109–119.

Lashley, K. S. (1951). The problem of serial order in behavior. In L. A. Jeffress (Ed.), *Cerebral mechanisms in behavior* (pp. 112–136). New York: Wiley.

Leckman, J. F., & Cohen, D. J. (1988). Descriptive and diagnostic classification of tic disorders. Chapter 1 in D. J. Cohen, R. D. Bruun, & J. F. Leckman (Eds.), *Tourette's syndrome and tic disorders: Clinical understanding and treatment.* New York: Wiley.

Lee, B. S. (1951). Artificial stutter. *Journal of Speech and Hearing Disorders, 16,* 53–55.

Lees, A. J. (1985). *Tics and related disorders.* London: Churchill Livingstone.

Lenneberg, E. H. (1967). *Biological foundations of language.* New York: Wiley.

Leonard, W. E. (1927). *The locomotive god.* New York: The Century Co.

Levelt, W. J. M. (1989). *Speaking: From intention to articulation.* London: MIT Press.

Levin, H., & Silverman, I. (1965). Hesitation phenomena in children's speech. *Language and Speech, 8,* 65–85.

Liberman, M., & Prince, A. (1977). On stress and linguistic rhythm. *Linguistic Inquiry, 8,* 249–336.

Lieberman, P. (1973). On the evolution of human language: A unified view. *Cognition, 2,* 59–94.

Lohr, F. (1969). *A study of the behavioral components of stuttered speech.* Unpublished doctoral dissertation, Western Michigan University, Kalamazoo.

Love, L. R., & Jeffress, L. A., (1971). Identification of brief pauses in the fluent speech of stutterers and non-stutterers. *Journal of Speech and Hearing Research, 14*, 229–240.

Ludlow, C. L. (1993). *Pathophysiology and treatment of speech disorders.* U.S. Department of Health and Human Services, National Institutes of Health, Institute on Deafness and Other Communication Disorders.

Luria, A. R. (1961). *The role of speech in regulation of normal and abnormal behavior.* Oxford: Pergamon Press.

Luria, A. R. (1970). *Traumatic aphasia.* The Hague: Mouton.

Luria, A. R. (1981). *Language and cognition.* New York: Wiley.

MacKay, D., & Bowman, R. (1969). On producing the meaning in sentences. *American Journal of Psychology, 82*, 23–39.

Maclay, H., & Osgood, C. E. (1959). Hesitation phenomena in spontaneous English speech. *Word, 15*, 19–44.

Mahl, G. F. (1956). Disturbances and silences in the patient's speech in psychotherapy. *Journal of Abnormal and Social Psychology, 53*, 1–15.

Mahl, G. F. (1958). On the use of "ah" in spontaneous speech: Quantitative, developmental, characterological, situational and linguistic aspects. *American Psychologist, 13*, 349.

Mahl, G. F. (1959). Measuring the patient's anxiety during interviews from "expressive" aspects of his speech. *Transactions of the New York Academy of Sciences, 21* (Series 11), 249.

Makuen, G. H. (1914). A study of 1000 cases of stammering, with special reference to the etiology and treatment of the affection. *Therapeutic Gazette, 38*, 385–390.

Malinowski, B. (1923). The problem of meaning in primitive languages. Supplement I in C. K. Ogden & I. A. Richards (Eds.), *The meaning of meaning.* London: Kegan Paul, Trench, Trubner & Co.

Marin, O. S. M. (1982). Brain and language: The rules of the game. Chapter 3 in M. A. Arbib, D. Caplan, & J. C. Marshall (Eds.), *Neural models of language processes.* New York: Academic Press.

Market, K. E., Montague Jr., J. C., Buffalo, M. D., & Drummond, S. S. (1990). Acquired stuttering: Descriptive data and treatment outcome. *Journal of Fluency Disorders, 15*, 21–33.

Martin, J. G., & Strange, W. (1968). The perception of hesitation in spontaneous speech. *Perception and Psychophysics, 3*, 427–438.

Max, L., & Caruso, A. J. (1998). Adaptation of stuttering frequency during repeated readings: Associated changes in acoustic parameters of perceptually fluent speech. *Journal of Speech, Language and Hearing Research, 41*, 1266–1281.

McCarthy, D. A. (1930). *The language development of the preschool child.* Minneapolis: University of Minnesota Press.

McGlone, J. (1980). Sex differences in human brain asymmetry: A critical survey. *Behavioral and Brain Sciences, 315*, 215–227.

McNeill, D. (1992). *Hand and mind: what gestures reveal about thought.* Chicago: University of Chicago Press.

McBride, C. (1969). *Silent victory.* Chicago: Nelson-Hall.

Meringer, R., & Mayer, K. (1985). *Versprechen und Verlesen.* Stuttgart: G. J. Goshen.

Milisen, R., & W. Johnson (1936). A comparative study of stutterers, former stutterers and normal speakers whose handedness has been changed. *Archives of Speech, 1,* 61–86.

Miller, G. A., Galanter, E., & Pribram, K. H. (1960). *Plans and the structure of behavior.* New York: Holt.

Miller, G. A., Newman, E. B., & Friedman, E. A. (1958). Length-frequency statistics for written English. *Information and Control, 1,* 370–389.

Miller, N. (1944). Experimental studies in conflict. Chapter 14 in J. McV. Hunt (Ed.), *Personality and the behavior disorders.* New York: Ronald.

Minifie, F. D., & Cooker, H. S. (1964). A disfluency index. *Journal of Speech and Hearing Disorders, 29,* 189–192.

Moeller, D (1975). *Speech pathology and audiology: Iowa origins of a discipline.* Iowa City: University of Iowa Press.

Moore, J. E. (1935). Annoying habits of college professors. *Journal of Abnormal and Social Psychology, 30,* 43–46.

Moore, W. E. (1946). Hypnosis in a system of therapy for stutterers. *Journal of Speech Disorders, 11,* 117–122.

Moore Jr., W. H. (1984). Central nervous system characteristics of stutterers. Chapter 4 in *Nature and treatment of stuttering.* San Diego: College-Hill.

Moore Jr., W. H., Flowers, P., & Cunko, C. (1981). Some relationships between adaptation and electromyographic activity at laryngeal and masseter sites in stutterers. *Journal of Fluency Disorders, 6,* 81–94.

Moser, E. (1932). Dysintegration of breathing and eye movements during silent reading and stuttering. *Psychological Monographs, 43,* 218–275.

Moser, H. M. (1938). A qualitative analysis of eye movements during stuttering. *Journal of Speech Disorders, 3,* 131–139.

Moser, H., Dreher, J. J., & Oyer, H. J. (1957). *One-syllable words.* Technical Report No. 41, Contract No. AF-19(604)-1577. Air Force Cambridge Research Center, Operational Applications Laboratory, Bolling Air Force Base, Washington, DC.

Mowrer, D. M. (1980). *A program to establish fluent speech.* Columbus, OH: Merrill.

Mowrer, O. H. (1952). The autism theory of speech development and some clinical applications. *Journal of Speech and Hearing Disorders, 17,* 263–268. (Reprinted as Chapter 4 in O. H. Mowrer (Ed.) (1980). *Psychology of language and learning.* New York: Plenum.)

Mowrer, O. H. (1956). Two-factor learning theory reconsidered, with special reference to secondary reinforcement and the concept of habit. *Psychological Review, 63,* 114–125.

Muir, F. L. (1964). *Case studies of selected examples of reticence and fluency.* Unpublished master's thesis, Washington State University.

Murphy, A. T., & Fitzsimmons, R. M. (1960). *Stuttering and personality dynamics.* New York: Ronald Press.

Murray, E. (1932). Dysintegration of breathing and eye movements during stuttering. *Psychological Monographs, 43,* 218–275.

Nadoleczny, M. (1914). *Disorders of speech and phonation in childhood.* New York: Lippincott.

Naylor, R. V. (1953). A comparative study of methods of estimating the severity of stuttering. *Journal of Speech and Hearing Disorders, 18,* 30–37.

Neelley, J. N. (1971). A study of the speech behavior of stutterers and nonstutterers under normal and delayed auditory feedback. *Journal of Speech and Hearing Disorders, Monograph Supplement 7,* 63–82.

Nice, M. M. (1920). Concerning all-day conversations. *Pedagogical Seminars, 17,* 166–177.

Nice, M. M. (1925). Length of sentences as a criterion of a child's progress in speech. *Journal of Educational Psychology, 16,* 370–379.

Nice, M. M. (1932). An analysis of the conversation of children and adults. *Child Development, 3,* 240–246.

Nicolosi, L., Harryman, E., & Krescheck, J. (1978). *Terminology of communication disorders: Speech, language, hearing.* Baltimore: Williams & Wilkins.

Nippold, M. A., & Rudzinski, M. (1995). Parents' speech and children's stuttering: A critique of the literature. *Journal of Speech and Hearing Research, 38,* 978–989.

O'Connell, D., & Kowal, S. (1980). Prospectus for a science of pausology. In H. W. Dechert (Ed.), *Temporal variables in speech* (pp. 1–10). New York: Mouton.

Oettinger, A. C. (1972). The semantic wall. Chapter 1 in E. E. David & P. B. Denes (Eds.), *Human communication: A unified view.* New York: McGraw-Hill.

Ojemann, G. (1983). Brain organization for language from the perspective of electrical stimulation mapping. *Behavioral and Brain Sciences, 6,* 189–230.

Ojemann, G. (1991). Cortical organization of language. *The Journal of Neuroscience, 11,* 2281–2287.

Oldfield, R. C. (1966). Things, words and the brain. *Quarterly Journal of Experimental Psychology, 18,* 340–353.

O'Neill, Y. V. (1980). *Speech and speech disorders in western thought before 1600.* Westport, CT: Greenwood Press.

Ong, W. J. (1982). *Orality and literacy: The technologizing of the word.* London: Methuen.

Orton, S. T. (1929). A physiological theory of reading disability and stuttering in children. *New England Journal of Medicine, 199,* 1046–1052.

Osgood, C. E. (1952). *Method and theory in experimental psychology.* Urbana: University of Illinois Press.

Osgood, C. E., & Seboek, T. A. (1959). *Psycholinguistics: A survey of theory and research problems.* Balitmore: Waverly.

Owen, W. (1963). In C. D. Lewis (Ed.), *Collected poems*. London: Chatto & Windus. (Originally published 1918.)

Paden, E. P. (1970). *A history of the American Speech and Hearing Association, 1925–1958.* Washington, DC: American Speech and Hearing Association.

Paget, J. (1902). Stammering with other organs than those of speech. No. III in *Selected essays and addresses*. London: Longmans, Green. (Published originally in the *British Medical Journal*, 1868.)

Pauls, D. (1990). A review of the evidence for genetic factors in stuttering. *ASHA Reports,* 18, 34–38.

Penfield, W., & Rasmussen, T. (1955). *The cerebral cortex of man*. London: Macmillan.

Penfield, W., & Roberts, L. (1959). *Speech and brain mechanisms*. Princeton: Princeton University Press.

Perkins, W. H. (1983). The problem of definition: Commentary on stuttering. *Journal of Speech and Hearing Disorders*, 48, 246–249.

Perkins, W. H., Kent, R. D., & Curlee, R. F. (1991). A theory of neurolinguistic function in stuttering. *Journal of Speech and Hearing Research*, 34, 734–752.

Peters, H. F. M., Hulstijn, W., & Starkweather, C. W. (Eds.) (1991). *Speech motor control and stuttering*. Amsterdam: Elsevier.

Phillips, J. (1973). Syntax and vocabulary in mothers' speech to young children: Age and sex comparisons. *Child Development*, 44, 182–185.

Phillips, M. (1968). Reticence: Pathology of the normal speaker. *Speech Monographs, 35*, 39–49.

Pick, A. (1973). *Aphasia*. Trans. J. W. Brown. Springfield, IL: Thomas. (Originally published 1931.)

Pinker, S. (1994). *The language instinct*. New York: William Morrow & Co.

Pintner, R. (1931). *Intelligence testing: Methods and results*. New York: Holt.

Pollock, J. L. (1982). *Language and thought*. Princeton: Princeton University Press.

Porter, H. von K. (1939). Studies in the psychology of stuttering, XIV: Stuttering phenomena in relation to size and personnel of audience. *Journal of Speech Disorders, 4*, 323–333.

Postma, A., & Kolk, H. (1993). The covert repair hypothesis: Prearticulatory repair process in normal and stuttered disfluencies. *Journal of Speech and Hearing Research, 36*, 472–487.

Postman, L., & Keppel, G. (Eds.) (1970). *Norms of word association*. New York: Academic Press.

Potter, J. M. (1980). What was the matter with Dr. Spooner? Chapter 1 in V. A. Fromkin (Ed.), *Errors in linguistic performance*. New York: Academic.

Prins, D., & Hubbard, C. P. (1990). Acoustical durations of speech segments during stuttering adaptation. *Journal of Speech and Hearing Research, 33*, 494–504.

Prins, D., Hubbard, C. P., & Krause, M. (1991). Syllabic stress and the occurrence of stuttering. *Journal of Speech and Hearing Research, 34*, 1011–1016.

Prosek, R. A., & Runyan, C. M. (1982). Temporal characteristics related to the discrimination of stutterers' and nonstutterers' speech samples. *Journal of Speech and Hearing Research, 25*, 29–33.

Ptacek, P. H., & Sander, E. K. (1966). Age recognition from voice. *Journal of Speech and Hearing Research, 9*, 273–277.

Quesal, B. (1995). Basic truths about stuttering therapy. *Letting Go*, Nov./Dec., p. 4.

Rauscher, F. H. (1997). Gesture, speech and lexical access: The role of movement in speech production. *Psychological Science, 7, 4*, 226–231.

Razdol'skii, V. A. (1965). State of speech of stammerers when alone. *Zhurnal Neuropatologika i Psikhiatrika im S. S. Korsakova, 65*, 1717–1720.

Rawson, H. (1981). *A dictionary of euphemisms and other doubletalk*. New York: Crown.

Reader's Digest (1982). Carol Burnett interview.

Records, M. A., Heimbuch, R. C., & Kidd, K. K. (1977). Handedness and stuttering: A dead horse? *Journal of Fluency Disorders, 2*, 271–282.

Reid, L. D. (1946). Some facts about stuttering. *Journal of Speech Disorders, 11*, 3–12.

Roberts, A. H. 1965). *A statistical analysis of modern English*. The Hague: Mouton.

Robbins, S. D. (1935). The role of rhythm in the correction of stammering. *Quarterly Journal of Speech, 21*, 331–342.

Rose, R. H. (1948). A physician's account of his own aphasia. *Journal of Speech and Hearing Disorders, 13*, 294–305.

Rubin, D. C. (1975). Within-word structure in the tip of the tongue phenomenon. *Journal of Verbal Learning and Verbal Behavior, 14*, 392–397.

Runyan, C. M., & Adams, M. R. (1978). Perceptual study of speech of "successfully therapeutized" stutterers. *Journal of Fluency Disorders, 3*, 25–39.

Runyan, C. M., & Adams, M. R. (1979). Unsophisticated judges' perceptual evaluations of the speech of "successfully treated" stutterers. *Journal of Fluency Disorders, 4*, 29–38.

Runyan, C. M., Bell, J. N., & Prosek, R. A. (1990). Speech naturalness ratings of treated stutterers. *Journal of Speech and Hearing Disorders, 55*, 434–438.

Sabin, E. J., Clemmer, E. J., O'Connell, D. C., & Kowal, S. (1979). A pausological approach to speech development. Chapter 2 in A. W. Siegman & S. Feldstein (Eds.), *Of speech and time*. Hillsdale, NJ: Lawrence Erlbaum Associates.

Sachs, J., Brown, R., & Salerno, R. (1976). Adult speech to children. In W. von Raffler-Engel & Y. Lebrun (Eds.), *Baby talk and infant speech*. Amsterdam: Swets and Zeitlinger.

Sackheim, H. A., Gur, R. C., & Saucy, M. C. (1978). Emotions are expressed more intensely on the left side of the face. *Science, 202*, 434–435.

Sakiey, E., & Fry, E. (1979). *3000 instant words*. Providence: Jamestown.

Sander, E. K. (1959). Counseling parents of stuttering children. *Journal of Speech and Hearing Disorders, 24*, 262–271.

Sanford, F. H. (1942). Speech and personality: A comparative case study. *Character and Personality, 10*, 169–198.

Savithri, S. R. (1988). Speech and hearing science in ancient India: A review of Sanskrit literature. *Journal of Communication Disorders, 21*, 271–317.

Schachter, S., Christenfeld, N., Ravina, B., & Bilous, F. (1991). Speech disfluency and the structure of knowledge. *Journal of Personality and Social Psychology, 60*, 362–367.

Schafer, K. (1973). *Kermit Schafer's blunderful world of bloopers* New York: Crown.

Schaltenbrand, G. (1965). The effects of stereotaxic electrical stimulation in the depth of the brain. *Brain, 88*, 835–840.

Schaltenbrand, G., Spuer, H., Wahren, W., & Rummler, B. (1971). Electro-anatomy of the thalamic ventral-oral nucleus based on stereotactic stimulation in man. *Zeitschrift für Neurologie, 199*, 259–276.

Schnider, P., Binder, M., Kittler, H., Steinhoff, N., & Auff, E. (1997). Uses of botulinum toxin: 1. *Lancet, 349*, 953.

Seashore, C. E. (1942). *Pioneering in psychology.* Iowa City: University of Iowa Press.

Seashore, R. H., & Eckerson, L. D. (1940). The measurement of individual differences in general English vocabularies. *Journal of Educational Psychology, 31*, 14–38.

Selmar, J. W. (1991). *Help! This child is stuttering.* Austin, TX: Pro-Ed.

Shapiro, C. W. (1970). *Phrasal stress patterns of the fluent speech of stutterers and nonstutterers.* Unpublished master's thesis, State University of New York at Buffalo.

Sheehan, J. G. (1953). Theory and treatment of stuttering as an approach-avoidance conflict. *Journal of Psychology, 36*, 27–49.

Sheehan, J. G. (1954). An integration of psychotherapy and speech therapy through a conflict theory of stuttering. *Journal of Speech Disorders, 19*, 474–482.

Sheehan, J. G. (1958a). Conflict theory of stuttering. In J. Eisenson (Ed.), *Stuttering: A symposium.* New York: Harper & Row.

Sheehan, J. G. (1958b). In E. F. Hahn (Ed.), *Stuttering: Significant theories and therapies.* Stanford: Stanford University Press.

Sheehan, J. G. (1958c). Projective studies of stuttering. *Journal of Speech and Hearing Disorders, 23*, 18–25.

Sheehan, J. G. (1970). Research frontiers. Chapter 8 in J. G. Sheehan (Ed.), *Stuttering: Research and therapy.* New York: Harper & Row.

Sheehan, J. G. (1974). Stuttering behavior: A phonetic analysis. *Journal of Fluency Disorders, 7*, 193–212.

Sherman, S. M., & Guillery, R. W. (2000). *Exploring the thalamus.* San Diego: Academic Press.

Siegman, A. W. (1978). The meaning of silent pause in the initial interview. *Journal of Nervous and Mental Disorders, 166*, 642–654.

Silverman, F. H. (1970). Concern of elementary school stutterers about their stuttering. *Journal of Speech and Hearing Disorders, 35*, 361–364.

Silverman, F., & Williams, D. (1967). Loci of disfluencies in the speech of stutterers. *Perceptual and Motor Skills, 24*, 1085–1086.

Skinner, B. F. (1957). *Verbal behavior.* New York: Appleton-Century-Crofts.

Smith, A. (1992). Commentary on "A theory of neurolinguistic functioning in stuttering." *Journal of Speech and Hearing Research*, 35, 805–809.

Smith, D. E. P., & Raygor, A. L. (1956). Verbal satiation and personality. *Journal of Abnormal and Social Psychology*, 52, 323–326.

Smith, H. L. (1959). Toward redefining English prosody. *Studies in Linguistics*, 14(3,4) (Buffalo, NY: University of Buffalo).

Smith, M. E. (1926). An investigation of the development of the sentence and the extent of vocabulary in young children. *University of Iowa Studies in Child Welfare*, 3, No. 5.

Smith, M. E. (1941). Measurement of the size of general English vocabulary through the elementary grades and high school. *Genetic Psychology Monographs*, 24, 311–345.

Snow, C. E. (1972). Mother's speech to children learning language. *Child Development*, 43, 549–565.

Snow, C. E., & Ferguson, C. A. (1977). *Talking to children: Language input and acquisition*. Cambridge: Cambridge University Press.

Snow, C. E., Arlman-Rupp, A., Hassing, Y., Jobse, J., Joosten, J., & Vorster, J. (1976). Mother's speech in three social classes. *Journal of Psycholinguistic Research*, 5, 1–20.

Speech Foundation of America (1962). *Stuttering: Its prevention*. Publication No. 3. Memphis, TN.

Springer, S., & Deutsch, G. (1998). *Left brain, right brain: Perspectives from cognitive science*. New York: W. H. Freeman.

Spurzheim, J. G. (1908). *Phrenology, or the doctrine of the mental phenomena*. Philadelphia: J. B. Lippincott. (Revised from the second American edition, in two volumes, published in Boston in 1833.)

Squire, J. C. (1961). Ballad of soporific absorption. In J. M. Cohen (Ed.), *The Penguin book of comic and curious verse*. London: Penguin Books.

Standen, A. (1950). *Science is a sacred cow*. New York: Dutton.

Stein, L. (1942). *Speech and voice* (p. 109). London: Methuen.

Stetson, R. H. (1951). *Motor phonetics*. Amsterdam: North-Holland.

St. Louis, K. O., & Lass, N. J. (1981). A survey of communicative disorders students' attitudes toward stuttering. *Journal of Fluency Disorders*, 6, 49–79.

Stromsta, C. (1965). A spectroscopic study of disfluencies labeled as stuttering by parents. *De Therapis Vocis et Loquelae*, 1, 317–320.

Strother, C., & Kriegman, L. (1943). Diadochokinesis of stutterers and nonstutterers, *Journal of Speech Disorders*, 8, 323–335.

Sussman, H. M., & MacNeilage, P. F. (1975). Hemispheric specialization for speech production and perception of stutterers. *Neuropsychologia*, 13, 19–26.

Taylor, A., & Moray, N. (1960). Statistical approximations to English and French. *Language and Speech*, 3, 7–10.

Terman, L. M., & Merrill, M. A. (1937). *Measuring intelligence*. Boston: Houghton Mifflin.

Thatcher, R. W. (1994). *Functional neuroimaging: Technical foundations.* San Diego: Academic Press.

Thorndike, E. L., & Lorge, I. (1944). *The teacher's word book of 30,000 words.* New York: Columbia University Press.

Throneberg, R., & Yairi, E. (1994). Temporal dynamics of repetitions during the early stage of stuttering. *Journal of Speech and Hearing Research, 37,* 1067–1075.

Toga, A. W., & Mazziotta, J. C. (1996). *Brain mapping: The methods.* San Diego: Academic Press.

Toga, A. W., & Mazziotta, J. C. (2000). *Brain mapping: The systems.* San Diego: Academic Press.

Trager, G. L., & Smith, H. L. (1951). An outline of English structure. *Studies in Linguistics.* Occasional Paper 3.

Travis, L. E. (1933). Speech Pathology. Chapter 16 in C. Murchison (Ed.), *A handbook of child psychology.* Worcester, MA: Clark University Press.

Travis, L. E. (1957). The psychotherapeutical process. Chapter 31 in L. E. Travis (Ed.), *Handbook of speech pathology.* New York: Appleton-Century-Crofts.

Treiman, R. (1995). Errors in short-term memory for speech: A developmental study. *Journal of Experimental Psychology: Learning, Memory and Cognition, 21,* 1197–1208.

Tweney, R. D., Tkacz, S., & Zaruba, S. (1975). Slips of the tongue and lexical storage. *Language and Speech, 18,* 388–396.

Van Lieshout, P. H. H. M., Peters, H. F. M., Starkweather, C. W., & Hulstijn, W. (1993). Physiological differences between stutterers and nonstutterers in perceptually fluent speech: EMG amplitude and duration. *Journal of Speech, Language and Hearing Research, 36,* 55–63.

Van Riper, C. (1937a). The effect of devices for minimizing stuttering on the creation of symptoms. *Journal of Abnormal and Social Psychology, 32,* 185–192.

Van Riper, C. (1937b). The preparatory set in stuttering. *Journal of Speech Disorders, 2,* 149–154.

Van Riper, C. (1954). *Speech correction: principles and methods* (3rd ed.). Englewood Cliffs, NJ: Prentice-Hall.

Van Riper, C. (1963). *Speech correction: principles and methods* (4th ed.). Englewood Cliffs, NJ: Prentice-Hall.

Van Riper, C. (1971a). Symptomatic therapy for stuttering. Chapter 38 in L. E. Travis (Ed.), *Handbook of speech pathology.* New York: Appleton-Century-Crofts.

Van Riper, C. (1971b). *The nature of stuttering.* Englewood Cliffs, NJ: Prentice-Hall.

Van Riper, C. (1973). *The treatment of stuttering.* Englewood Cliffs, NJ: Prentice-Hall.

Van Riper, C. (1992). Stuttering? *Journal of Fluency Disorders, 17,* 81–84.

Van Riper, C., & Hull, K. (1955). The quantitative measurement of the effect of certain situations on stuttering. Chapter 8 in W. Johnson and R. R. Leutenegger (Eds.), *Stuttering in children and adults.* Minneapolis: University of Minnesota Press.

Vennard, W., & Irwin, J. W. (1966). Speech and song compared in sonograms. *National Association of Teachers of Singing Bulletin, 23,* 18–23.

Villarreal, J. J. (1950). Two aspects of stuttering therapy. *Journal of Speech Disorders, 15,* 215–220.

Viswanath, N. S., & Neel, A. T. (1995). Part word recognition by people who stutter: Fragment types and their articulatory processes. *Journal of Speech, Language, and Hearing Research, 38,* 740–750.

Voelker, C. H. (1938). An experimental study of the comparative rate of utterance of deaf and normal hearing speakers. *American Annals of the Deaf, 83,* 274–284.

Voelker, C. H. (1944). A preliminary investigation for a normative study of fluency, a clinical index to the severity of stuttering. *American Journal of Orthopsychiatry, 14,* 285–294.

Vygotsky, L. S. (1934). *Myshlenie i rech'.* Moscow: Sotsekriz. (English translation: *Thought and language.* Cambridge: MIT Press, 1962.)

Wall, M., & Meyers, F. (1984). *Clinical management of childhood stuttering.* Baltimore: University Park Press.

Wallach, J. (1992). *Interpretation of diagnostic tests.* Boston: Little, Brown.

Warren, E. (1837). Remarks on stammering. *American Journal of Medical Science, 21,* 75–99.

Watkins, R. V., Yairi, E., & Ambrose, N. G. (1999). Early childhood stuttering, III: Initial status of expressive language abilities. *Journal of Speech, Language, and Hearing Research, 42,* 1125–1135.

Watson, B. C., & Freeman, F. J. (1997). Brain imaging contributions. Chapter 7 in R. F. Curlee & W. H. Perkins (Eds.), *Nature and treatment of stuttering: New directions* (2nd ed.). San Diego: College-Hill Press.

Watson, C. S., & Love, L. (1965). Distribution of silent periods in speech: Stutterers versus nonstutterers. *Journal of the Acoustical Society of America, 38,* 935.

Webster, E. J. (1966). Parent counseling by speech pathologists and audiologists. *Journal of Speech and Hearing Disorders, 31,* 331–340.

Wechsler, D. (1944). *The measurement of adult intelligence.* Baltimore: Williams & Wilkins.

Weinberg, B. (1964). Stuttering among blind and partially sighted children. *Journal of Speech and Hearing Disorders, 29,* 322–326.

Weintraub, W. (1981). *Verbal behavior: Adaptation and psychopathology.* New York: Springer.

Weiss, D. M. (1992). Fluency enhancing systems ... for free! *Letting Go, 12,* 2, 4–5.

Wendahl, R. W., & Cole, J. (1961). Identification of stuttering during relatively fluent speech. *Journal of Speech and Hearing Research, 4,* 281–286.

Wertheimer, M. (1934). On truth. *Social Research, 1,* 135–146.

West, R. (1943). The pathology of stuttering. *Nervous Child, 2,* 96–106.

West, R. (1958). An agnostic's speculations about stuttering. In J. Eisenson (Ed.), *Stuttering: A symposium.* New York: Harper & Row.

West, R., Ansberry, M., & Carr, A. (1957). *The rehabilitation of speech* (3rd ed., p. 15). New York: Harper.

Wilder, J., & Silbermann, J. (1927). Beitrage zum Tic-problem. In: *Abhandlungen aus der Neurologie, Psychiatrie, Psychologie, und ihren Grenzgebeiten.* Berlin: S. Karger.

Wingate, M. E. (1962a). Evaluation and stuttering, I: Speech characteristics of young children. *Journal of Speech and Hearing Disorders, 27,* 106–115.

Wingate, M. E. (1962b). Evaluation and Stuttering, II: Environmental stress and critical appraisal of speech. *Journal of Speech and Hearing Disorders, 27,* 244–257.

Wingate, M. E. (1962c). Evaluation and stuttering, III: Identification of stuttering and the use of a label. *Journal of Speech and Hearing Disorders, 27,* 368–377.

Wingate, M. E. (1964). Recovery from stuttering. *Journal of Speech and Hearing Disorders, 29,* 312–321.

Wingate, M. E. (1965). A standard definition of stuttering. *Journal of Speech and Hearing Disorders, 30,* 101–102.

Wingate, M. E. (1966a). Prosody in stuttering adaptation. *Journal of Speech and Hearing Research, 9,* 550–556.

Wingate, M. E. (1966b). Stuttering adaptation and learning, I: The relevance of adaptation studies to stuttering as "learned behavior." *Journal of Speech and Hearing Disorders, 31,* 148–156.

Wingate, M. E. (1966c). Stuttering adaptation and learning: II. The adequacy of learning principles in the interpretation of stuttering. *Journal of Speech and Hearing Disorders, 31,* 211–218.

Wingate, M. E. (1971). The fear of stuttering. *Asha, 13,* 3–5.

Wingate, M. E. (1972). Deferring the adaptation effect. *Journal of Speech and Hearing Research, 15,* 543–546.

Wingate, M. E. (1975). Expectancy as basically a short-term process. *Journal of Speech and Hearing Research, 13,* 31–42.

Wingate, M. E. (1976). *Stuttering: theory and treatment.* New York: Irvington-Wiley.

Wingate, M. E. (1977a). Criteria for stuttering. *Journal of Speech and Hearing Research, 20,* 596–607.

Wingate, M. E. (1977b). The relationship of theory to therapy in stuttering. *Journal of Communication Disorders, 10,* 37–44.

Wingate, M. E. (1979a). The first three words. *Journal of Speech and Hearing Research, 22,* 604–612.

Wingate, M. E. (1979b). The loci of stuttering: Grammar or prosody? *Journal of Communication Disorders, 12,* 283–290.

Wingate, M. E. (1982). Early position and stuttering occurrence. *Journal of Fluency Disorders, 7,* 243–248,

Wingate, M. E. (1983). Speaking unassisted: Comments on a paper by Andrews *et al. Journal of Speech and Hearing Disorders, 48,* 255–263.

Wingate, M. E. (1984a). A rational management of stuttering. Chapter 7 in M. Peins (Ed.), *Contemporary approaches in stuttering therapy.* Boston: Little, Brown & Co.

Wingate, M. E. (1984b). Fluency, disfluency, dysfluency and stuttering. *Journal of Fluency Disorders, 9,* 163–168.

Wingate, M. E. (1984c). Pause in stuttered and normal speech. *Journal of Fluency Disorders, 9*, 227–235.

Wingate, M. E. (1984d). Stutter events and linguistic stress. *Journal of Fluency Disorders, 9*, 295–300.

Wingate, M. E. (1986a). Adaptation, consistency and beyond: I. Limitations and contradictions. *Journal of Fluency Disorders, 11*, 1–36.

Wingate, M. E. (1986b). Adaptation, consistency and beyond: II. An integral account. *Journal of Fluency Disorders, 11*, 37–53.

Wingate, M. E. (1986c). Physiologic and genetic factors. Chapter 3 in G. E. Shames & H. Rubin (Eds.), *Stuttering: Then and now*. Columbus: Charles E. Merrill.

Wingate, M. E. (1987). Fluency and disfluency: Illusion and identification. *Journal of Fluency Disorders, 12*, 70–101.

Wingate, M. E. (1988). *The structure of stuttering*. New York: Springer-Verlag.

Wingate, M. E. (1997). *Stuttering: A short history of a curious disorder*. Westport, CT: Greenwood Press.

Wingate, M. E. (1998). Phoneme vs. letter count in the first one thousand words of *3000 Instant Words*. Unpublished research.

Wingate, M. E. (2001). SLD is not stuttering. *Journal of Speech, Language, and Hearing Research, 44*, 381–383.

Wischner, G. J. (1947). *Stuttering behavior and learning: a program of research*. Unpublished doctoral dissertation, Iowa State University.

Wischner, G. J. (1948). An experimental approach to stuttering as learned behavior. *American Psychologist, 3*, 278–279.

Wischner, G. J. (1950). Stuttering behavior and learning: a preliminary theoretical formulation. *Journal of Speech and Hearing Disorders, 15*, 324–335.

Wolff, W. (1943). *The expression of personality*. New York: Harper.

Wolk, L., Conture, E. G., & Edwards, M. L. (1990). Coexistence of stuttering and disordered phonology in young children. *South African Journal of Communication Disorders, 37*, 15–20.

Wolpe, Z. S. (1957). Play therapy, psychodrama, and parent counseling. Chapter 32 in L. E. Travis (Ed.), *Handbook of speech pathology*. New York: Appleton-Century-Crofts.

Wulf, H. H. (1973). *Aphasia: My world alone*. Detroit: Wayne University Press.

Wyke, B. (1970). Neurological mechanisms in stammering: An hypothesis. *British Journal of Disorders of Communication, 5*, 6–15.

Wyrick, D. R. (1949). *A study of normal nonfluency in conversation*. Unpublished master's thesis, University of Missouri, Columbia.

Yairi, E. (1996). Applications of disfluencies in measurements of stuttering. *Journal of Speech and Hearing Research, 39*, 402–403.

Yairi, E., & Ambrose, N. (1992). A longitudinal study of stuttering in children: A preliminary report. *Journal of Speech and Hearing Research, 35*, 755–760.

Yairi, E., & Lewis, B. (1984). Disfluencies at the onset of stuttering. *Journal of Speech and Hearing Research, 27*, 154–159.

Yairi, E., Ambrose, N., & Cox, N. (1996). Genetics of stuttering: A critical review. *Journal of Speech and Hearing Research, 39*, 771–784.

Yarmey, A. D. (1973). I recognize your face but I can't remember your name: Further evidence on the tip-of-the-tongue phenomenon. *Memory and Cognition, 1*, 287–290.

Yaruss, J. S. (1999). Utterance length, syntactic complexity, and childhood stuttering. *Journal of Speech, Language, and Hearing Research, 42*, 329–344.

Yaruss, J. S. & Conture, E. G. (1996). Stuttering and phonological disorders in children: Examination of the Covert Repair Hypothesis. *Journal of Speech, Language, and Hearing Research, 39*, 349–364.

Yorkston, K. M., & Beukelman, D. R. (1980). An analysis of connected speech samples of aphasic and normal speakers. *Journal of Speech and Hearing Disorders, 45*, 27–36.

Zangwill, O. (1975). Excision of Broca's area without persistent aphasia. K. J. Zülch, O. Creutzfeldt, & G. C. Galbraith (Eds.), *Cerebral localization* (pp. 258–263). New York: Springer-Verlag.

Zerbin, R. W. (1973). Erfassung der symptomatik stotternder. *Die Sprachheilarbeit, 18*, 174–185.

Zimmerman, G. (1980). Stuttering: A disorder of movement. *Journal of Speech and Hearing Disorders, 23*, 122–136.

Index

ISBN 0-12-759451-5